INSIDE TERADOME

AF681976

CREATION BOOKS

London • San Francisco

CREDITS

Inside Teradome
An Illustrated History Of Freak Film
Written, edited and compiled by:
Jack Hunter
ISBN 1 871592 41 0
CREATION CINEMA COLLECTION, VOLUME 2
© Jack Hunter 1995, 1998
First published 1995 by:
CREATION BOOKS
This new revised edition published 1998
Design/layout/typesetting:
PCP International
Design technician:
Bradley Davis

Acknowledgements

The publishers and author wish to extend deepest thanks to all the people and organisations who have made the compilation of this book possible.
Stills credits:
AIP, Allied Artists, Avco-Embassy, the BFI, the Cannon Group, CIC, Columbia/Tri-Star, Dreamland Productions, EMI, Rank Film Distributors, Richard Kern, Mainline, MGM, New Line, New World Pictures, Orion, Paramount Pictures, Pathé, Jack Stevenson, Twentieth Century-Fox, United Artists, Universal Pictures, Warner Bros, Nick Zedd.
Any omissions will be credited in future editions.
Cover still:
Santa Sangre, by courtesy of Mainline Pictures.
This book is dedicated to:
Hate and chaos (thanks for everything).

CONTENTS

INSIDE TERADOME

"Whosoever runs with monsters, beware lest he become one; for when you peer into the abyss, the abyss peers into you."

– NIETZSCHE

FOREWORD

What is Freak Film?

The ultimate strain of bizarre cinema, a psycho-sexual fusion of the grotesque and the perverse, haunted by primal spectres of deformity and mutilation. This study of Freak Film gravitates around the one movie which, more than any other, can serve to define the parameters of the genre: Tod Browning's *Freaks*.

As a starting-point for Freak Film, a fulcrum where sideshow and cinema fuse into their most perfect union, *Freaks* leads us not only forward through 60 years of bizarre movies, to recent works such as *Santa Sangre* and *Boxing Helena*, but also back, through the very origins of cinema itself, to the first recorded freakshows; forcing us to examine the mythological and scientific, political and psycho-geographical history of 'freaks' – or human anomalies, as they might rather be called.

As cinema, *Freaks* displays a series of motifs which feature regularly in the bizarre film:

i) the dark underbelly of the carnival sideshow or travelling circus as an arena for deceit, sexual compulsion and violence;

ii) deformed or disfigured characters ostracized because of their 'otherness' and driven to desperate acts of revenge;

iii) a 'family' of outsiders presented as a grotesque and telling reflection of the social 'norm';

iv) sadism, specifically the deliberate creation of 'freaks' by surgery, mutilation or disfigurement;

v) the use of genuine human anomalies to enhance an *outré*, horrific or menacing atmosphere (with its attendant implications of voyeurism).

For the purposes of this book, the definition of Freak Film is that which includes any, or indeed all, of the above themes in a story set *within the realms of the physically or psychologically possible* (although the ultimate mutilation of Olga Baclanova in *Freaks* seems an unlikely accomplishment, we must ultimately believe that the freaks achieved it through their own skill and ingenuity). It is this grounding in reality, however black that reality may be, which sets bizarre cinema apart from its more fantastic relatives. Works set in a supernatural, fantasy or science-fictional milieu have not generally been included for comment in the main body of text, save where they either centre around a carnival setting, or involve the participation/exploitation of genuine human anomalies.

NB: This book is also written from the viewpoint that 'bizarre' films and other films of intense imagination, rather than constituting some sort of sub-genre in the history of film, do in fact represent the pinnacle of cinematic art, since any artistic medium can only be explored to its full potential when used to express imaginative extremes.

PART ONE:

HELL ON EARTH

A Brief History Of Teratology And Freakshows

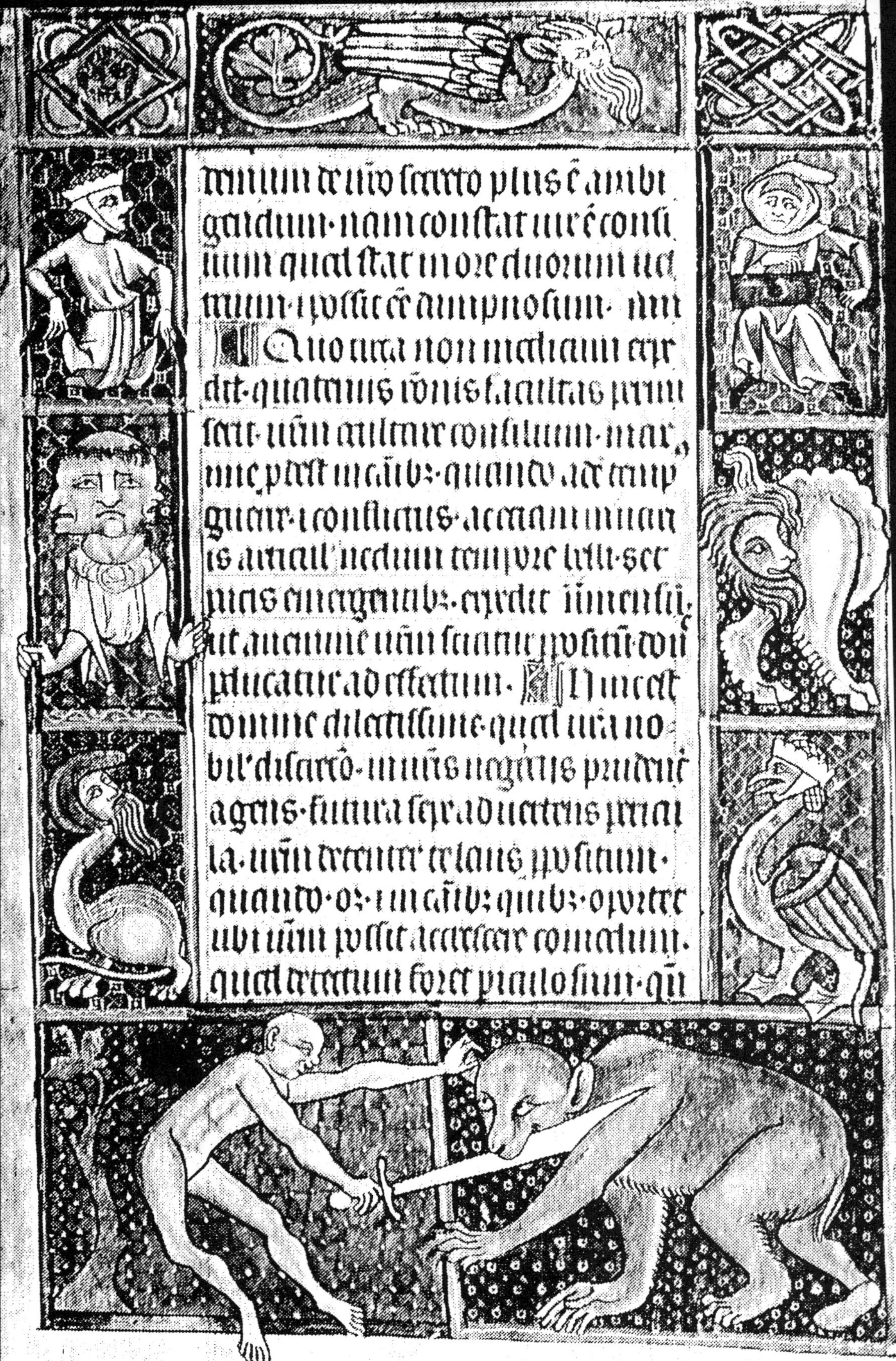

Chapter One:

THE ATROCITY EXHIBITION

(From Myth To Millennium)

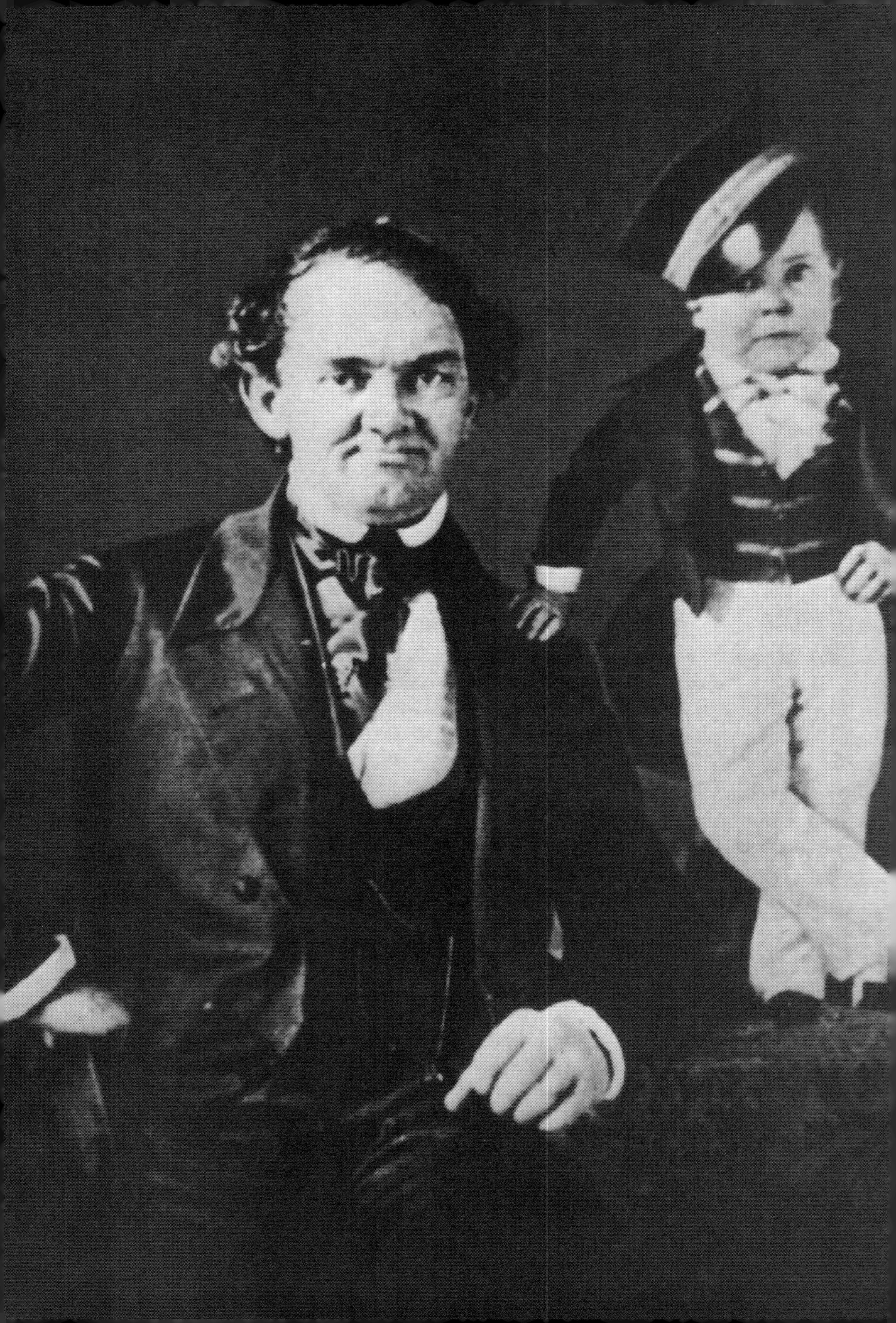

TERADOME

Man has always distorted his world. In the skies and the sea and far places, he has always imagined monsters and demons, mythological beasts and misshapen men. In his religions, he has conceived a weird descent of man from god and demi-god, from human folly and divine incest. Particularly, he has invented man-beasts to haunt himself, lexicons of dead souls recording hellish hybrids – minotaurs and mermen, goat-boys and gorgons, sirens and centipede-men, subterranean or amphibious cults spawned in profane antediluvian nuptial chambers. He has made half-real the terrors of his nightmares.

In classical times, Greek legends and travellers' tales peopled the earth with fantastic creatures. Heroes rode on winged horses to the rescue of maidens, killing dragons on the way. Voyagers were tempted by the deathly love and chanting of sirens. There were whole races of freakish men, some with faces sunk in their chests, others with a single foot so large it could shade them from the sun when they were not hopping upon it. From the most primitive cave-drawings, through to the medieval demonography and infernal visions of Bosch and Grünewald and beyond, the dreams – and fears – of mankind created a phantasmagoric zoo of weird beings, the walking demons of a Hell on Earth.

Until the dawn of rationalism in the 18th century, and the beginning of classification for all species, there was little or no scientific method to distinguish between the fable and the fact. Commentators as diverse as Homer, Herodotus, Ktesias, Megasthenes, Pliny, Aristotle (who coined the term *lusus naturae*, 'jokes of nature'), through to Albrecht Dürer and Sebastian Brant with woodcuts of eight-legged sows and other monstrous births, Hartmann Schedel in his *Liber Chronicarum* (1493), Grien in the *Büch Granatapfel* (1511), Alhazred in the *Necronomicon*, Pontoppidan, Olaus Magnus in his *Historia De Gentibus Septentrionalibus* (1555), Julius Obsequens' *Des Prodiges* (1555), André Thevet in *La Cosmographie Universelle*, Pierre Boaistuau in his *Histoires Prodigieuses* (1560), Ambroise Paré in his *Animals, Monsters And Prodigies* (1573), Lycosthenes' *Prodigiorum Ac Ostentorum Chronicon*, Jacob Rueff in his *De Conceptu Et Generatione Homines* (1587),

Schenck von Grafenberg in his *Monstrorum Historia* (1609), Fortunius Licetus in his *De Monstris* (1616), and Ulisse Aldrovandi in his *Monstrorum Historia* (1642), had clouded the boundaries of myth and reality almost beyond recognition. Gaspar Schott's *Miscellanea Curiosa Medica Physica* (1662) even contains instructions on how to make infants into freaks by witch-like artifice. Human monsters were otherwise attributed to the wrath of God, or punishment for the sins of sodomy (cf. Paracelsus' *De Animalibus Natis Ex Sodomia* [1493]). Paré's list of alleged causes of human monsters still reflect this superstitious viewpoint nearly a century later:

"The first is the glory of God. The second, His wrath. The third, too great a quantity of semen. The fourth, too small a quantity. The fifth, imagination. The sixth, the narrowness or smallness of the womb. The seventh, the unbecoming sitting position of the mother, who, while pregnant, remains seated too long with her thighs crossed or pressed against her stomach. The eighth, by a fall or blows struck against the stomach of the mother during pregnancy. The ninth, by hereditary or accidental illness. The tenth, by the rotting or corruption of the semen. The eleventh, by the mingling or mixture of seed. The twelfth, by the artifice of wandering beggars. The thirteenth, by demons or devils."

The first steps toward a clearer picture came from France. C. L. L. de Buffon, in his *Varieties Of The Human Species, Of Monsters* (1749), declared a new dictum which would be followed by most of his immediate successors in identifying types of human anomaly:

"All possible monsters can be reduced to three categories: the first is that of monsters by addition, *the second, monsters* by omission, *and the third, those that are such* by reason of the reversal or wrong positioning of parts.*"*

Upon these general ground-rules, a history of human teratology would be founded.

C. E. Hoppius' *Anthropomorphia* (1760) was an early attempt to trace an evolution of beast into man; then in 1775, Regnault published his *Freaks Of Nature* (subtitled *A Collection Of The Principal Monstrosities Produced By Nature In The Animal World*). This was a collection of forty plates, drawings of 'freaks' which were all amazingly true to life. The collection was diluted only by the inclusion of a number of specimens from the animal kingdom, such as a cyclopian cat. Meanwhile various non-scientific accounts were also starting to appear, autobiographical texts such as William Hay's *Deformity: An Essay* (1755), and Joseph Boruwlaski's *Memoirs Of A Polish Dwarf* (1788).

A more exact and specific science of teratolgy was ushered in by Haller's *De Monstris*; this was the start of a period which would also see the publication of two milestones in the field: *Anatomical Philosophy* (1822) by Etienne Geoffroy Saint-Hilaire, and *Treatise On Teratology* (1837) by Isodore Geoffroy Saint-Hilaire. J. G. Milligan's *Curiosities Of Medical Experience* appeared in 1839, and at around this same time F.-E. Guerin published his encyclopaedic, 14-volume *Illustrated Dictionary Of Natural History And The Phenomena Of Nature*.

The later 19th, and early 20th centuries, would see a veritable deluge of books and treatises on human anomalies; the blood-gates had opened on the second Golden Age of Monsters. France was still at the heart, its medical bookshops filled with such tomes as Camille Dareste's *Research Into The Artificial Production Of Monstrosities*, Edward J. Wood's *Giants And Dwarfs* (1868, an early 'showbusiness' account), Lancereaux' *Atlas Of Pathological Deformity* (1871), John Davenport's *Curiositatis Eroticae Physioligiae* (1875), Jules Guérin's *Research Into Deformities* (1880), E. Martin's *History Of Monsters From Antiquity To The Present Day* (1880), Charcot and Richer's *The Deformed And The Diseased In Art*, Paul Moreau's *Fous Et Bouffons* (1885), Cordier's *Monsters In Legend And In Nature* (1890), Guinard's *Summary Of Teratology*, Blanc's *Anomalies Of Man And Mammals* (1893), George M. Gould and Walter L. Pyles' *Anomalies And Curiosities Of Medicine* (1896), *ad infinitum*. At the same time, the theatres, circuses and sideshows were brimming with live exhibits from across the globe; it seemed that the public could not get enough of them.

Although this mad passion for real 'monsters' abated somewhat with the turn of the century, with sideshows fading in popularity as cinema developed its own fantastic themes and attractions, textbooks continued to appear regularly until the '30s; most notable amongst them being Chauvin's *Summary Of Teratology* (1920), Dr. Dubreuil-Chambardel's *Variations Of The Human Body* (1925), Lesbre's *Treatise On Teratology* (1927), C. J. S. Thompson's *Mystery And Lore Of Monsters* (1930), and Binet-Sanglé's *Ancestors Of Man* (1931). One year after this, across the world in America, Tod Browning's misunderstood film *Freaks* was released to almost universal revulsion; it seemed that the public's appetite for human anomalies had, finally, reached saturation point.

The 'freakshow' itself – in other words the recognition, treatment and display of human anomalies as special beings (whether for better or for worse) – is an institution which actually dates back in one form or another to the beginnings of recorded history, in every civilization across the world. In King Assurbanipal's library in Nineveh, a tablet was found and deciphered which describes an array of recognizable human monsters; both the Assyrians and Babylonians (*c.*2800 BC) used anomalies to make predictions. Fetomancy involved telling the future from aborted foetuses, while teratoscopy was the art of divination from deformed births.[1] The Egyptians made gods of dwarfs, such as Bes, Ita, and Ptah, and set their images on altars.[2] Mutu, the two-headed god, was worshipped in temples consecrated to his name, as were the jackal-headed Anubis and ibis-headed Thoth. So great was their passion for dwarfs that many children were deliberately deformed, made to grow up confined in boxes or with limbs bound into distorted shapes. Pnumhotpu, a misshapen dwarf who became master of the Pharaoh's wardrobe, was acclaimed by poets and immortalized by court sculptors; even the corpse of Tutankhamen was floated across the waters of death on a raft crewed by naked achondroplasic dwarfs. One of the first dwarf court jesters was also an Egyptian, named Danga (*c.*2600 BC); equally renowned was Bahalul, jester to the Persian Caliph Haroun-al-Rashid.

The Greeks deified hermaphrodites and other androgynous creatures, though reputedly scorned hunchbacks and cripples; the Spartans left all their deformed offspring out to perish; the Romans, on the other hand, derived the utmost pleasure from all manner of malformed beings – as befits the originators of the circus. Like the Egyptians before them, they were not averse to creating freaks by the purposeful twisting and dislocation of infant bodies. Nero, Tiberius, Caligula and the other megalomaniac emperors were constantly surrounded by retinues of strange anomalies; Domitian sent his private legion of achondroplasic dwarf-gladiators into the arena to do battle with ferocious Amazon women, and it is reported that the finest ladies of Rome would wait in hiding to watch these naked warriors train, so great was the phallic power accredited to dwarfs (who could be bought in a special market, the *Forum Morionium*). Augustus Caesar had a pet dwarf named Lucius. Heliogabalus, maddest of them all, adored the company of his dwarfs, and gave them the power over life and death. Sulla went so far as to gather a bizarre harem of female hunchbacks, dwarfs, cripples, and the limbless, all of whom he lusted after without surcease; likewise Julia, grand-daughter of Augustus, who assembled a similar throng of gargoyles for the sole aim of pleasuring her in unparalleled orgies of sexual gratification and cruelty. Hsuan Tsany, emperor of old China, was said to have been madly in love with a two-headed courtesan, who embraced and caressed him with her four arms. Chinese women were also ritually subjected to foot-binding, a practice which stunted and rounded their feet so they might be used as pseudo-vaginas by their masters.

Human anomalies had something of a worse time with the rise of Christianity; in the Middle Ages, Christians persecuted and burnt at the stake anything and everything which they feared or did not understand, including cats and other animals, women and 'witches', gypsies, even books. In this genocidal environment, 'monsters' had no chance; their twisted bodies were sure sign that they were the progeny of Satan. Even normal twins were roasted as things of evil. Not until the rise of Nazism – with which Christianity bears closest comparison – in the 20th century would there be such an exterminating purge declared on the physically impaired or mentally retarded.

The Renaissance signalled a general return to favour for anomalies, and this period was soon to establish itself as the second 'golden age' of monsters. Astronomer Tycho Brahe, for one, relied exclusively on the prognostications of his dwarf advisor, Zep. The courts of Europe thronged with dwarfs and hunchbacks, giants, pinheads, and the limbless, becoming veritable menageries. Often used as executioners, dwarfs payed for the privileges of court by having their tongues cut out and eardrums run through with hot wires lest they repeat state secrets. The Medicis had a special 'dwarf-pit' constructed, in which naked male and female achondroplases were set to fornication, fellation and sodomy for the voyeuristic delight of the officials; the twisted servitors of Philip II, who sought out dwarfs both male and female for his pleasures, are immortalized on the façade of the Prado; Louis II of

Bavaria collected madmen; while King Adolphus Frederick of Sweden kept a harem of amputee lovers. Other dwarf-collectors included King Sigismund-Augustus of Poland, the Roman Cardinal Vitelli – who had a retinue of 39 specimens –, and Peter the Great, who in 1710 threw a wedding banquet for no less than 70. Catherine the Great, conversely, hankered after giants. Eventually disillusioned by their poor bedroom performances, she resorted to copulating with stallions and was reputedly killed by one such beast when it burst from harness.

Victor Hugo tells of James II and his monster-factories, where normal people were butchered and mutilated to be churned out as deformed playthings, or beggars, to order. Sculptors in human flesh held sway, and charlatans could make a fortune selling ointments to promote dwarfism or other lucrative handicaps in infants.

Chiefs in this field were the *Dacianos* (later referred to as *Comprachicos* ['child-buyers'] by Hugo in his novel *L'Homme Qui Rit*), a nomadic and mendicant sect descended from migrant Hindustani tribesmen. The manufacture of cripples and freaks was their stock-in-trade. Dr Carlos Garcia in his *La Desordenada De Los Bienos Agenos* (1619) confirms: *"The Dacianos kidnap young children and cripple and disfigure them so they may be sold to beggars and blind men."* A common trick was to slash a child's mouth open from ear to ear, giving him the permanent grin of a clown. Such mutilations were also commonplace in China and India, where priests earned a living as travelling eunuch-makers. Castration was also practised in Europe to produce young boy sopranos, *castrati* whose vocal range could not be matched by women. Even in England, court tradition called for the cutting of a man's larynx to turn him into a human cock whose hideous crowing marked the passage of night.

This mania for human anomalies scarcely abated with the dawn of the 18th and 19th centuries. Jan Bleu opened his legendary *House Of Monsters* in Amsterdam; the French Royal Court was scandalized by the sexual exploits and bizarre tastes of Petit-Pépin, a phocomelian midget whose image appears in Regnault's *Freaks Of Nature*; the Duke of Lorraine, Stanislas Leczinski, favoured his hideous midget Nicholas Ferry above all other, nick-naming him 'Baby' and indulging his murderous assaults on dogs and the other court dwarfs alike; Frederick I collected giants – dead or alive; Frederick II followed suit, and went so far as to create a regiment of them – in doing so bankrupting the treasury.

One of the last famous English dwarfs in private service was 'Nanibus', the outlandishly-caparisoned retainer of the eccentric William Beckford, author of the Gothic masterpiece *Vathek*. Meanwhile, the progress of medical research had engendered a proliferation of 'resurrectionists' – professional grave-robbers, employed by the likes of surgeon *extraordinaire* John Hunter ("the father of British surgery") to retrieve the finest teratological specimens fresh from the earth. Hunter, author of *On Monsters* (1775), was renowned not only for his extensive collection of human skulls and other exotica, but also for the notorious iron melting-pot in which he boiled away the meat and fat from anomalous human bones.

Another Englishman, Sergeant-Major Philip Ashby, born in 1742, was reputedly responsible for establishing the format of the "Three-Ring" circus; he also inaugurated the sideshow, setting up exhibitions of both human and animal anomalies as well as ghoulish artefacts such as the guillotine (complete with wax heads). Then, across the Atlantic, came the greatest showman of them all, the man who would make the freakshow a way of life – Phineas Taylor Barnum (1810-91).

Barnum founded his American Museum in 1841, a New York establishment boasting many 'freak' attractions. From this base, he was to set up his fabled travelling circus. Barnum's first major attraction was the legendary midget, Tom Thumb. Born Charles S. Stratton in Bridgeport, Connecticut, in 1838, this tiny human being was discovered by Barnum, taken to New York and introduced as General Tom Thumb from England. Tom soon became world-famous, and also incredibly wealthy (he started to collect the diamonds and other riches showered on him by high society), even entering a scandalous affair with the actress Cora Pearl. He eventually married the midget Lavinia Warren in 1863; the wedding was the event of the social season, with gifts from the likes of the Rockefellers, the Vanderbilts, and even President Lincoln, being put on display by Barnum. Tom Thumb retired a very rich man, aged 20. When Barnum made some bad investments, Tom came out of retirement to bail him out, making himself another small fortune – despite having grown to nearly 3 feet tall – in the process. Tom Thumb died in 1883, but the global mania for freakshows and outlandish theatricals raged on for the rest of the century.

This cult of deformity culminated in the giant Barnum and Bailey show in Paris in 1901, in which a massive retinue of "living phenomena and human prodigies" was advertised and displayed, comprised of both genuine anomalies and music-hall attractions alike. The full billing read as follows:

BARNUM AND BAILEY

Giant American Museum of Human Prodigies and Phenomena

An extraordinary and unique collection of bizarre human beings

GIANTS, DWARFS, PERFORMERS

who work without hands and others who support themselves without feet. Human beings endowed by nature with limbs that others do not possess. Others deprived by nature.

A happy colony of privileged beings who live, work, suffer and enjoy all the feelings common to mortals, who are in some cases happier than their fellow-men more favoured by nature.

These phenomena draw high salaries, make good investments, and many of these strange beings depicted on our posters and exhibited on our stages ought to be envied rather than pitied by all.

The Japanese Conjuress

MISS SHIMAKURI is one of the very rare feminine exponents of the art of the famous Robert Houdini.

However, her conjuring tricks and feats of prestidigitation are quite different from those of that master; they have an Oriental flavour that sometimes borders on occultism. This is more than skill; it is sorcery.

The Microscopic Japanese Juggler

An atom of humanity. A fragment of Oriental grace, and expert in the art of juggling.

The Hercules With The Elastic Chest

MASTER HERMAN is gifted with an astonishing power. Merely by breathing, that is to say, by the expansive power of his lungs, he breaks the solid steel chains and strong iron rings that are bound round his chest.

The Poodle Man

JO-JO is a rare example of the whims of nature: an unbelievable and insoluble mystery. He seems to combine everything that is shocking and unpleasant. The most perceptive mind in the head of a dog. The mouth of a dog speaking four languages. This young Russian is known as the Poodle-Man because of the long, silky hair that covers his face, eyes, nose, ears, chin, and neck. Several names have been given to him, but the 'Poodle-Man' seems to be the most appropriate, for his physiognomy most resembles this breed of dog.

The Sword Swallower

MISS CLIFFORD must surely be the oddest and most original performer ever seen. The capacity of her throat amazes everyone. She puts big, sharp swords, daggers and bayonets into her mouth and pushes them gently down until no more than the hilt can be seen. She completes these extraordinary feats by swallowing gold and silver wrist-watches, and other indigestible objects.

The Fry Brothers

are the most entertaining performers. They play the 'Marimba', a very resonant musical instrument that has never been mentioned in musical history and is, nevertheless, widely played among the natives of Guatemala and the South American countries.

The Man With The Ostrich Stomach

ALFONSO is known as the 'African Phenomenon' because of his enigmatic powers of swallowing and digestion. He is an absolutely exceptional human being. He chews up glass, pebbles, and other hard substances, swallows nails and sharp, pointed sheets of metal; he eats cotton wool for his second course and ordinary soap for his hors d'oeuvres, washing down this strange menu with frequent mouthfuls of petrol and ammonia.

The Magnetic Woman

MISS ZOLINO, a young lady of striking beauty, has some most unusual talents. In particular, we should mention the sword-climbing. This exercise consists in climbing barefoot up and down a ladder with steps made of razor-sharp swords; in addition, she has extraordinary magnetic qualities which give her unheard-of strength, which confounds the combined efforts of ten strong men.

The Leopard Girl

This remarkable little girl was born to an American negress in the State of Louisiana. She presents one of the greatest oddities that nature, in her peculiar vagaries, can produce, that is to say, a skin of two distinct colours. Her skin, which should properly be black all over, has large white patches rather like piebald horses, leopards' skin, or tortoise-shell, or certain kinds of marble.

The Albino

ROB ROY gives the strangest performances in the world. Medical science can find no explanation for them. He is a perfect example of the human variety known as 'Albinos'; in addition, he has the rare ability to dislocate every bone in his body.

The Armless Man

CHARLES TRIPP is a phenomenon. He was born without arms and, in default of hands, uses his feet so cleverly that he can even thread needles; he writes superbly, uses a penknife to sharpen his pens or pencils, and is, in a word, as skilful with his feet as other people are with their hands.

The Midget

QUEEN MAB. A pretty, microscopic little person, perfectly formed in every respect, except in size, she weighs only 19 lb 13 oz and is only 22¾" tall. She speaks several languages fluently and has a great many accomplishments, doubly remarkable in such a small person. She so much resembles a living doll that children often want to take her home with them to play with her.

The Tattooed Man

FRANK HAYES has his whole body completely tattooed with a thousand designs in Indian ink. These tattoos, which are very fine, and very artistically executed, represent strange figures, flowers, birds, and wild animals. They are like the tattoos cannibals used to inflict on their victims, and convey an idea of the customs of primitive peoples.

The Skeleton Dandy

Certainly the thinnest man in the world, a real skeleton. He is the world champion for light weight in adults; his legs and arms are real pins, and his body looks like an X-ray photograph. Nothing but skin and bones!

The Woman With Long Hair

MISS MABEL, a pretty young American, has phenomenally long and beautiful hair, which covers the floor when she stands upright.

Tomasso, The Human Pincushion

This strange man has a remarkable power which has hitherto been observed only in the Fakirs of the East. He sticks all kind of pointed instruments into his skin. One of the most astounding tricks in his repertoire consists in allowing a threaded needle to be passed through his naked arm by a member of the audience.

The Lightning Calculator

SOL STONE is a most peculiar man who has a miraculous gift for mathematics. His propensities and his conception of numbers defy description. He adds up enormous columns of figures with unbelievable speed, and takes no more than a second to make calculations that would take trained mathematicians whole hours.

The Man With The Unbreakable Head

BILLY WELLS certainly has the most extraordinary skull. This remarkable man places enormous blocks of granite on his head and holds them there with his own hands, while a member of the audience beats the granite with a blacksmith's hammer, until the block falls to pieces.

The Mastodon Man

One of the biggest men ever seen; his bulk, corpulence, and weight are enormous. There may possibly have been taller men, but surely none whose all-over measurements were as phenomenal as this.

The Telescope Man

This exhibit is a young man born in America. He has an exceptionally strong constitution. But his chief distinction, which has earned him a place in this brotherhood of exceptional human beings, is his ability to lengthen or shorten his spinal column at will. In so doing, he considerably increases or decreases his height. This oddity, due to anatomical reasons that would take too long to explain here, can be compared to the reptiles' ability to stretch and contort themselves.

The Rubber Man

JAMES MORRIS is an unparalleled phenomenon. His skin is as elastic as rubber, and can stretch enormously. The skin on his nose, cheeks, arms, chest and legs can be stretched 20" away from his body, while he can cover his whole face with the skin of his chin and neck.

The Girl With The Mossy Hair

is a delightful young person. She has a magnificent head of hair which, unlike that of most girls, looks like a tuft of moss, so very thick that it stands straight up on her head like a spear.

The Bearded Woman

MISS ANNIE JONES is another example of the whims of nature. She is an extremely pretty person, but has a long beard. She also has very beautiful hair: it is 4' 10" long. This young lady is indeed an interesting figure and has been the subject of scientific research.

> *The Armless Japanese Girl*
> MISS OGURI, a native of Japan, is a most prepossessing person. Like her colleague, Mr. Charles Tripp, she has no arms, but like him she has learned to use her feet with amazing skill. Few people could do with their hands what this clever, though incomplete, Japanese girl does with her feet.

Some of these acts may seem less than remarkable, but the crowds came nonetheless. As Barnum himself proclaimed:

"If my puffing was more persistent, my advertising more audacious, my posters more glaring, my picture more exaggerated, my flags more patriotic and my transparencies more brilliant than they would have been under the management of my neighbours, it was not because I had less scruple than they, but more energy, far more ingenuity, and a better foundation for such promises."

Though Barnum died in 1910, his circus continued to promote prodigies throughout the world, emulated in America by scores of travelling carnivals and sideshows which relentlessly criss-crossed the continent, seeking out new recruits as they went until no stone was left unturned. Deformed children, kept under lock and key for years, were suddenly seen as valuable commodities and eagerly rented out or sold by their parents. In the sideshows they found a true home, living and working with their own kind, creating a dark parallel society whose attraction never failed to pull in the leering crowds, 'normal' folk unwittingly gazing into the mirror of their hidden selves.

Other top retinues included the Ringling Bros. Circus, the Clyde Beatty Circus, and Al G. Barnes' Circus, and famous sideshows were to be found at Dreamland, Coney Island, and in Robert L. Ripley's itinerant *Believe It Or Not!*. Freaks were imported from all over the world for these revues, and America sustained its appeal as the global mecca for Nature's outsiders.

Nate Eagle, an impresario who specialised in handling midgets and dwarfs, had a troupe of around 300 members, whom he housed in a travelling series of 'midget villages', where the houses and streets were all scaled down to size, culminating with an exhibition at the 1934 Chicago World's Fair. In Gibsonton, Florida, successive seasons of carnival folk using the town as winter quarters led to it becoming a veritable haven for sideshow performers, and it earned the reputation of containing 'more freaks per square mile' than any other area in the world.

Meanwhile, as demand for human oddities grew, more and more 'self-made' freaks joined the ranks of those created by Nature. Koo-Koo, the "Bird Girl", and Betty Green, the "Stork Woman", who both appeared in *Freaks*, were notable examples (acquiring a grotesque persona by costume, make-up and exaggeration); another was Mortado, the "Human Fountain", who actually had holes bored through his hands and feet so that water could pass through them, or he could be 'crucified'. Wooden plugs kept the holes from sealing. These acts, along with the likes of Pujol, the Parisian petomane, or others who swallowed swords, or fish and lizards like Mac Norton, or drank petrol, or made their eyes stand out on stalks like "Popeye" Perez, were really not far removed from the lowest of the low in the unspoken hierarchy of carnival acts – the geek.

The geek was a generally down-and-out, often alcoholic or simple-minded man (or woman) whose act consisted of them sitting in a stinking bone-pit, dressed like deranged nightmare children, where they would draw a crowd of horrified/fascinated onlookers by biting the heads off live rats, chickens, or even snakes. While some geeks were so wasted they needed to be fed by hand, others prided themselves on catching and tearing apart their prey with their bare hands (these were known as "glommin' geeks"). Top geeks, not content with the kill, would then eat the animal raw, crunching the bones between their teeth and smearing their faces with hot blood and viscera, or vomiting back undigested fur, feathers and gristle. One such geek was the infamous Bosco, who reportedly ate live snakes. More recently, one Veronica Shant achieved wide renown for her feral appetites; she was reportedly a virginal, church-going saint outside the pit. Geeking, unsurprisingly, was among the first carnival acts to be outlawed as the 20th century unfurled.

The largest group of self-made freaks remains the tattooed men and ladies, those who have had themselves 'illustrated' from head to foot to create a new, almost living, skin. As early as 1890, the American Irene Woodward (1863-1916) was touring as "The Beautiful Irene". Other tattooed ladies included Sylvia, Surita, Emma de Burgh, Englishwoman Anny Frank, the German Marie Theissen ("The Pearl of the Rhein"), Maud Arizona, Alwanda, Wallona Aritta, Creola, Angelika, Celly d'Astra, Arabella, and Anetta Nerona. Then there were tattooed men such as Don Manuelo, Rasmus Nielson, and Richardo, the "Living Tapestry". None of these, however, could surpass the achievement of Sir Horace Rider, the Englishman who, in 1922, submitted his entire body to the needle of the famous London tattooist George Burchett and emerged, 150 hours and 100 plastic surgery operations later, as The Great Omi. A former army officer, the man had apparently inherited and then squandered a fortune after World War I. Unable to re-enter the army, he drew one last inspiration from carnival life, his abiding interest, and had himself tattooed in a unique and extraordinary way – having every inch of his skin, including eye cavities, throat and genitals, etched with dark, one-inch wide zebra-like stripes and swirls. The Great Omi travelled the world with a succession of shows and circuses, becoming one of the highest-paid acts ever to appear and also exhibiting himself for war charities and other causes.

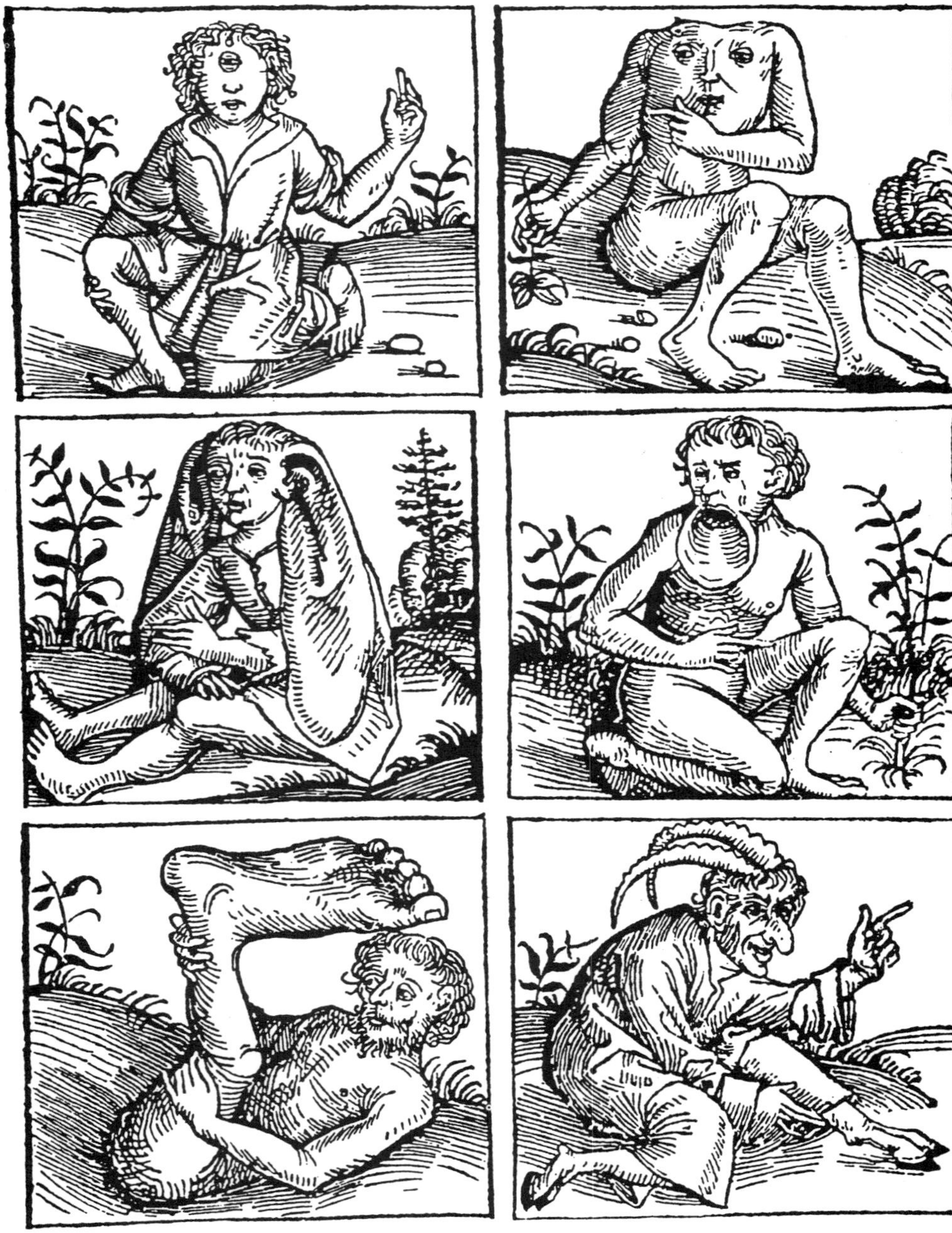

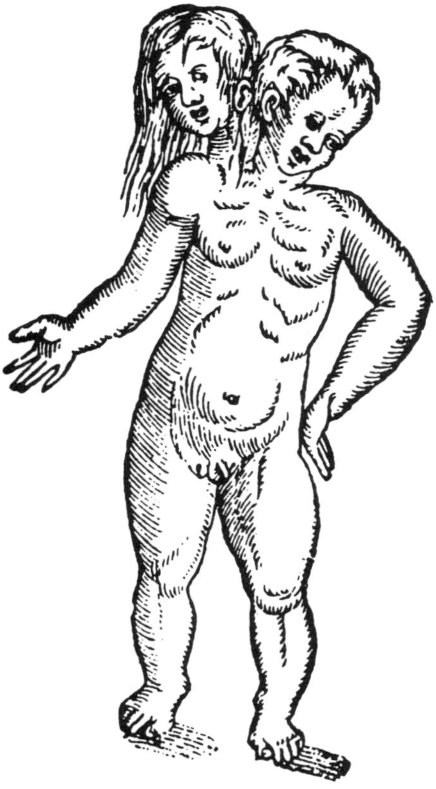

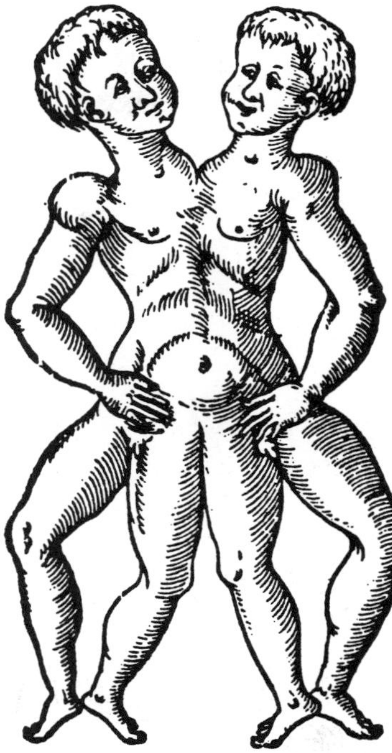

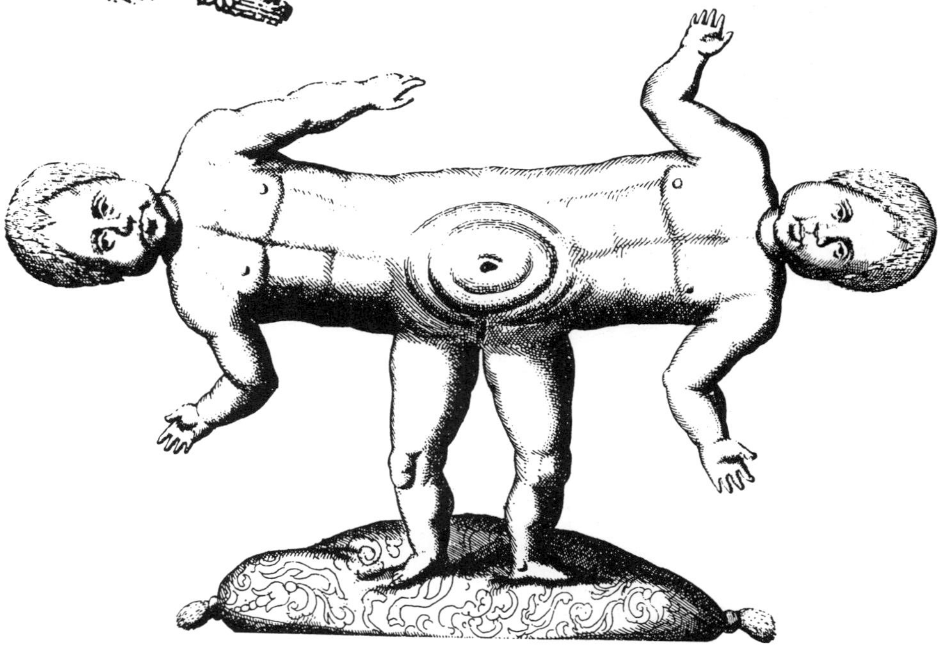

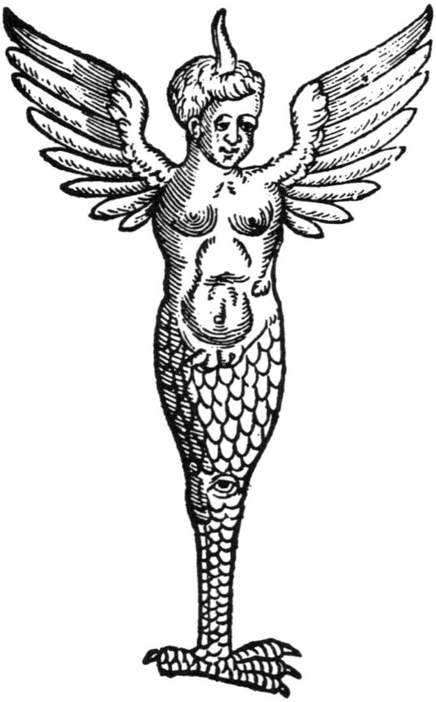

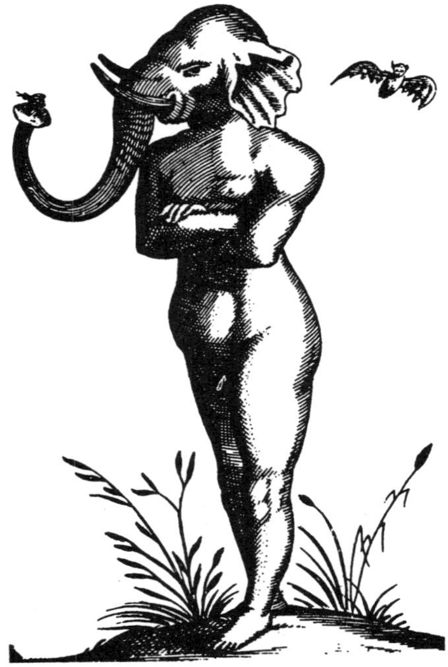

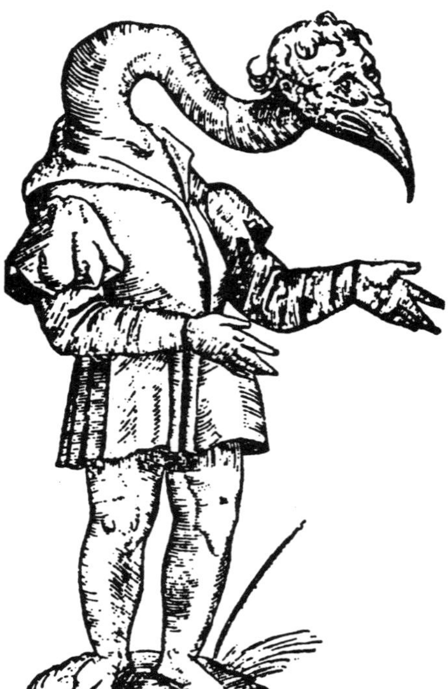

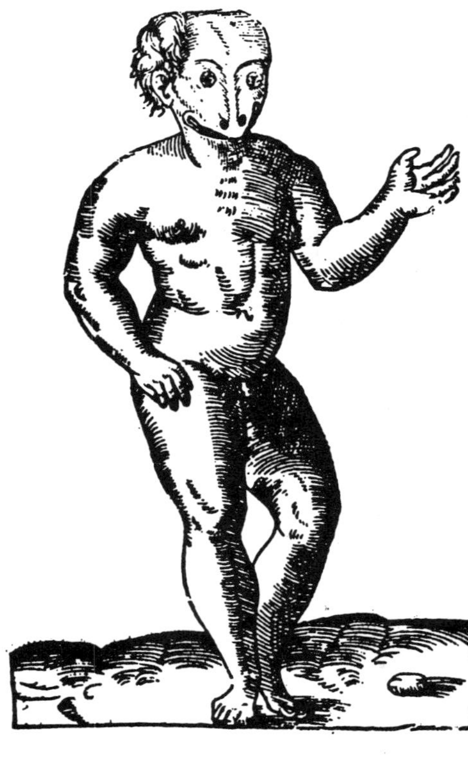

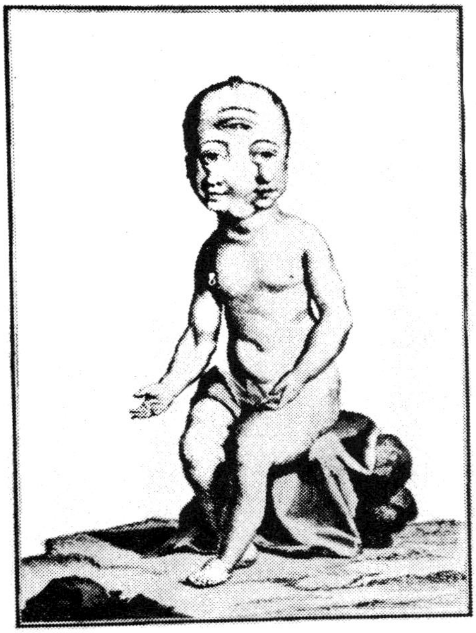

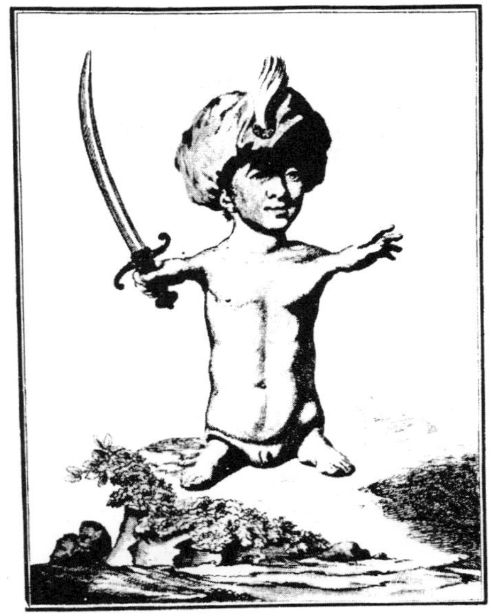

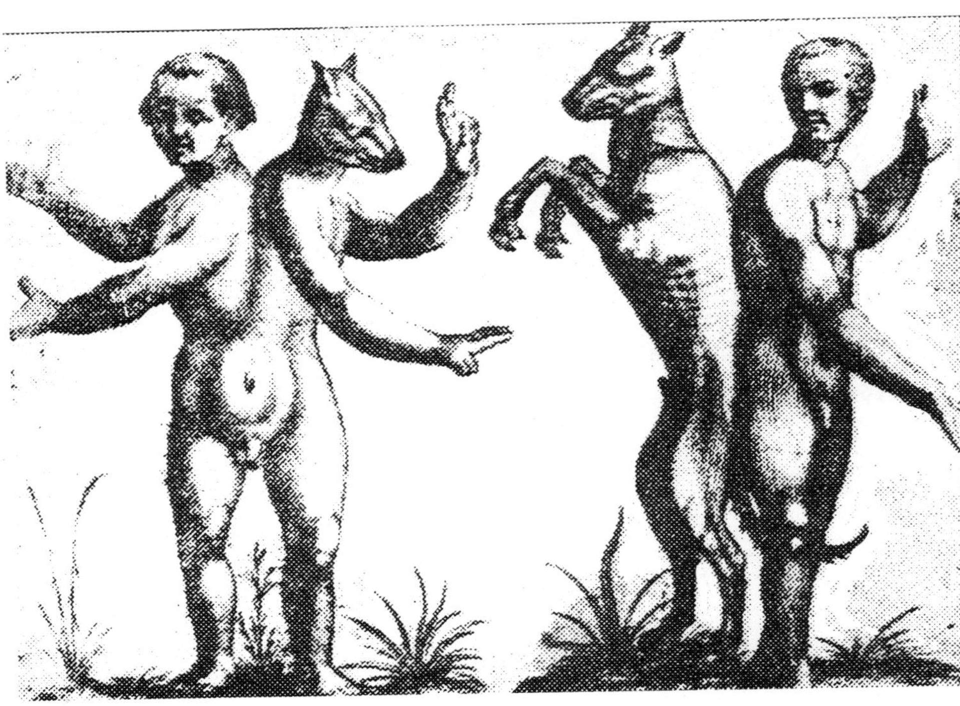

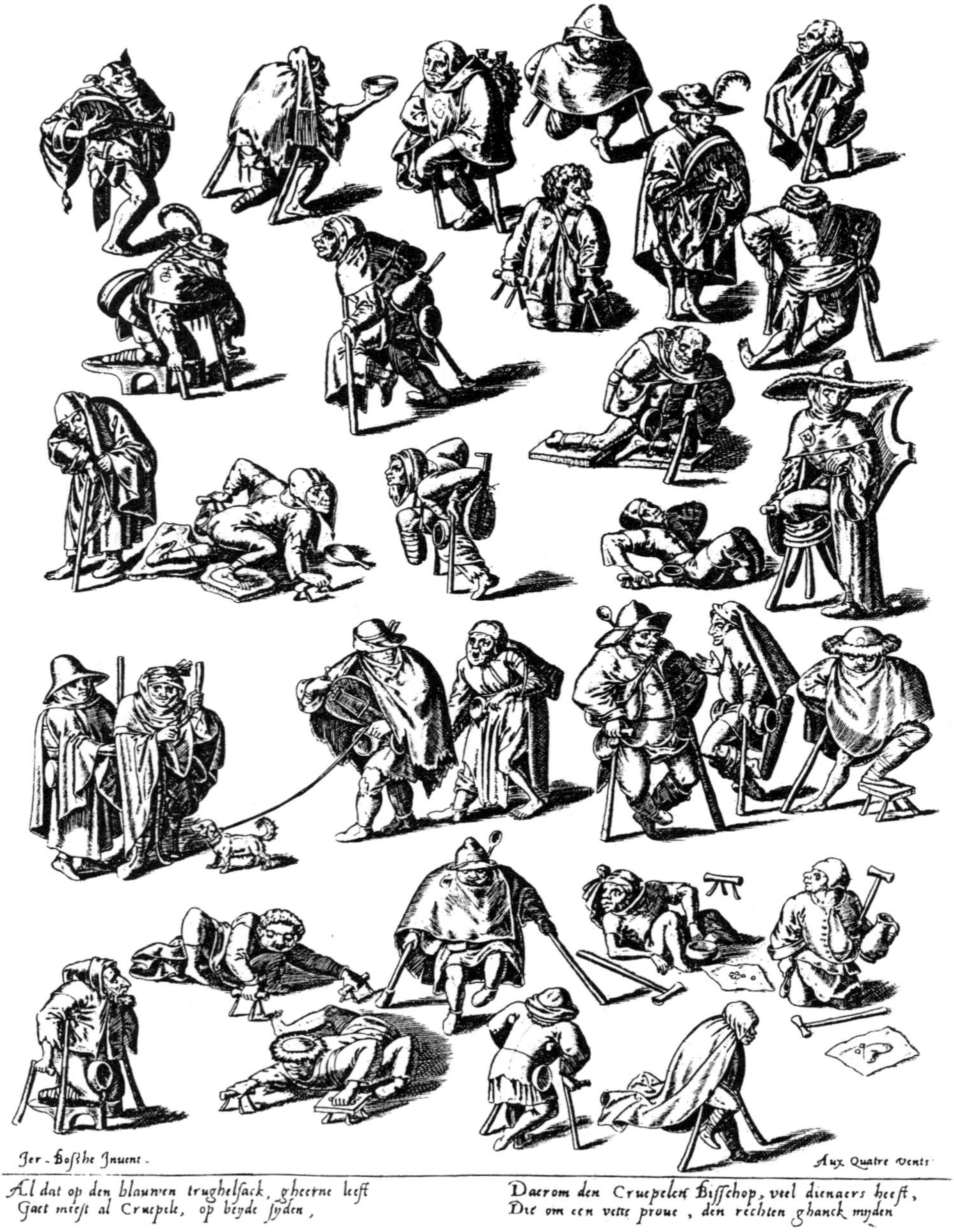
Jer. Bosche Inuent.
Aux Quatre Vents
Al dat op den blauwen trughelsack, gheerne leeft
Gaet meest al Cruepele, op beyde syden,
Daerom den Cruepelen Bisschop, veel dienaers heeft,
Die om een vette proue, den rechten ghanck myden

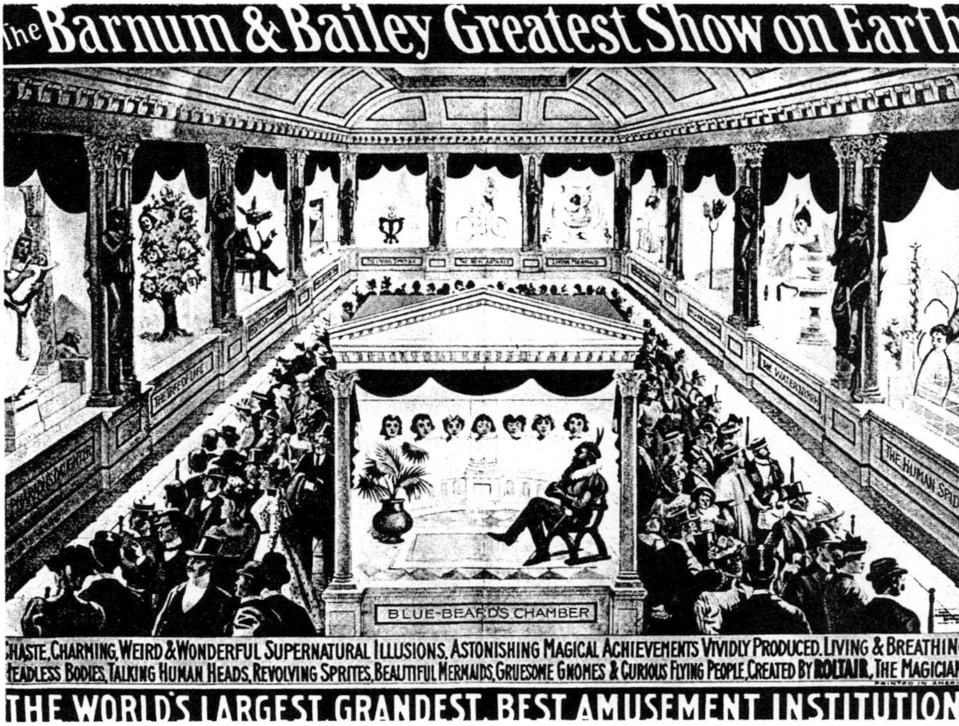
The Barnum & Bailey Greatest Show on Earth
BLUE-BEARD'S CHAMBER
HASTE, CHARMING, WEIRD & WONDERFUL SUPERNATURAL ILLUSIONS. ASTONISHING MAGICAL ACHIEVEMENTS VIVIDLY PRODUCED. LIVING & BREATHING
EADLESS BODIES, TALKING HUMAN HEADS, REVOLVING SPRITES, BEAUTIFUL MERMAIDS, GRUESOME GNOMES & CURIOUS FLYING PEOPLE, CREATED BY ROLTAIR, THE MAGICIAN.
THE WORLD'S LARGEST GRANDEST BEST AMUSEMENT INSTITUTION

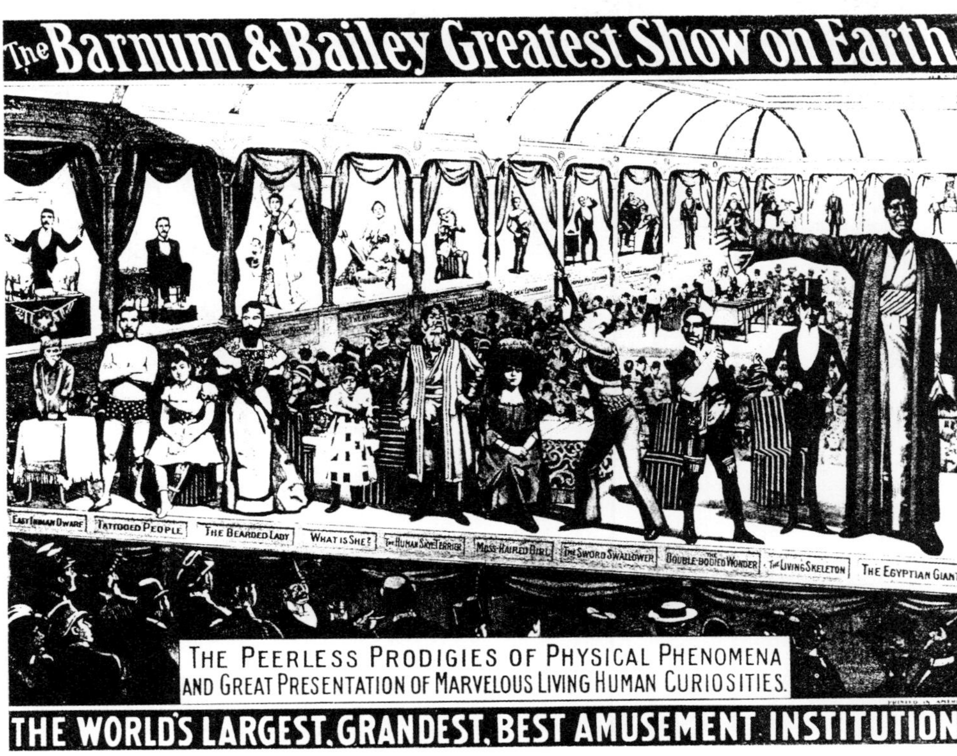
The Barnum & Bailey Greatest Show on Earth
East Indian Dwarf
Tattooed People
The Bearded Lady
What is She?
The Human Skye Terrier
Moss-Haired Girl
The Sword Swallower
The Double-Bodied Wonder
The Living Skeleton
The Egyptian Giant
THE PEERLESS PRODIGIES OF PHYSICAL PHENOMENA
AND GREAT PRESENTATION OF MARVELOUS LIVING HUMAN CURIOSITIES.
THE WORLD'S LARGEST, GRANDEST, BEST AMUSEMENT INSTITUTION.

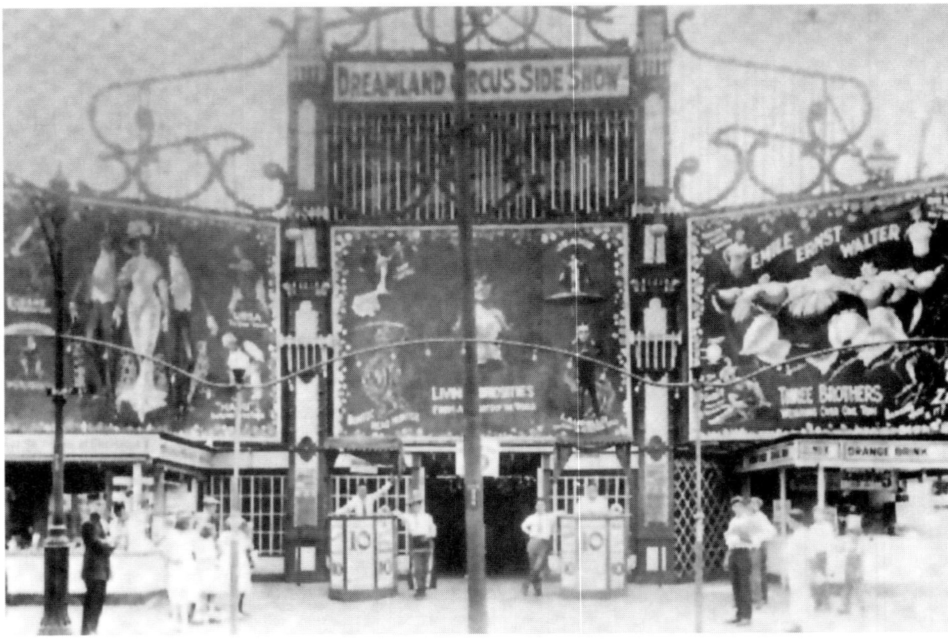
EMILE ERNST WALTER
THREE BROTHERS
ORANGE DRINK

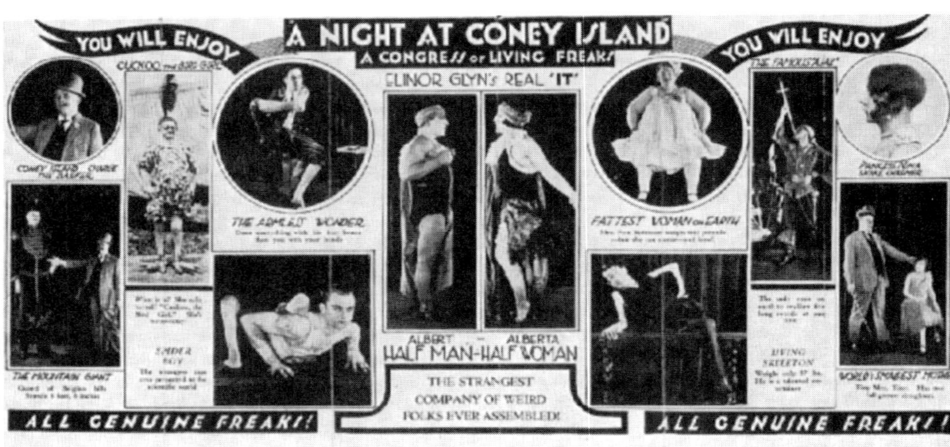
YOU WILL ENJOY
A NIGHT AT CONEY ISLAND
A CONGRESS OF LIVING FREAKS
YOU WILL ENJOY
ELINOR GLYN'S REAL 'IT'
THE ARMLESS WONDER
FATTEST WOMAN ON EARTH
ALBERT - ALBERTA
HALF MAN-HALF WOMAN
THE STRANGEST COMPANY OF WEIRD FOLKS EVER ASSEMBLED!
THE MOUNTAIN GIANT
ALL GENUINE FREAKS!
ALL GENUINE FREAKS!

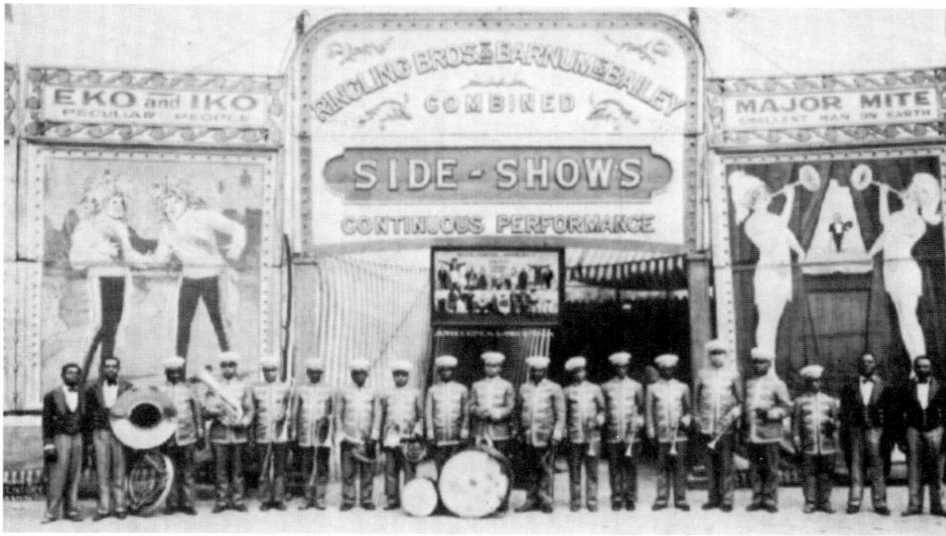
EKO and IKO
PECULIAR PEOPLE
COMBINED
SIDE-SHOWS
CONTINUOUS PERFORMANCE
MAJOR MITE
SMALLEST MAN ON EARTH

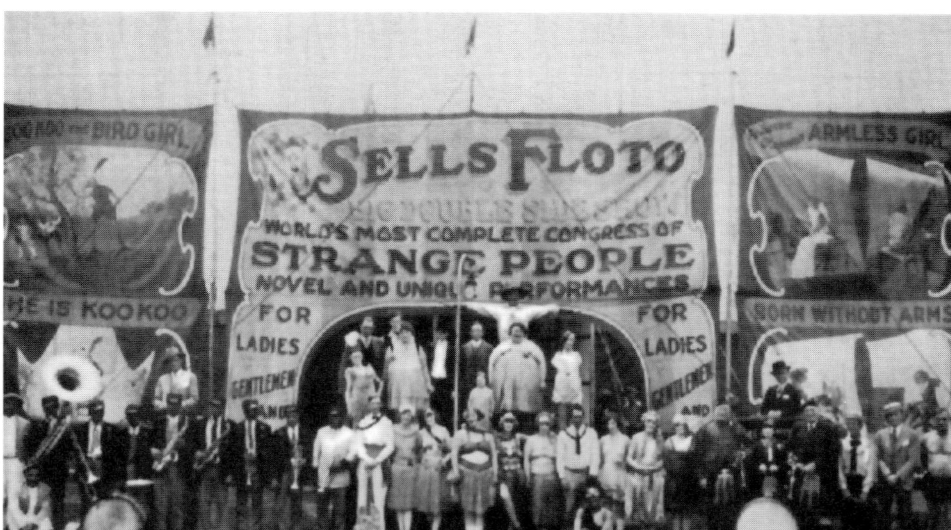
BIRD GIRL
SELLS FLOTO
WORLD'S MOST COMPLETE CONGRESS OF
STRANGE PEOPLE
FOR LADIES
GENTLEMEN
FOR LADIES
GENTLEMEN
AND
ARMLESS GIRL
BORN WITHOUT ARMS

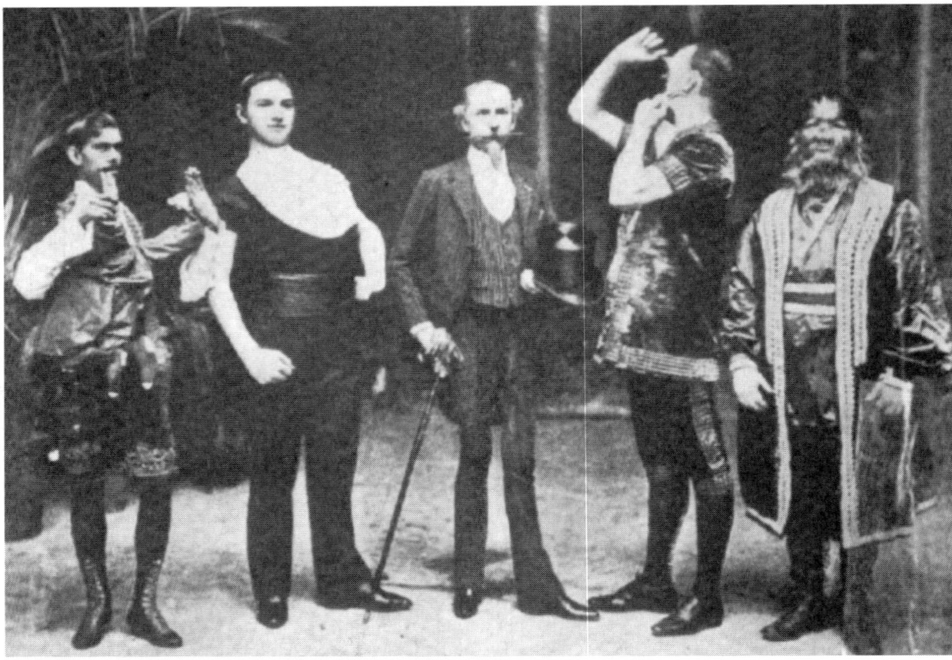

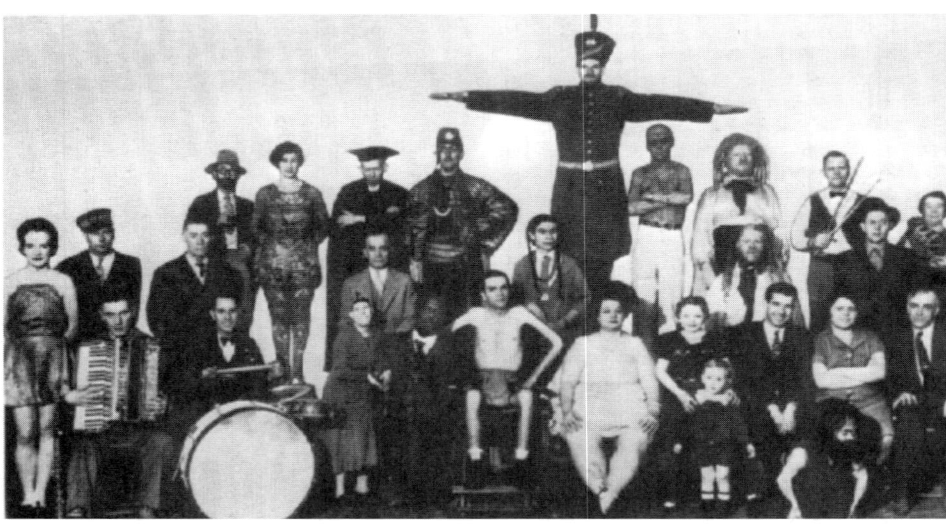

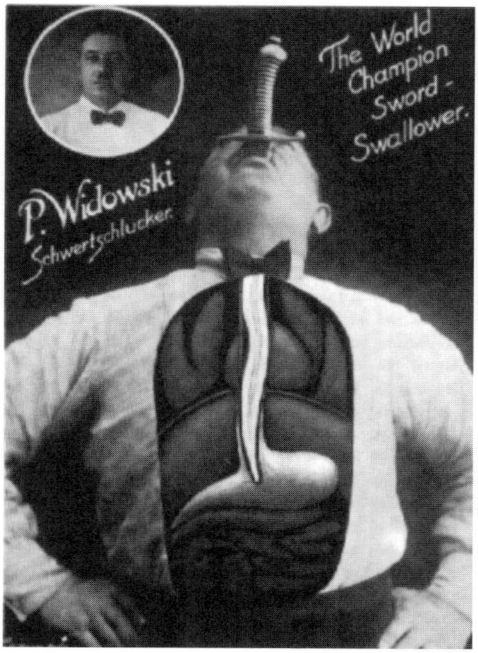
The World Champion Sword-Swallower.
P. Widowski
Schwertschlucker.

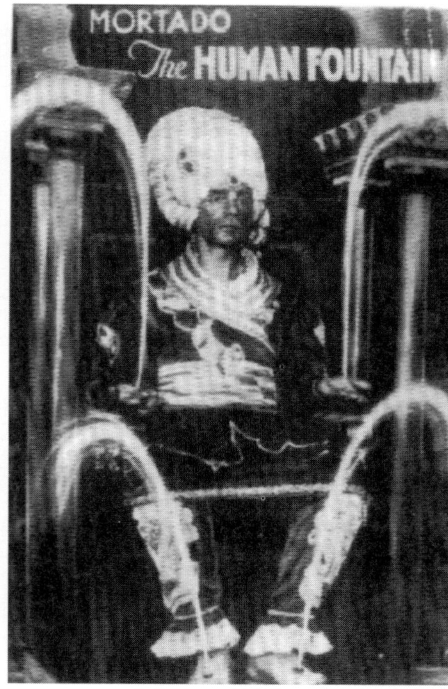
MORTADO
The HUMAN FOUNTAIN

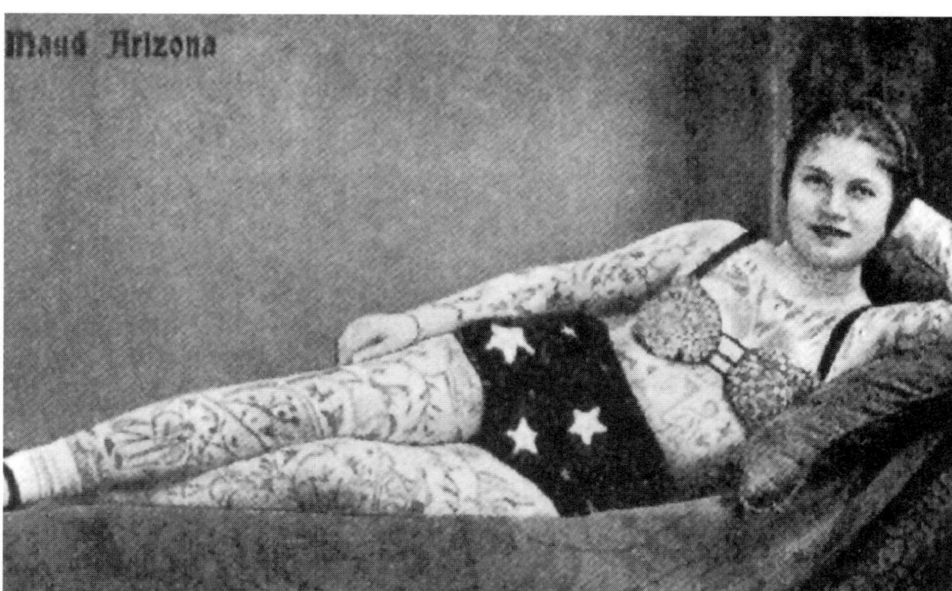
Maud Arizona

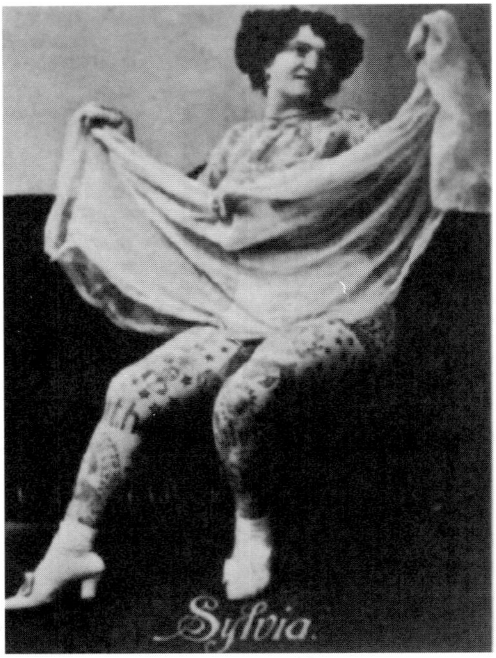

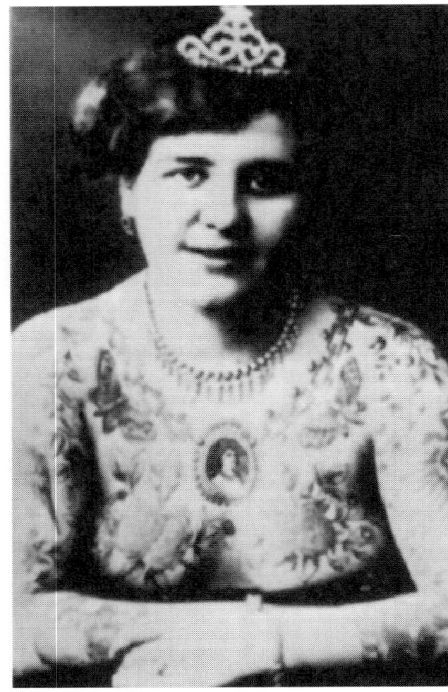

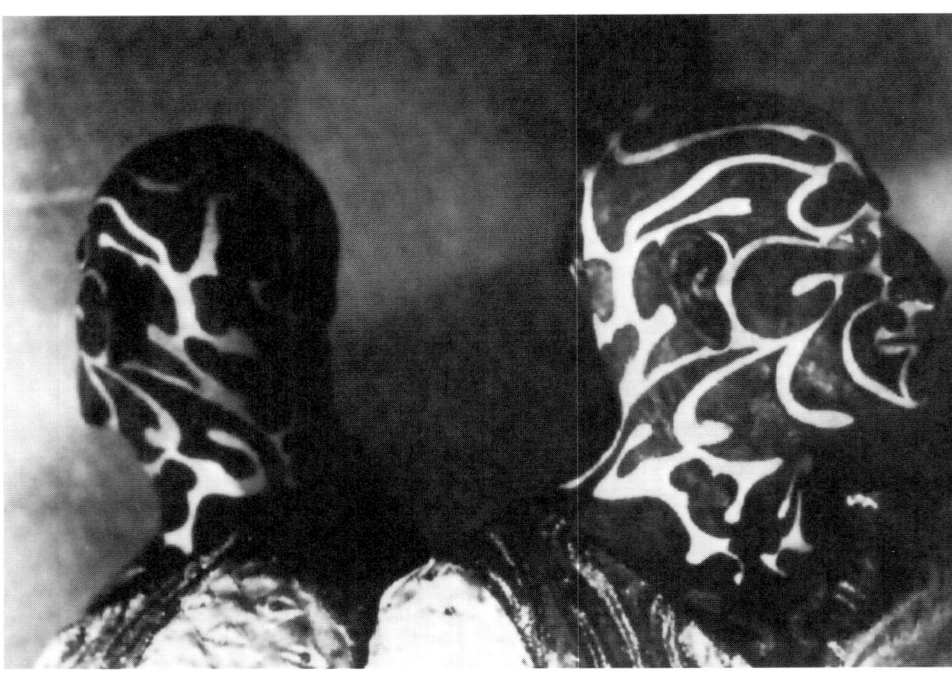

The Great Omi

TAXONOMY

When science eventually overtook superstition in the categorisation and diagnosis of prodigies and marvels, the old myths were discarded and the remaining 'monsters' finally became 'human anomalies'. Among the main types of anomaly and condition identified in this new teratology were:

Hypertrichosis (and sundry zoomorphism):
Those suffering from this condition are the 'dog-men' and 'ape-women'; unfortunates born with an acute, bestial surplus of hair on their faces and bodies. Famous examples have included Horace Gonzales, an Italian living in Rome in the early 17th century, whose features were recorded for posterity in a celebrated engraving by the Florentine engraver Stephano Della Bella (1610-64). One of the earliest and most exact known representations of hypertrichosis, it ensured Gonzales' place in the annals of teratology. Another immortalised effigy is that of Tognina d'Ambras, the 'lion-faced girl', from the legendary family of hypertrichotics, by courtesy of the artist Giacomo Franco (c1580).

Among their famous successors were Jojo (1870-1903), the 'dog-faced boy', also known as the 'Poodle-Man' during his stint with Barnum; Lionel (1890-1932), the 'lion-man', real name Stéphane Bibrowski; Adrian Jerticheff, the 'dog of the Caucasus', who was first exhibited in Paris around 1873, sired an identical son, and believed himself the victim of a satanic curse; and the Malphoons, a whole family of Burmese 'dog-men' spanning three generations, who were exhibited in Paris throughout 1889.

Perhaps the strangest (and saddest) case of all was that of Julia Pastrana, the 'Gorilla-woman'. Alternatively known as the 'dog woman' or the 'ugliest woman in the world', Pastrana was born in Mexico in 1832 and, despite her looks, was very sensitive and intelligent. She was discovered by an impresario, Theodore Lent, who became her manager and inducted her into show business. She soon became famous – and extremely profitable – and in order to keep his prize exhibit, Lent finally decided to marry her. Julia became pregnant, and eventually gave birth to a hairy, grimacing monster baby. Both mother and infant died in child-birth, and her last words are quoted as being:

"I die happy, for I know I have been loved for myself alone." Yet the tragic tale does not end there. Lent, determined to get his money's worth, had the two corpses embalmed, attired them in extravagant finery and toured them around Europe in a double crystal glass coffin. When the badly-preserved corpses started to rot, Lent had them stuffed and mummified like hunting trophies; after several more years touring these grisly remains, he eventually sold them off. The bodies now belong to an American collector. Lent also found a living replacement for Julia; discovering Marie Bartels, a similarly hairy woman from Karlsbad, he re-christened her Zenora Pastrana and whisked her away to be his latest money-spinning exhibit. Lent died in 1884. [The extraordinary story of Julia Pastrana was filmed nearly a century later as *La Donna Scimmia*]

In Pastrana's footsteps came another female oddity: Krao, the 'chimpanzee-girl'. Born in Laos in 1872, she was discovered by one Karl Bock, and a description of her in *Nature* magazine, May 12 1883, reads:

"Her whole body is covered with smooth, straight black hair; her jaw is very prominent; her ability to push the lips out is developed to almost the same extent as a chimpanzee, and the set of her mouth, when she is annoyed, is quite characteristic; lastly, she has a prehensile foot, which she uses to pick the smallest objects off the ground."

Krao went on to star in Barnum and Bailey's circus before dying in New York, in 1926. Other hairy women, or 'bearded ladies', have included Helena Anthonia (c1600), Margareta von Parma, Magdeleine Ventura (painted by Ribera in 1631), Josephine Clofullia, Madame Clémentine Delait (1865-1939), Anna Kritch (the bearded dwarf), Juliane Sleebus, Madame Adriana, Milly Muro, Annie Jones (1865-1902, a Barnum exhibit), peroxide-whiskered Grace Gilbert (1880-1925) and Olga Roderick (who appeared in the film *Freaks*). Most recent of all was Puerto Rican Percilla Santher, who formed the bearded half of a bizarre marriage when she wed Emmett Bejano, the 'alligator-man' from Barnum in the '40s. She appears in Robert Kaylor's *Carny* (1980).

Similar in appeal to the hypertrichotics, and usually billed as 'wild people', were the albinos, those with white hair, white skin and red eyes – sometimes referred to as the "night people" or "ice people". In America, Ada Russel (1873-1921) was an albino of great renown, as was Rob Roy (born 1866), who toured Europe with Barnum and Bailey in 1898, and Rolla, the 'albino princess'. Best known of them all was Tom Jack The Ice King, born Karl Breu c.1876. Tom Jack toured the world with Barnum and Bailey, was at one time assistant to Houdini, and later changed his name again to Toya, touring with his albino "Ice Family". Others of note included: Eliane Turnery, Princess Mitty, the Norwegian Mella Knudsen, Maud Mills (born 1899, Wyoming), Liliane (born in 1907, married the giant Peter Tom in 1929), albino twins Thelma and Doris, and last but not least the brothers Eko and Iko, a pair of negroid albinos from Ecuador who were regularly billed as the "sheep-headed cannibals". Albino negroes were also exhibited for their patchy pigmentation, and given such appellations as the "Leopard-boy" and the "Tiger-women".

Other 'jungle people' were rather less convincing; Waino and Plutano, the so-called "Wild Men of Borneo", were in reality a pair of hirsute midget grapplers from Long Island. True feral children, those raised in the wild by animals, have seldom been authenticated; alleged examples have included Amala and Kamala (the "Wolf-girls of Midnapore"), Lucas (the Baboon boy), and various "gazelle boys".[3]

Another group often presented as wild people (although they are almost invariably child-like and harmless) are microcephalics: in other words, Pinheads (sometimes called "bird-heads"). The only group of show freaks who are congenitally mentally retarded, they have 'owners' as opposed to 'managers' and are usually asexual, the males and females often attired alike in dresses, hair shaved to a beribboned top-knot (a trend instigated by P. T. Barnum). They can behave erratically, and are sometimes kept chained to their keepers for their own safety. The most historically famous pinhead was named Triboulet, court jester to Francis I of France in the 1500s. He is said to have resembled a monkey, and his tall pointed hat is the model for the traditional 'dunce's cap'. Show pinheads have included: Bartola and Maximo, the Aztec Children; Godino and Apexia; Hattie and Tain; Assra, the amazing dwarf pinhead; Zip, Barnum and Bailey's "missing link" (habitually attired in a furry jumpsuit), teamed with Pip for *Freaks*, which also featured the Snow Twins Jennie and Elvira, and the famous Schlitzie. Schlitzie (mental age: 3) also appeared in the film *Meet Boston Blackie* (1941).

Aside from the dog-boys, monkey-girls, bird-people and others, a whole range of different zoomorphs have cropped up in the carnival pantheon, most notably: "pig-boys" with snouts, tusks or curly tails; "spider-boys", scurrying crab-like across the midway; the legendary "biped armadillo"; Irma Lousteau, the "panther-woman" marked with random outcrops of fur; Hoppie, the "Frog-boy"; Grace McDaniel, the "mule-headed" woman, so named for her spectacular facial deformity (resulting from a birthmark); Miss Violet (born 1888) and Lucy Elvira Jones, the double-jointed "Camel-girls", and their male counterpart Pony Boy; Miss Mignon, the "Penguin-lady"; Serpentina, the "snake-girl" with no bones other than in her head and neck; ectrodactylac Grady Stiles, the "Lobster Boy", proud to descend from five generations of Lobster People;[4] Mrs. Banks, the "bear-cub"; Sealo, the "Seal Boy", named for his flipper-like arms; "alligator-men" such as Emmett Bejano and John H Williams, who suffer from a condition known as *ichthyosis*; and "elephant-skinned" people such as the Englishman John Merrick ("The Elephant Man"), Anna C. Schmidt and Miss Susie (born Vienna, 1904). Legend even tells of a "shark-boy", a repugnant fish-skinned hermaphrodite deemed too hideous to even be exhibited.

Other skin conditions have included "elastic skin", as exhibited by Peter Spanner, James Morris, Harry Haag, Etta Lake and Arthur Loose, and have also accounted for grotesque 'one-offs' such as the "Knotty Man".

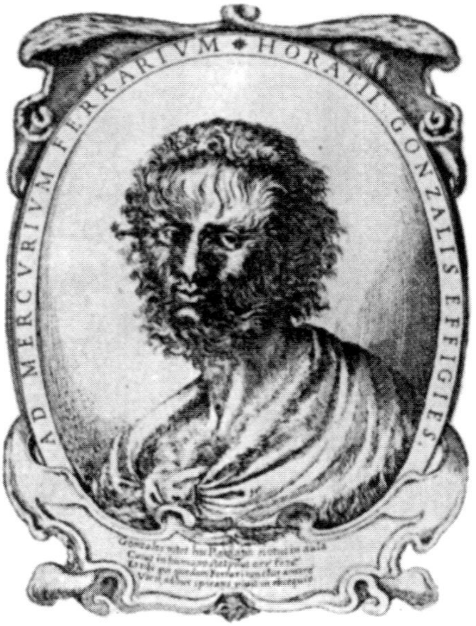

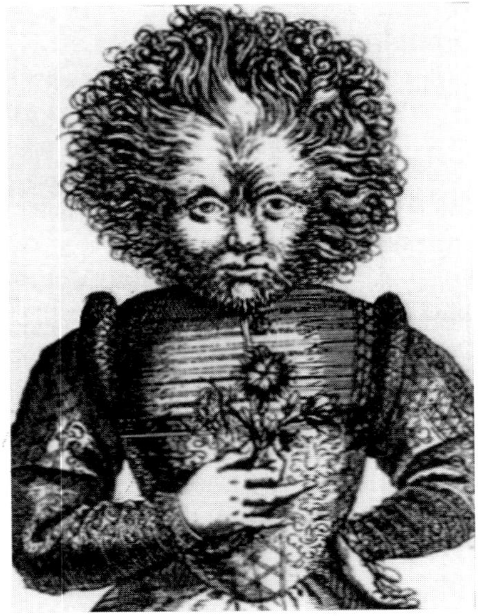

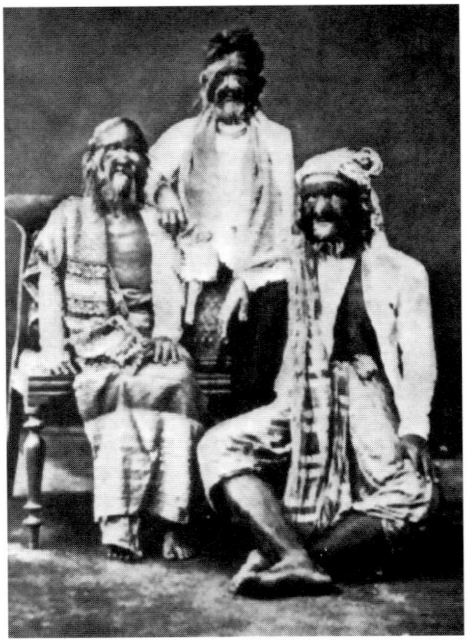

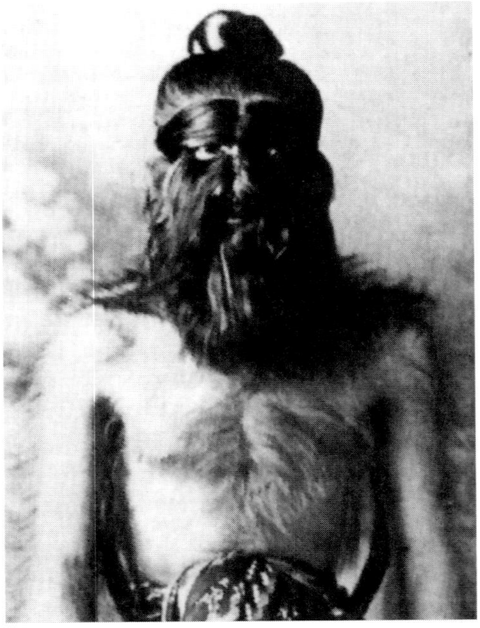

The Malphoons

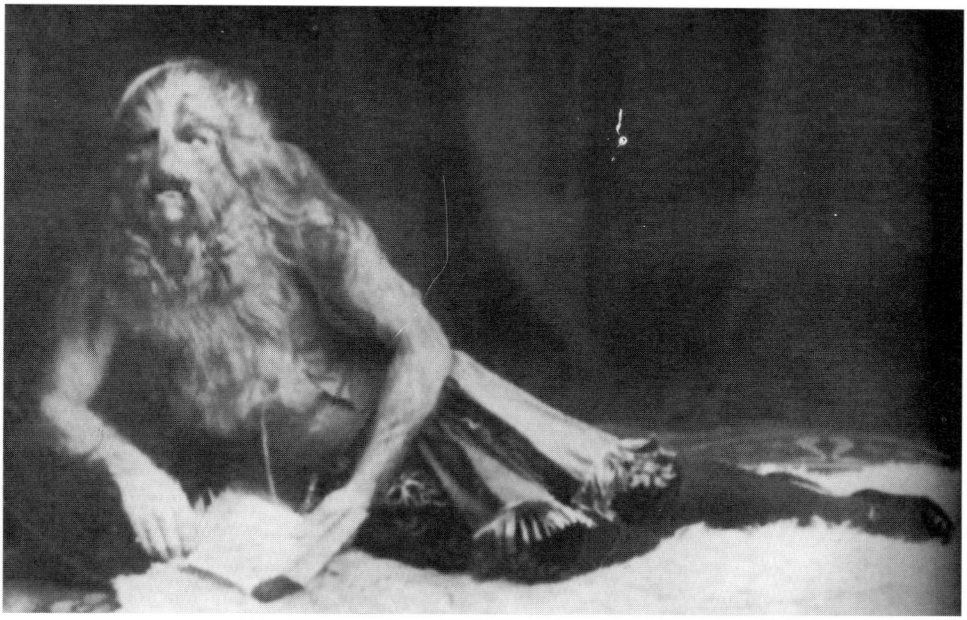

Lionel

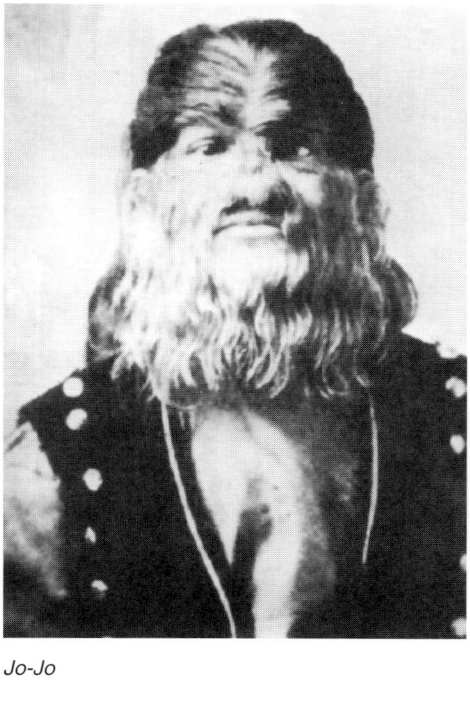

Jo-Jo

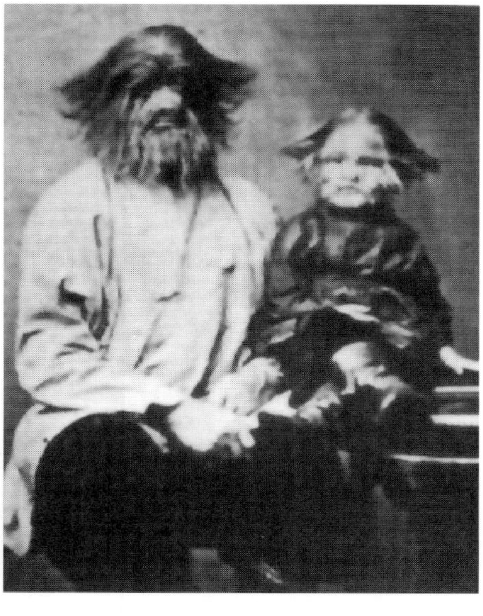

Adrian Jerticheff & Son

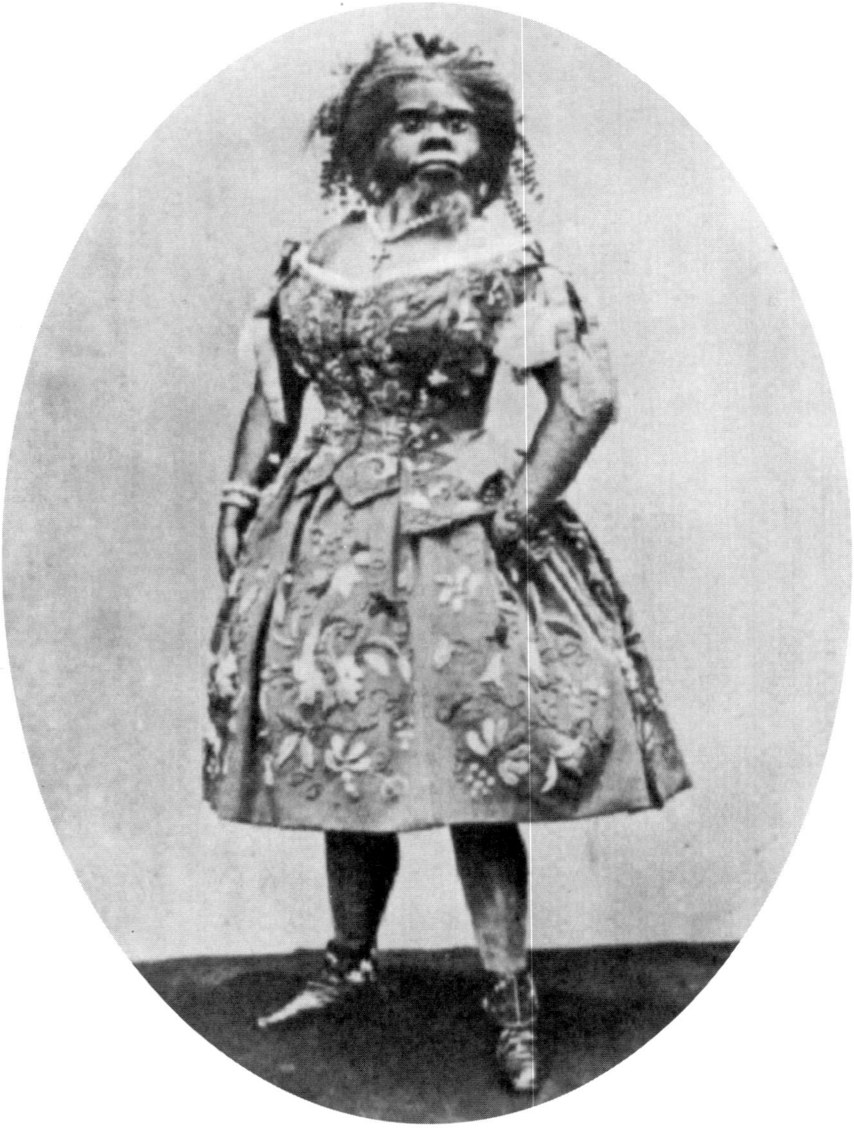

Julia Pastrana

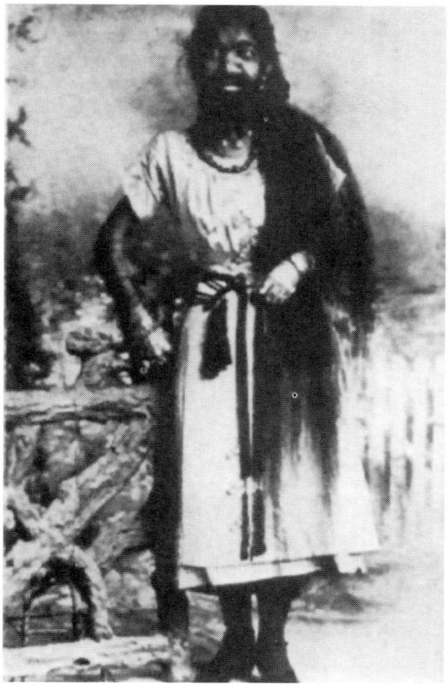

Zenora Pastrana

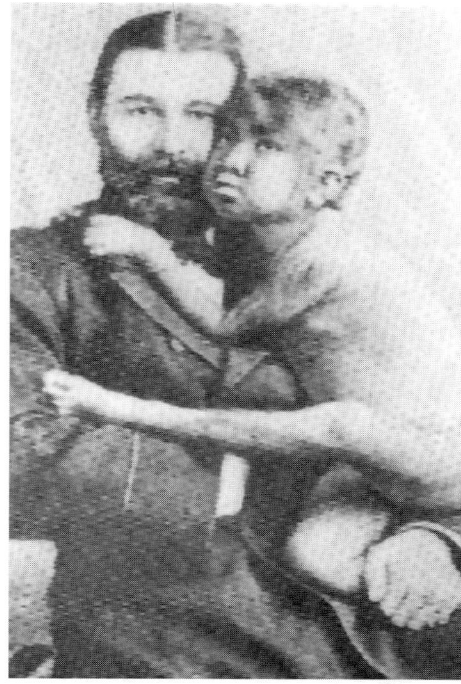

Krao

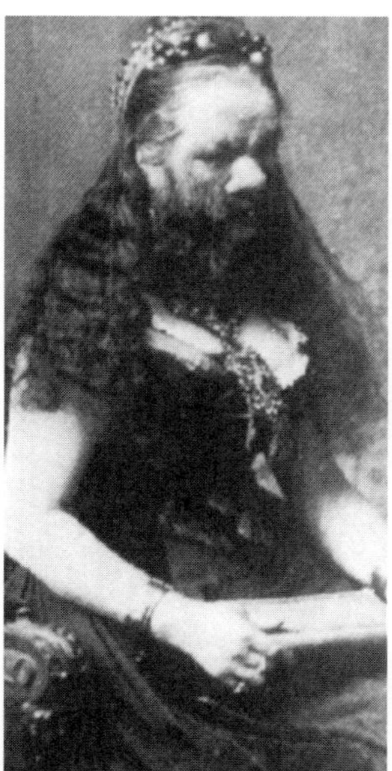

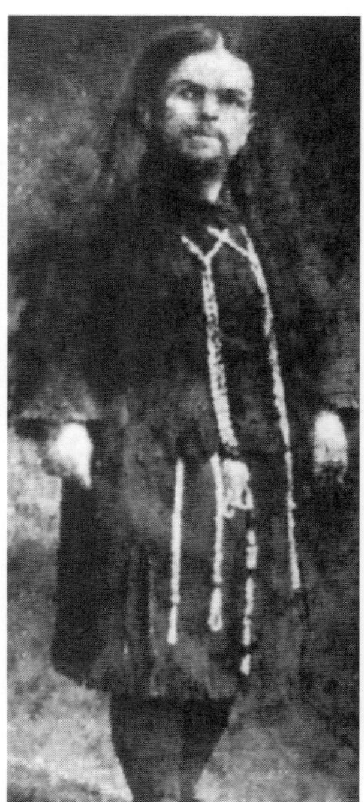

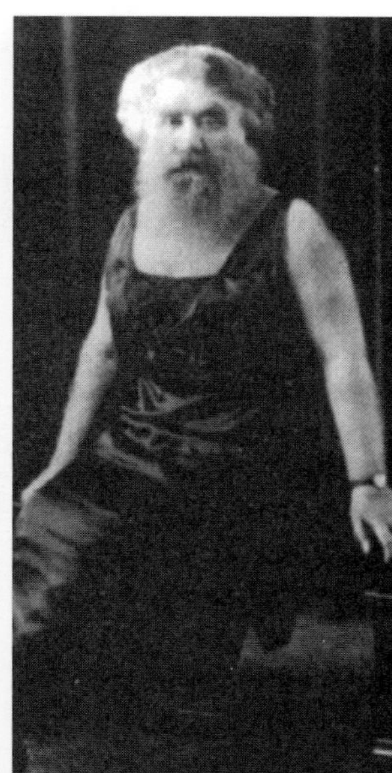

Anna Kritch

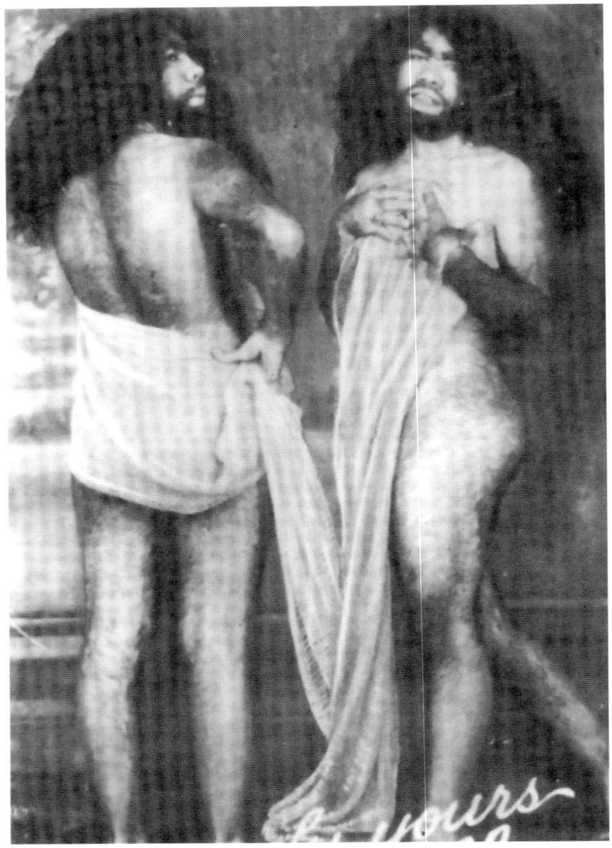

Percilla

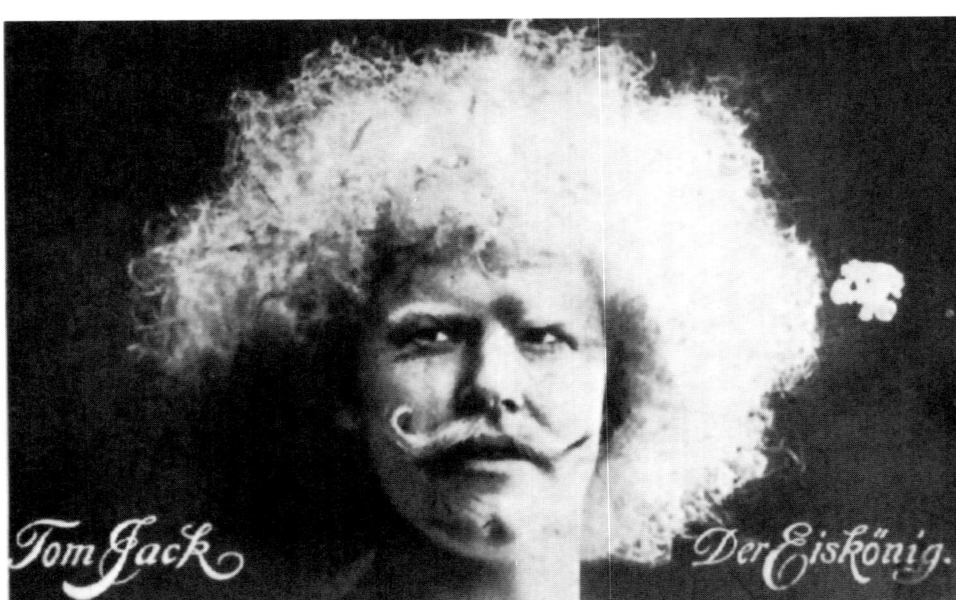

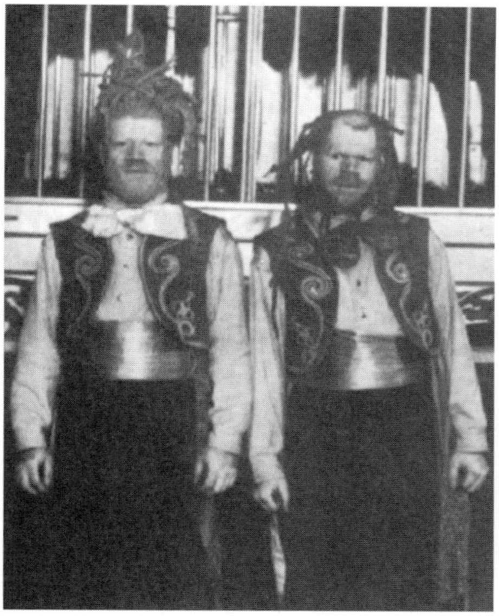

Iko and Eko

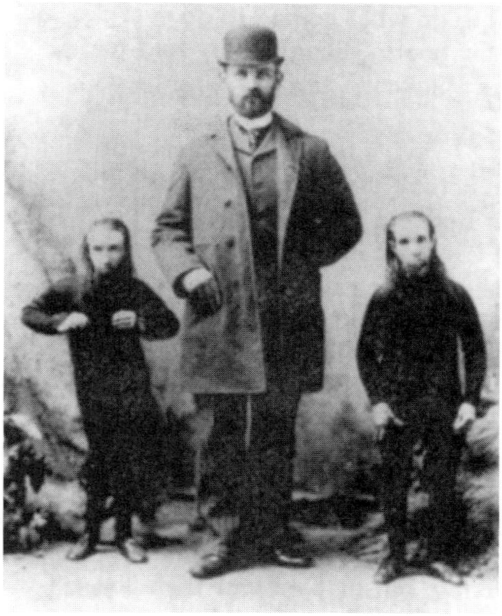

Waino and Plutano

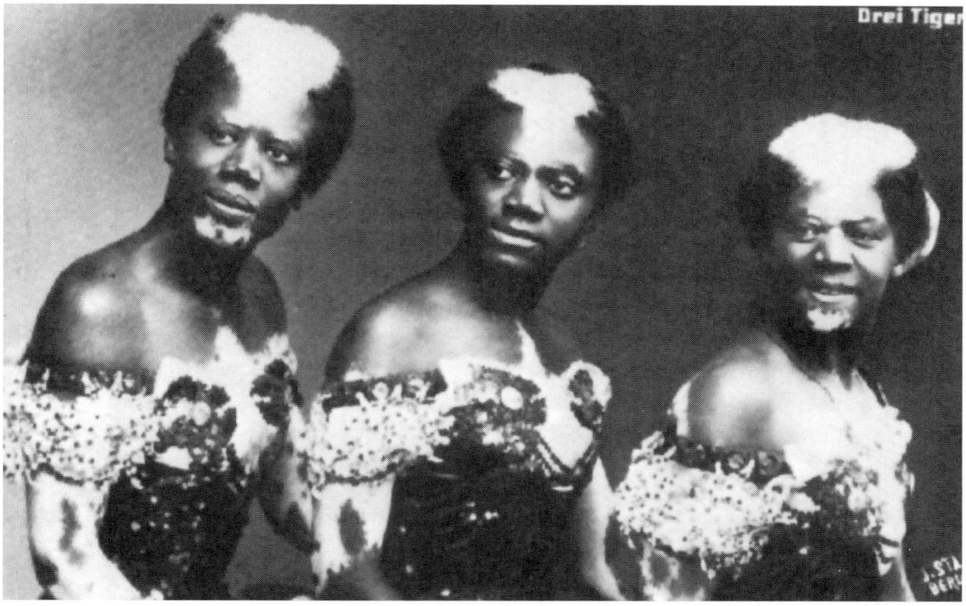

The Tiger Ladies

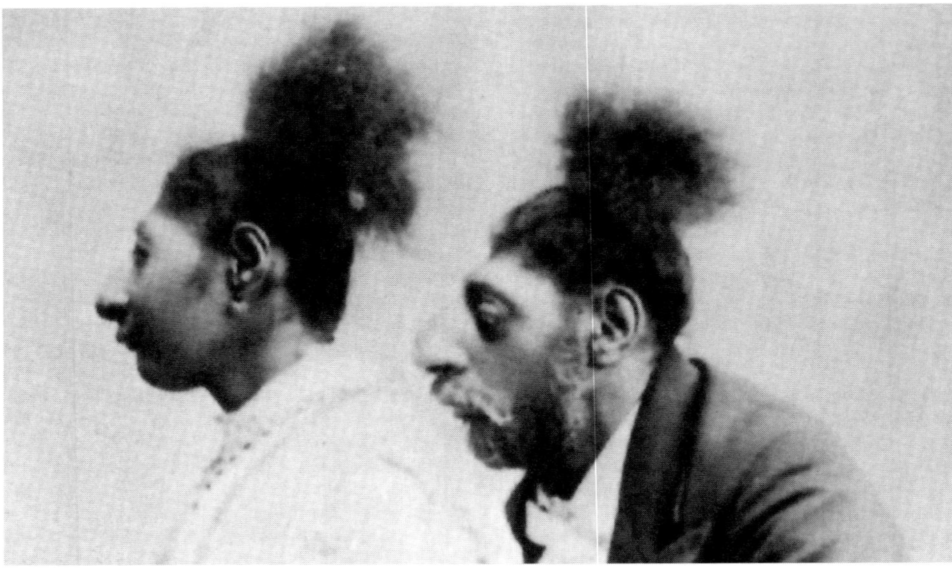

Hattie and Tain

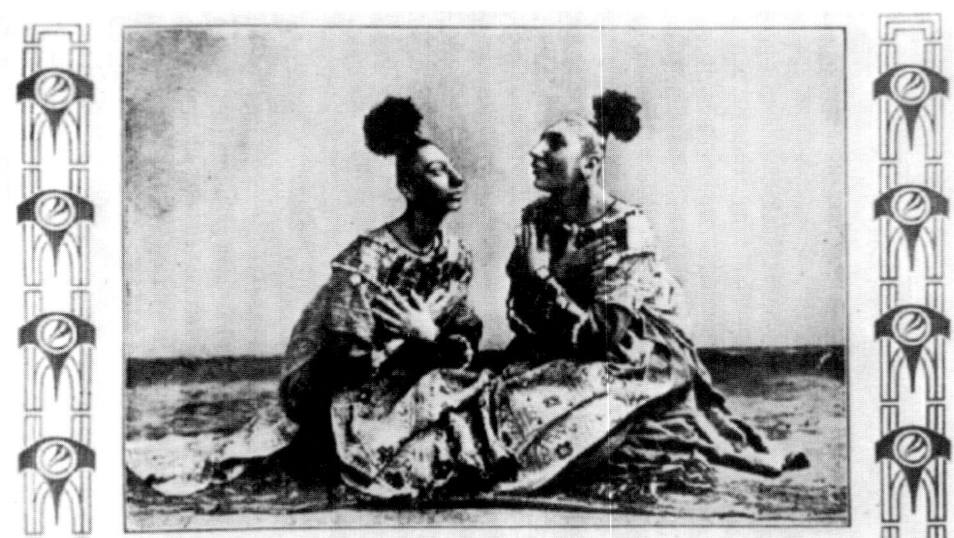

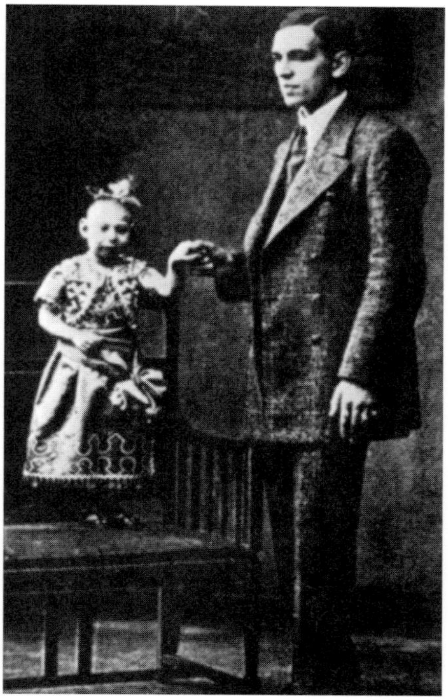

Assra

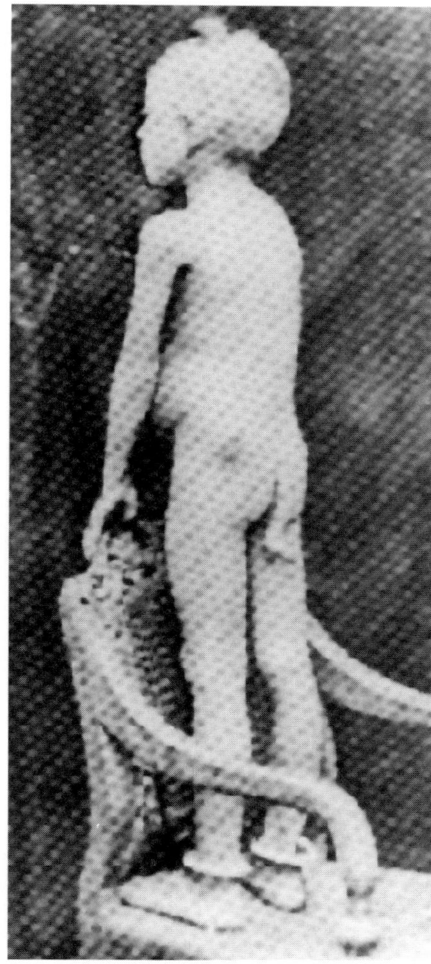

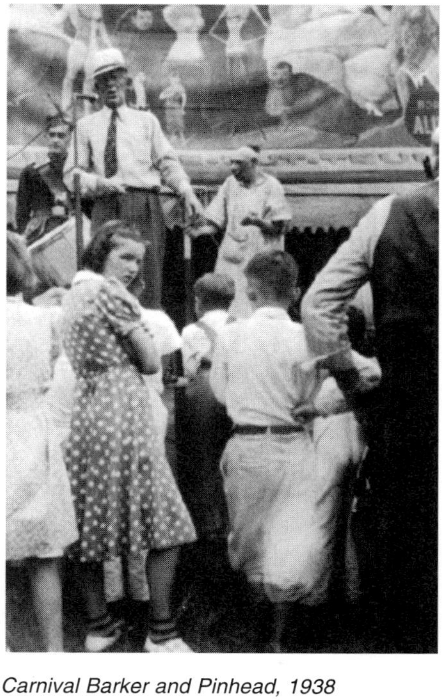

Carnival Barker and Pinhead, 1938

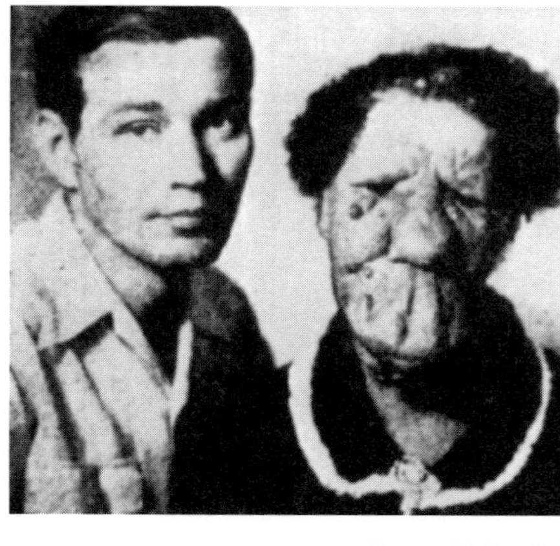

Grace McDaniels

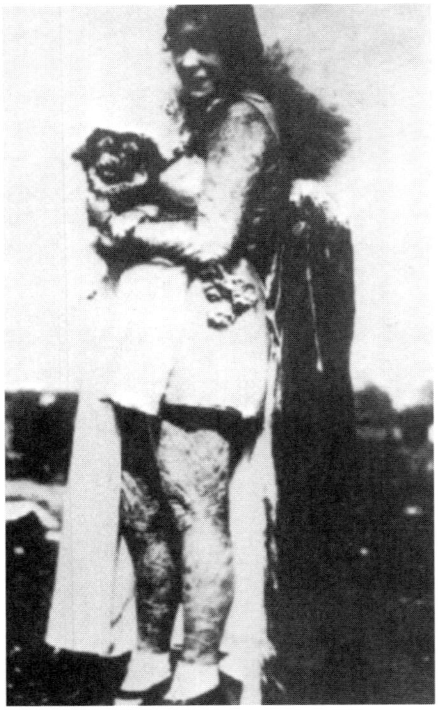

Miss Suzie

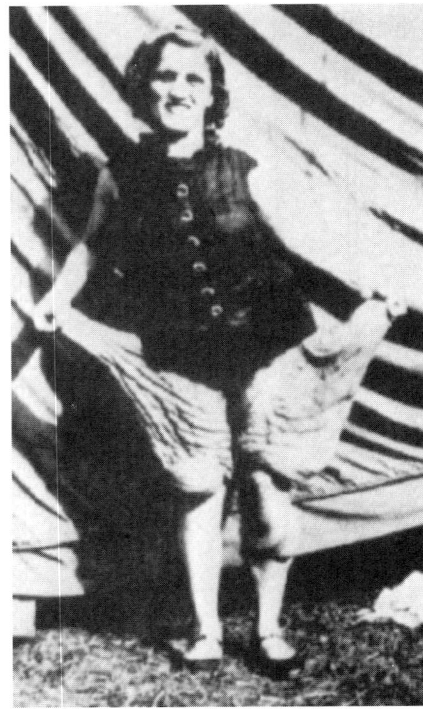

Agnes Schmidt

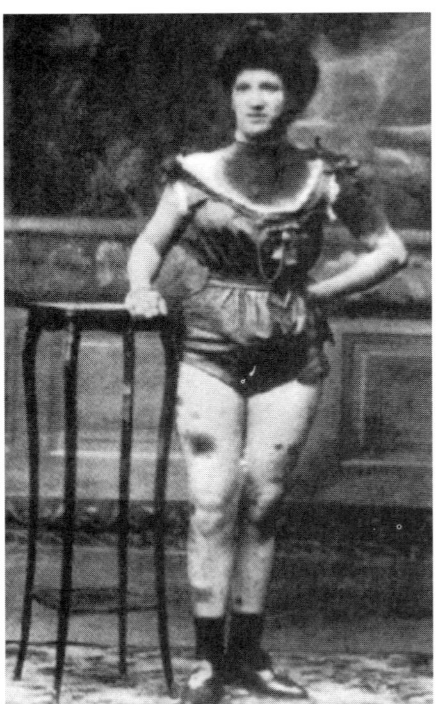

Irma Lousteau

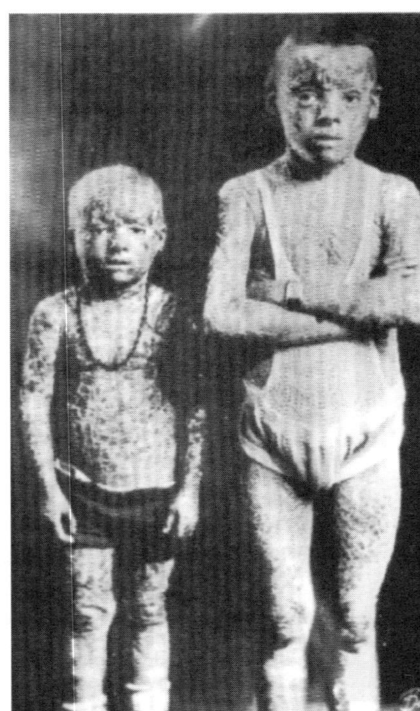

Alligator Boys

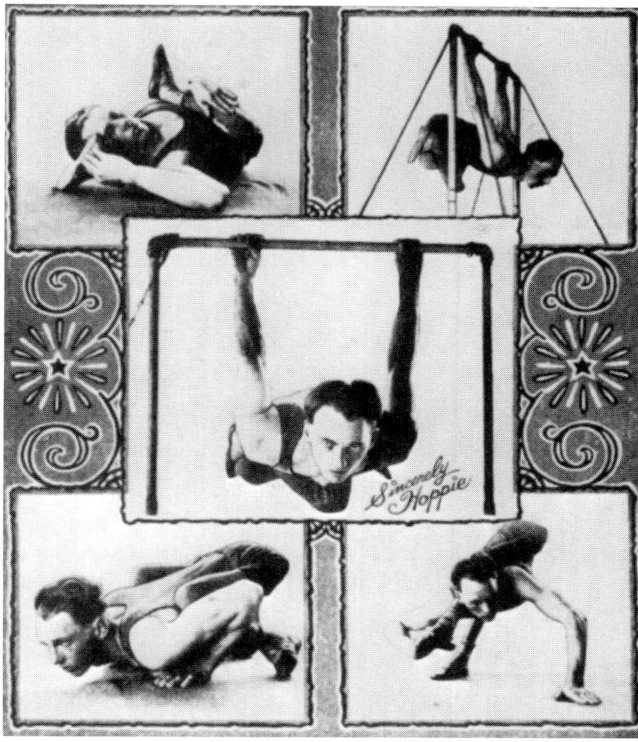

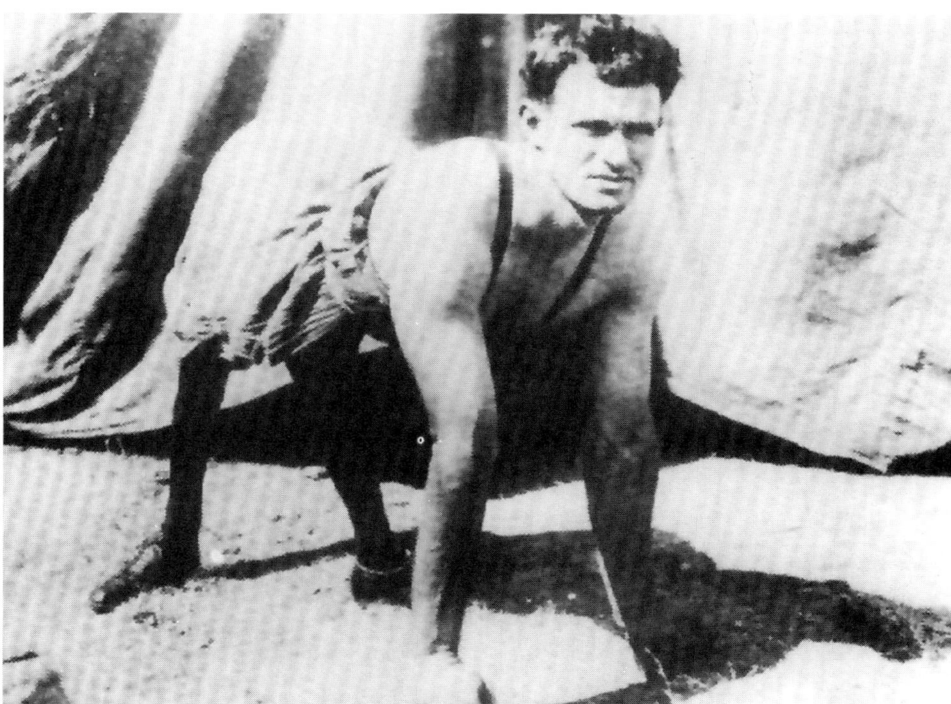

Ponyboy

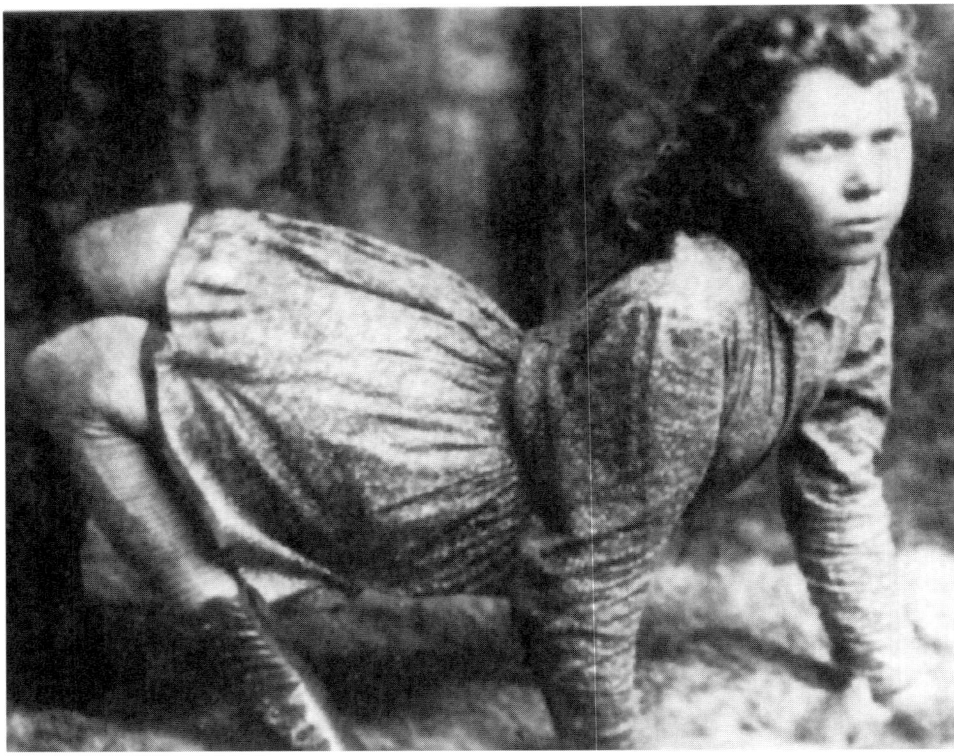

Lucy Elvira Jones

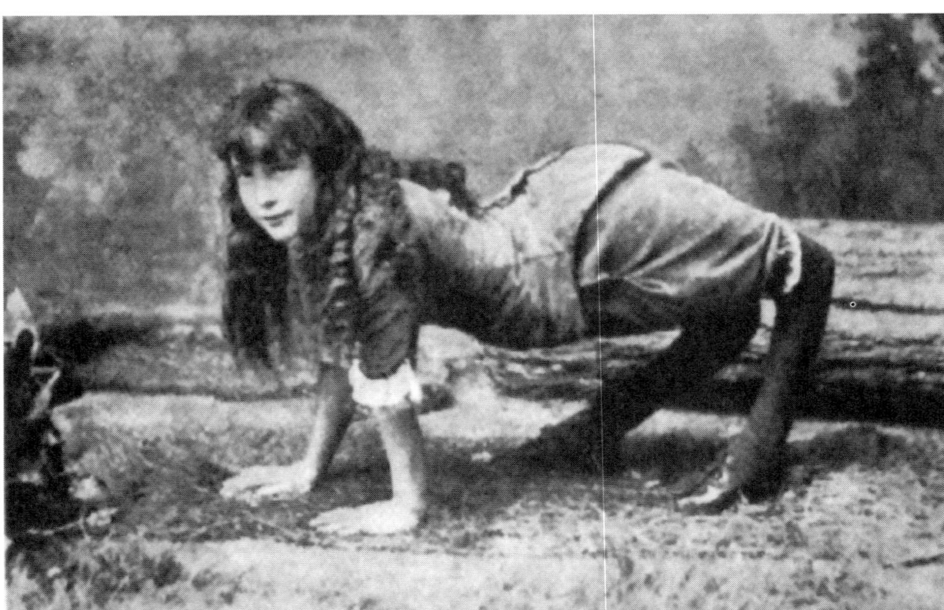

Miss Violet

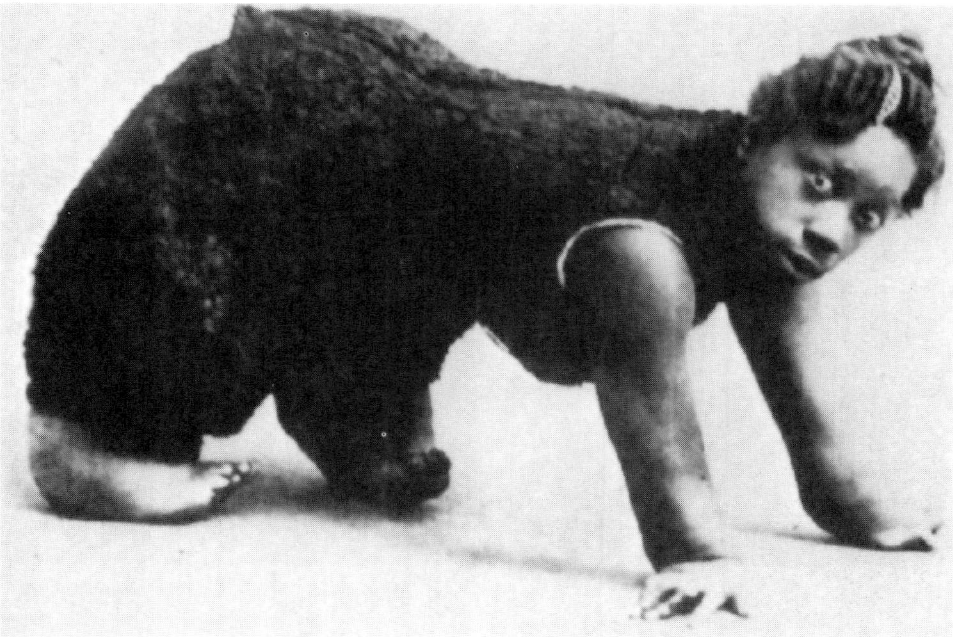

Mrs Banks

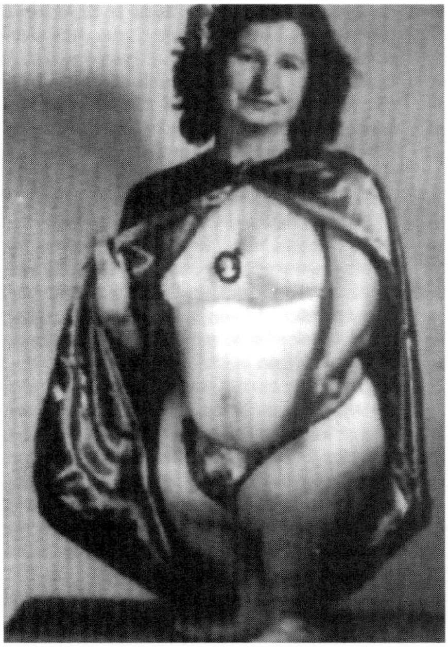

Miss Mignon

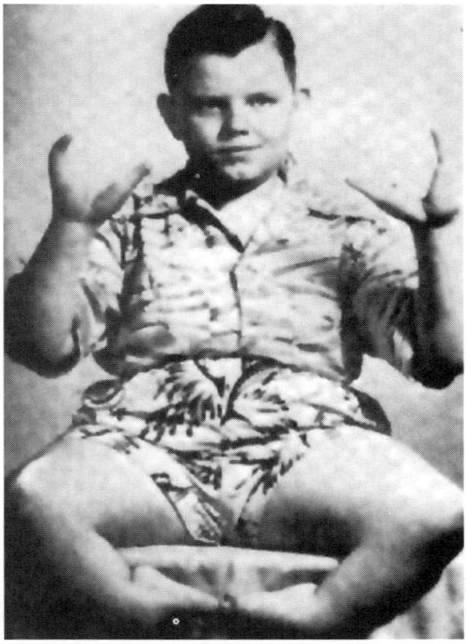

Grady Stiles

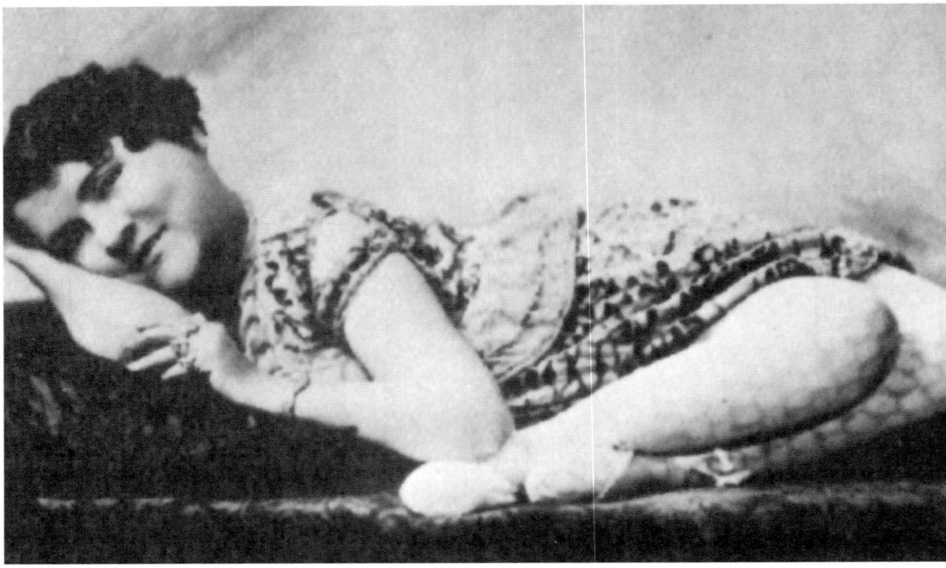

Serpentina

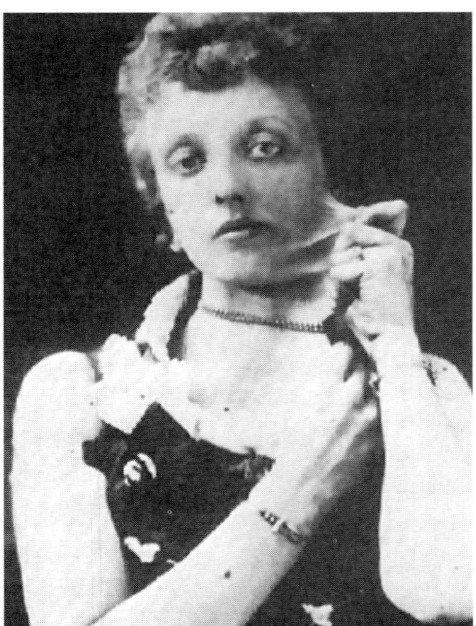

Etta Lake

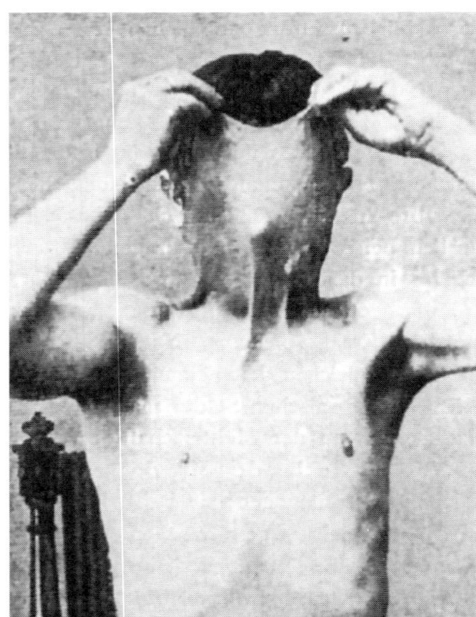

Peter Spanner

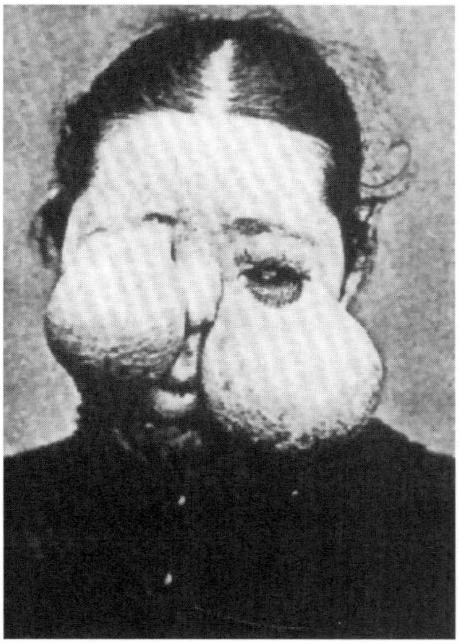

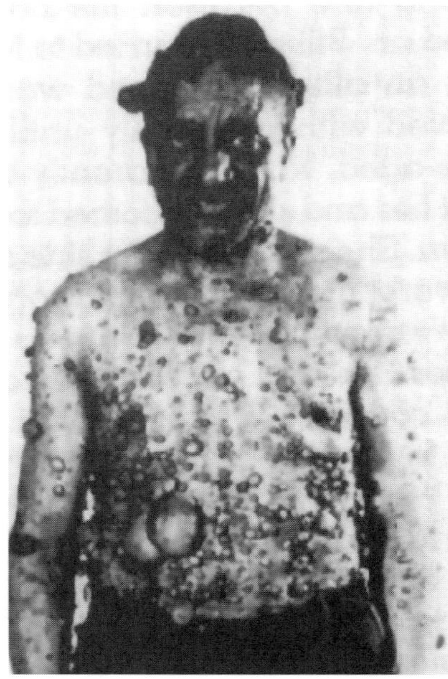

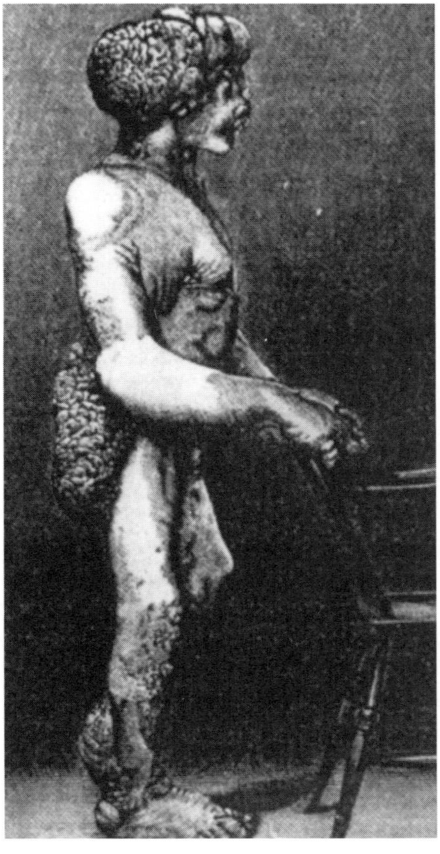

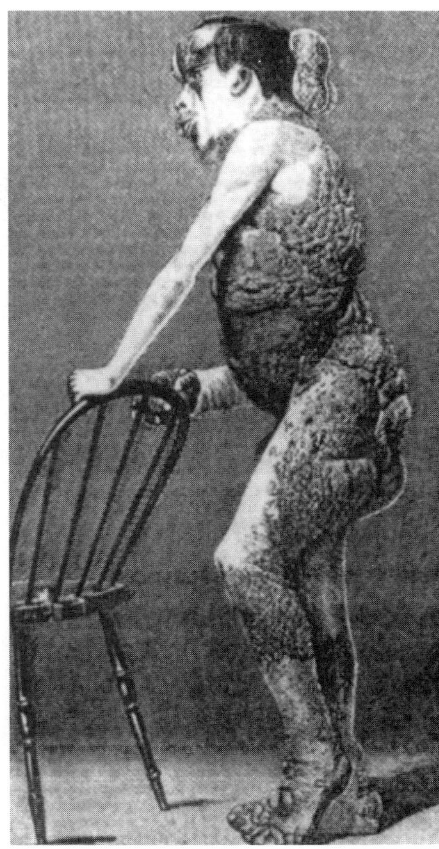

The Elephant Man

Autository, or 'double' monsters:
In other words, Siamese twins. Common types of Siamese twins include craniopages (joined at the head), xiphopages (joined at the side or chest), gastropages (joined at the stomach) and pygopages (joined at the pelvis). Less common are ischiopages, bodies totally fused into one to give the impression of a two-headed, eight-limbed human spider, whose incredibly complex nature renders separation impossible. Always of the same sex, there have been unsubstantiated reports of hermaphrodite Siamese twins, each twin being of both male and female gender.

The term 'Siamese twins' actually originates from the famous xiphopages Chang and Eng, born in Siam in 1811 (their names simply mean 'left' and 'right' in Chinese), although the earliest authenticated case dates right back to 1100, a pair of sisters born in England by name of Helisa and Mary Chulkurst. The anatomist Luigi Galvani reputedly possessed a pickled, three-headed foetus, while it is reported that King James IV of Scotland greatly favoured a certain subject whose body was 'single below, with only two legs, but had two chests and two heads'. Sebastian Münster recorded an unusual case in his *Cosmographiae Universalis* (1544), but the first to be scrutinized scientifically appear to have been Hélène and Judith, born in 1701, who feature in Buffon's *Histoire Naturelle*. When they died in 1723, an autopsy revealed that they had but a single anus, and two vaginas which merged into a single vulva. Such physical anomalies have since been found to be common in Siamese Twins; one pair of baby girls separated in 1974 having no fewer than four vaginas between them.

Other famous examples have included Elizabeth Bedbury, a two-headed lady born in 1842 in Surrey (exhibited at the notorious Bartholomew's Fair in Smithfield, London), the Indians Gangalai and Gourabai, the Russians Macha and Dacha, the Cubans Kenerado and Rivero, the gastropage brothers Liou-Tang-Sen and Liou-Seng-Sen (Barnum & Bailey exhibits), multi-talented English pygopages Violet and Daisy Hilton (who appear in Tod Browning's *Freaks*), pygopages Josepha-Rosa Blazek (performers at the *Théâtre de la Gaité* in 1890's Paris), the Mexican gastropages Mary and Arrita, black American sisters Millie and Christine (born in slavery and otherwise known as the "United African Twins"), and Lucio and Simplicio Godina. These last two were brothers born in 1906 in the Phillipines, and came to Europe in 1930. They married normal twin sisters, and danced the tango as a foursome, becoming champion ice-skaters. But one brother got drunk at the wheel, and knocked over a child. He escaped a prison sentence, since it was deemed unfair to also incarcerate the innocent twin, and a hefty fine was imposed instead. His brother then refused to perform any longer, to which the other responded with a suicide threat. In the end, Simplicio died first, in 1936. Lucio had the corpse surgically removed, but perished 11 days after. It is reported that Chang and Eng were dogged by similar problems, being forced to quit America to escape the attentions of one Miss Gloria, a raving nymphomaniac obsessed with the potential of their double genitalia. They eventually married two women who disliked each other, and had to visit them in turn, riding to their separate homes which each boasted a king-sized bed for three; they nonetheless sired a reputed twenty-two children between them.

Probably the most remarkable of 'double-monsters' was a derodym, the strange being known as Giovanni and Giacomo Tocci. Born October 4th 1877 in Sardinia, the Toccis consisted of two identical heads atop a splayed, V-shaped torso fitted with four arms, supported by a single pelvis and two legs. They also sported a third buttock, and were generally incapable of perambulation due to atrophy. Each head was duly baptised; Giovanni, on the right, was lively and intelligent, while Giacomo, to the left, was more slow-witted. In 1892, aged 15, they went to America, where the Scientific Academy pronounced them "the most remarkable double-monster to have ever reached maturity". In 1897 the Toccis returned to Italy and built themselves a high-walled house near Venice, and lived there having married two sisters (since they had two heads but only one penis, it would seem that each enjoyed the other's bride). They lived until 1940, and died age 63. Another example was Rita-Christina, born in 1829 in Sardinia; but this double creature, with two heads and bodies joined to a single lower half (a condition known as *dicephalus*), only lived to eight months.

More recent cases of united twins have included Mary and Margaret Gibb, Lotti and Rosemarie Knaack, Donald and Ronald Gaylon, Santina and Giuseppina Foglia, Clara and Alta Rodriguez, and black American craniopages Yvonne and Yvette, born in Los Angeles in 1949, whose parents held a party in 1961 to celebrate the first million dollars earned from exhibiting their offspring.

Separating Siamese twins surgically has always been a pre-occupation amongst doctors and surgeons. The main problem is that twins of this nature often have only one heart, one liver, one set of intestines etc, so that there are insufficient organs to support two separate entities. The first recorded attempt dates from 1701, when a certain Dr. Treyling operated on two sisters, Magdelena and Suzanna, joined at the base of the spine. They died. Most notorious of all was the attempt made in Paris in 1892 by Dr. Doyen to separate the famous Indian xiphopages Radica and Doodica Orissa. Born in 1888, these sisters had been hounded from their native home by the locals, who believed their affliction to be a divine curse. Priests gave them sanctuary, believing them to be demi-goddesses, but eventually sold them to a London impresario who exhibited them in the Tuileries in 1892. When Doodica succumbed to tuberculosis, Dr. Doyen of the Trousseau hospital announced that he would operate to part them. The operation become a public spectacle, a grand event with Doyen – quickly dubbed the "Barnum of surgery" by his rivals – performing before the cameras in what could perhaps be regarded as the first genuine exploitational photography of human anomalies. The operation was not a success; Doodica succumbed under the knife, and Radica was dead within two years. The first successful separation was achieved in 1952; it is now a commonplace and generally safe practice.

An extraordinary type of Siamese twins are 'parasitic monsters'. These fall into two main categories: heteradelphians and pygomelians. Both are born with half-formed siblings extruding from their own bodies. Early recorded examples of the former were Hans Kaltenbrunn, born in 1525 with a parasitic brother hanging from his belly, and Lazarus-Johannes Batista Colleredo, born in Genoa in 1617. Colleredo's parasite, unusually, had a head. Michel Montaigne, who witnessed one of these creatures first-hand, left the following account amongst his essays:

"This tale shall speak for itself, for I shall leave its discussions to the physicians. Two days ago I saw a child being led about by two men and a nurse, who said they were his father, his uncle, and his aunt, in order to make a few pence by displaying him, because of his strangeness. In all else, he conducted himself normally, he stood on his feet, walked, and chattered more or less like all children of his age: he had never taken nourishment, except at his nurse's breast; and what was put in his mouth in my presence, he chewed a little, and put out again: his cries did indeed seem rather peculiar: he was exactly fourteen months old. Under his nipples he was fastened and joined to another child, which had no head, and had the conduit of its back stopped, the rest being whole; one of his arms was indeed shorter than the other, but it had been broken accidentally at birth: they were joined face to face, as if a younger child were trying to embrace another, older, one. The joint and space where they were joined was but four inches across, or thereabouts, so that if you lifted the imperfect child up, you could see under the other's navel: so the joint was between his nipples and his navel. The navel of the imperfect one could not be seen, but all the rest of his belly could. So what was not joined, such as the arms, buttocks, thighs and legs of the imperfect one, hung free and swinging against the other, and could reach half-way down his leg. The nurse told us that he made water in both places, so the other one's limbs were nourished and living, and in the same state as his own, except that they were smaller and thinner."

One of first show-heteradelphians was the Indian boy Laloo (1869-1902), who came to London in 1882 to exhibit his headless twin. Though billed as a female, the twin was actually male and capable of urination and of sustaining an erection. Laloo perished in a Mexican train crash, in 1905. Another Indian was Perumal, who modestly exhibited in Europe with his headless parasite (named Sami) dressed in silks. Jean Liberra, born in Rome in 1884, became famous with Barnum & Bailey. His parasitic twin, Jacques, was very well developed, and whilst Liberra was in Berlin, a certain Professeur Berdenheimer X-rayed him. His conclusion was that the twin had a head-cage inside its host, and that technically it was alive. Liberra married, had four normal children, and died in 1946. Betty Lou Williams, a black American, was born in Atlanta with the remains of her twin sister protruding from her side. As she grew up, the twin (unusually) grew in proportion. By 1950, Betty Lou was earning $5,000 a month as an exhibit. She died in 1958, reputedly of a broken heart.

Famous pygomelians – in whom only the legs or lower half of their twin is externalised – have included the American Myrtle Corbin, who boasted an extra pair of underdeveloped legs and two vaginas; Elsie Linn, who sported a third, deformed leg; the Cuban Jean Baptista dos Santos, born in 1845, who had extra sets of legs *and* fully-functional genitals; and, most renowned of all, Francesco A. Lentini, born in 1889 with an extra leg, virtually full-sized, sprouting from his right buttock. This leg also carried the atrophied remains of a vestigial fourth limb, giving him sixteen toes in all. He could control all three legs perfectly, and could ride a bicycle with ease. Lentini too was blessed with an extra (though reputedly underdeveloped) set of genitals. He came to America in 1898 and soon found fame and fortune, also marrying and siring four children. The creation of the three-legged stool was, reputedly, inspired by him. He died in Florida in 1964.

Other odd configurations have come to light. Exceptionally grotesque was the case of Edward Mordake, who is said to have been cursed with a "devil twin" – the shrunken head and face of a girl appended to the back of his head. The face was reputedly animated, and the thought of it drove him to an early suicide. The Mexican Pasqual Piñon was also apparently born with a small extra face, this one growing out of his forehead. Again, the eyes moved and the mouth would open and close, though it withered in later life. A famous historical example is the so-called "Home's case", the double-skulled skeleton of an Indian infant.

Related to these individuals is the case of Bill Durks, an American born in 1930. Durks' extraordinary face shows the arrested beginnings of becoming two heads, or perhaps twins; he became a celebrated carnival attraction, and even took to painting a third eye in the gap between his divided nose. Durks died in 1976.

Finally, and most perhaps bizarre of all, comes the enigma of epignathic parasites, virtually formless pieces of human matter usually extruding from the host's mouth. They are a form of teratoma, very much like foetuses *in fetu*. These latter are thought to be tiny, macerated, barely-developed embryos lodged completely inside their living twins. In 1951, the case was reported of a male child found to be housing no less than five such vestigial siblings *within his cranium*. Two years later, Algerian doctors operating on a young boy for a 'stomach tumour' finally removed a six-inch-long male foetus; a number of similar cases have since been recorded.

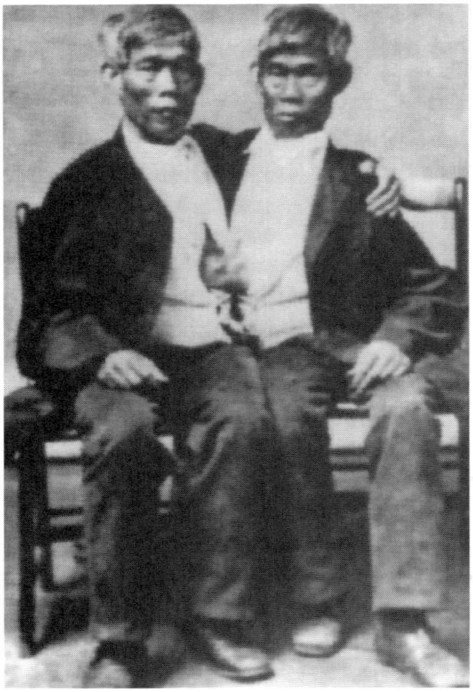

Chang and Eng

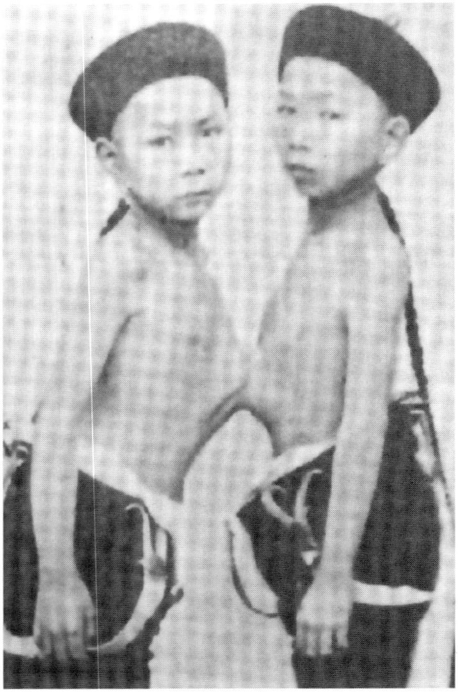

Liou-Tang-Sen and Liou Seng-Sen

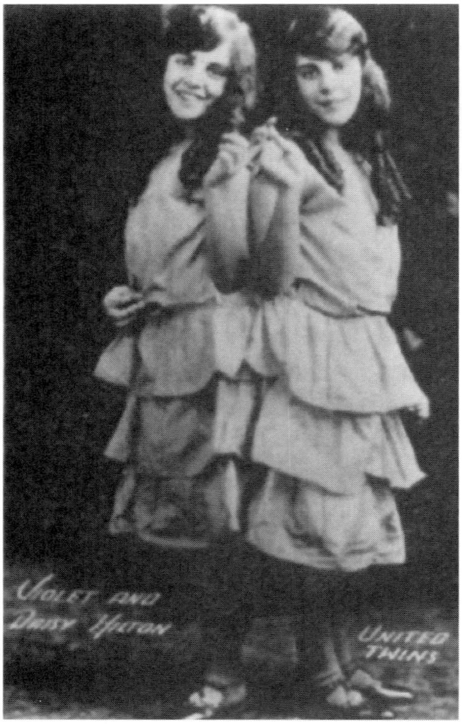

The Hilton Sisters

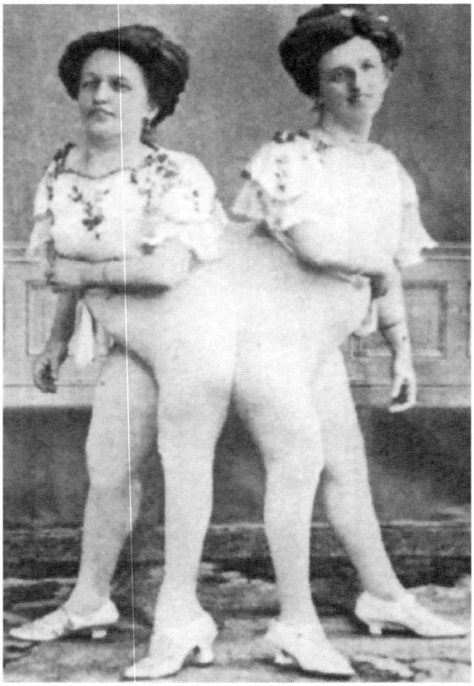

Rosa-Josepha

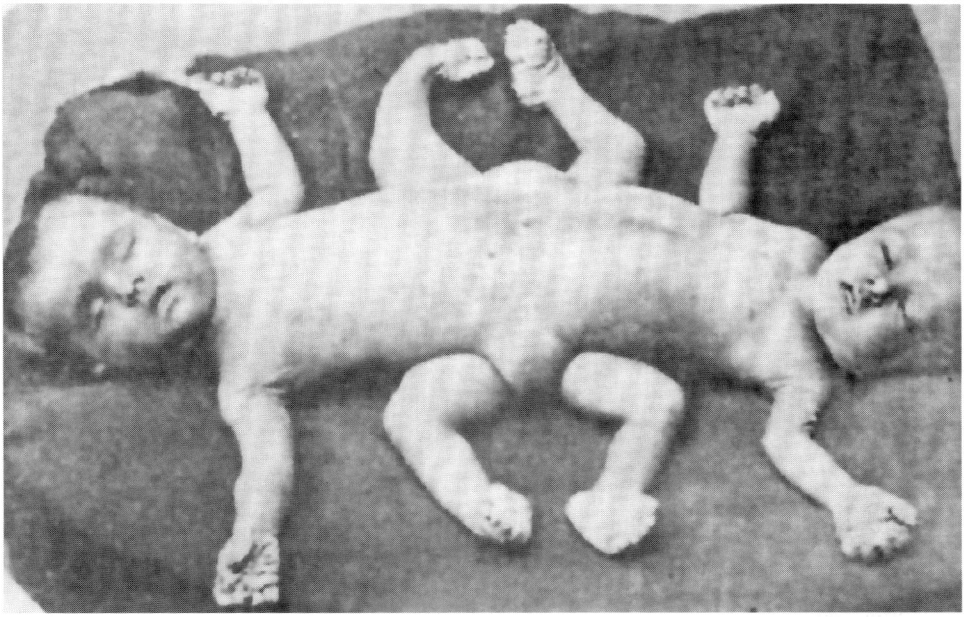

Ischiopages

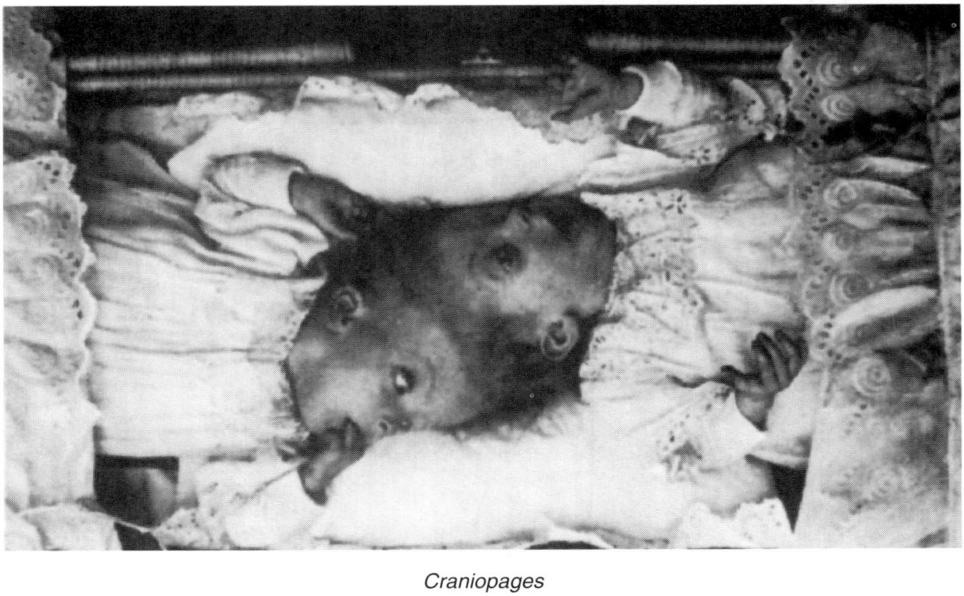

Craniopages

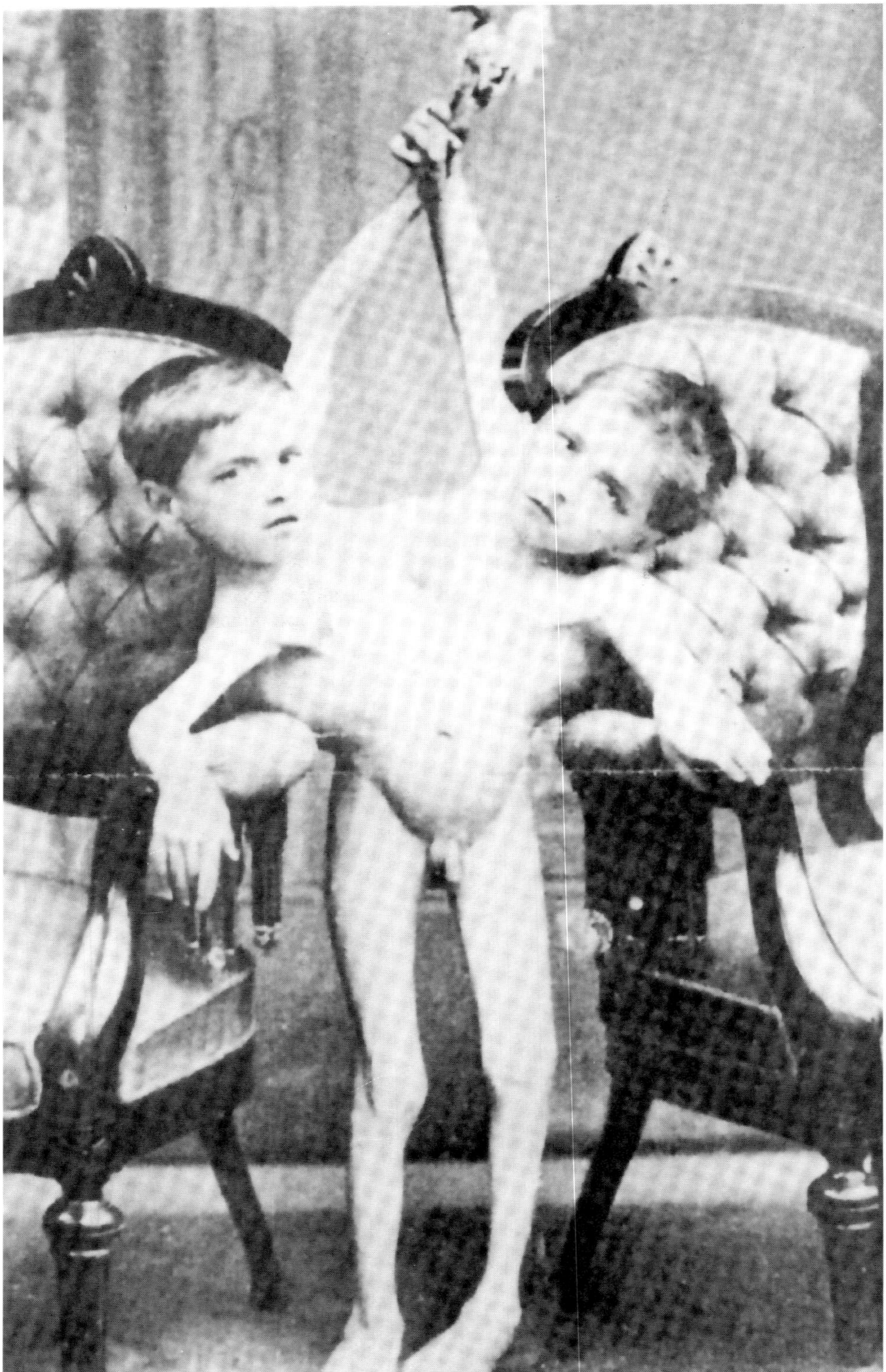

The Toccis

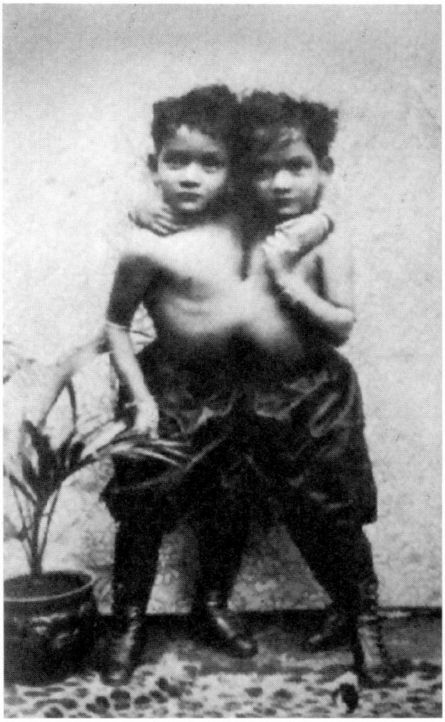

Radica and Doodica

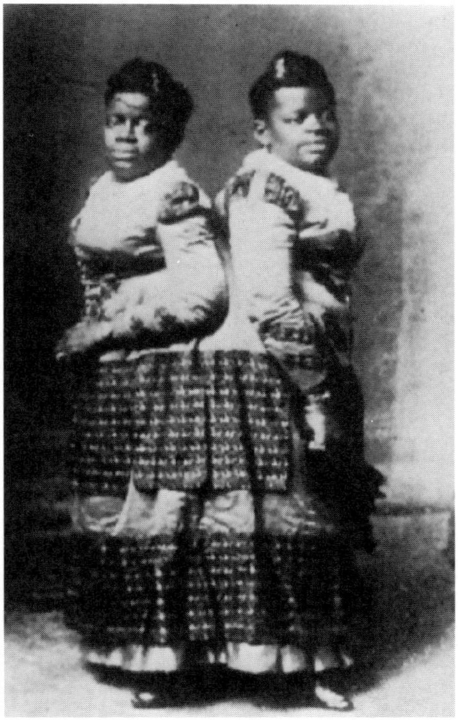

Millie-Christine

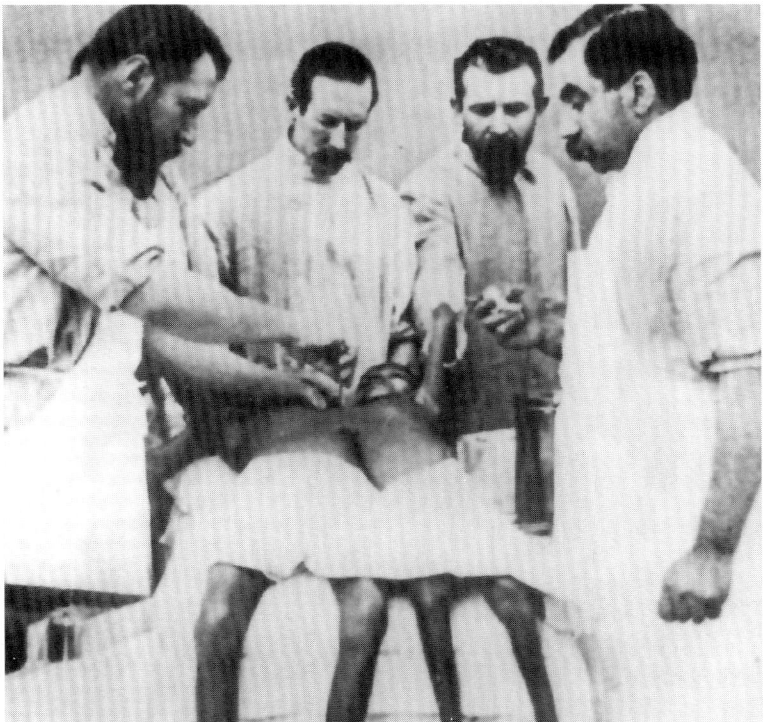

Dr. Doyen operates

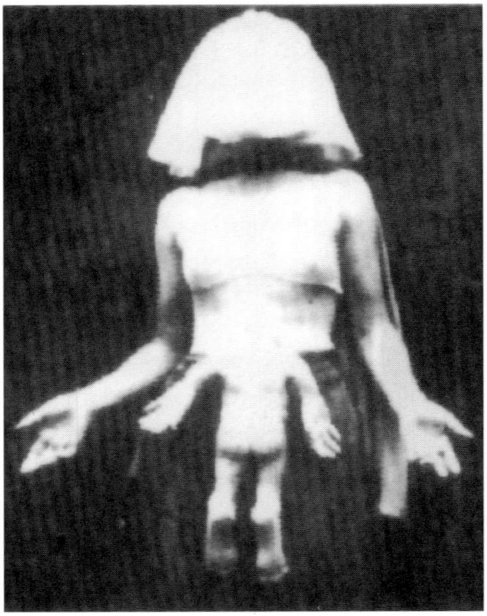

Margarete Clark

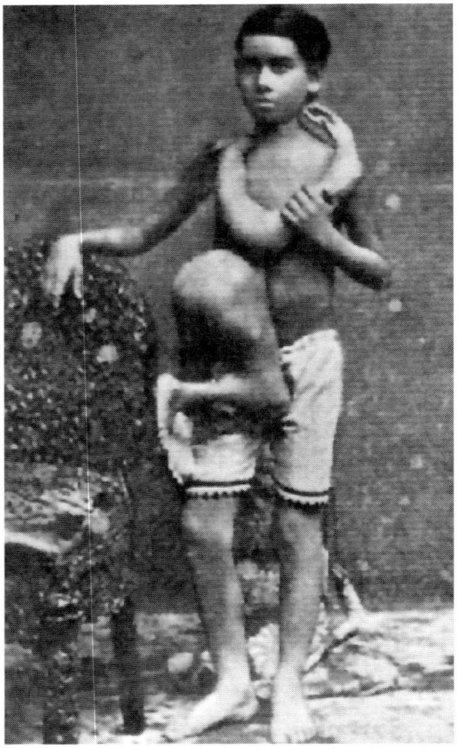

Laloo

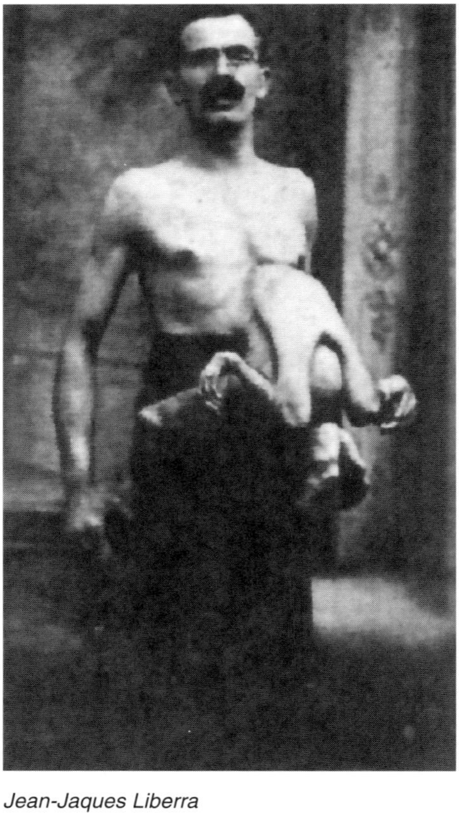

Jean-Jaques Liberra

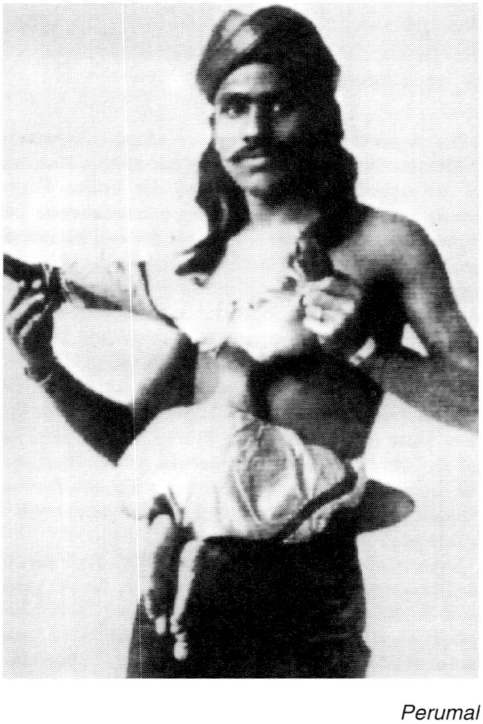

Perumal

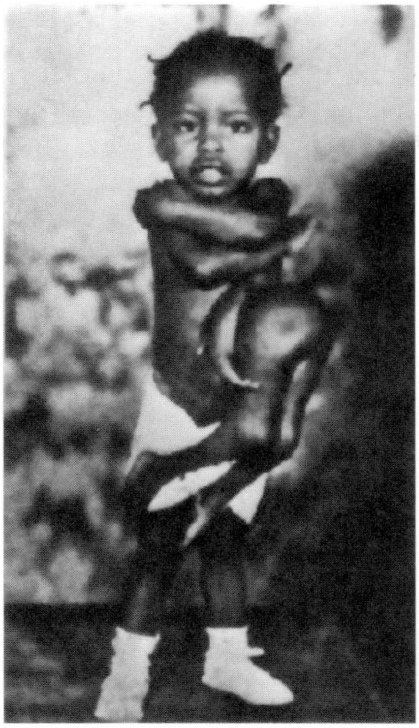

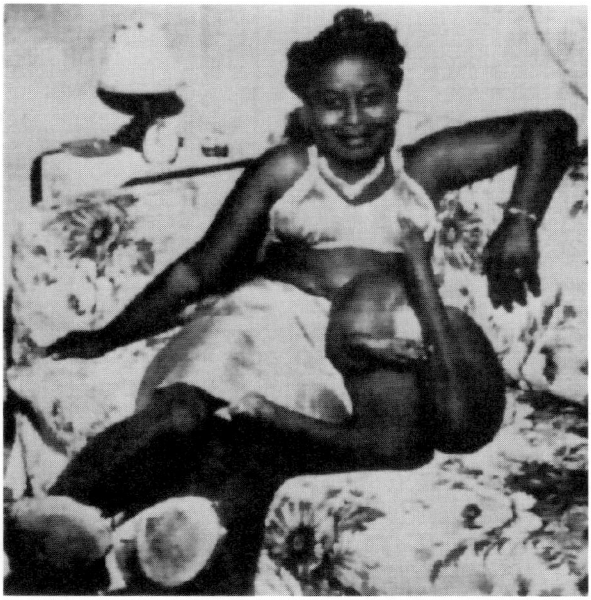

Betty Lou Williams

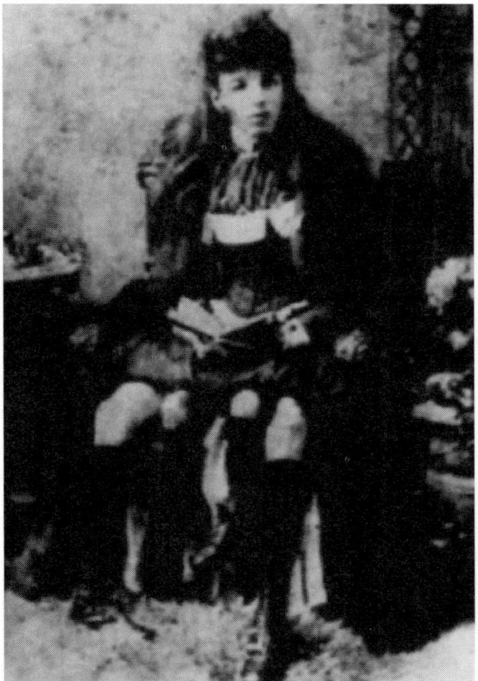

Myrtle Corbin

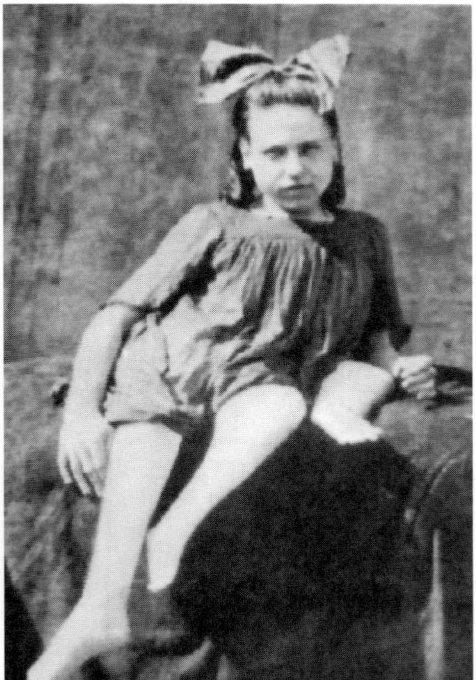

Elsie Lynn

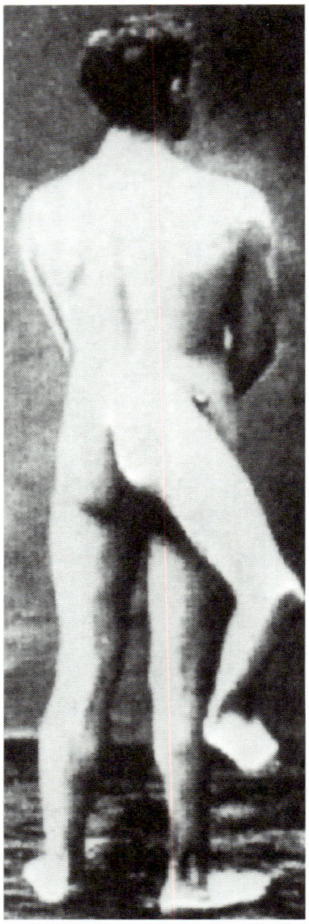

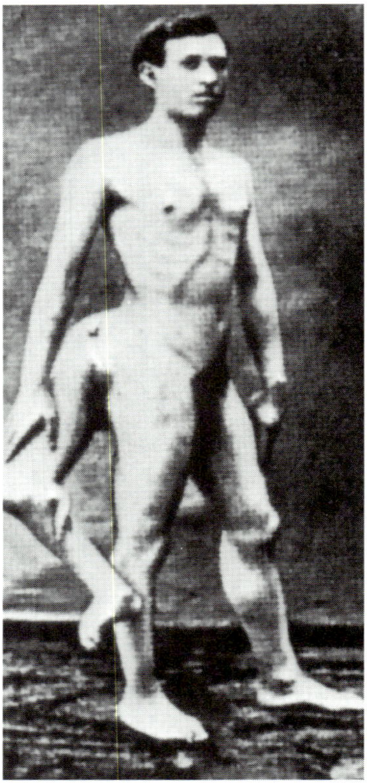

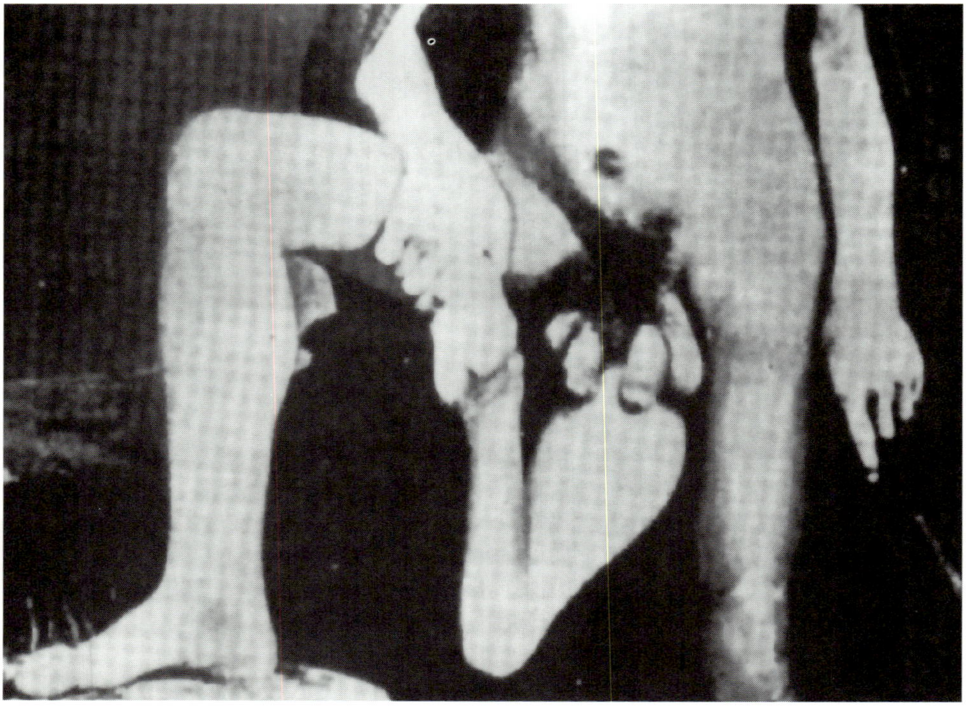

The Great Lentini

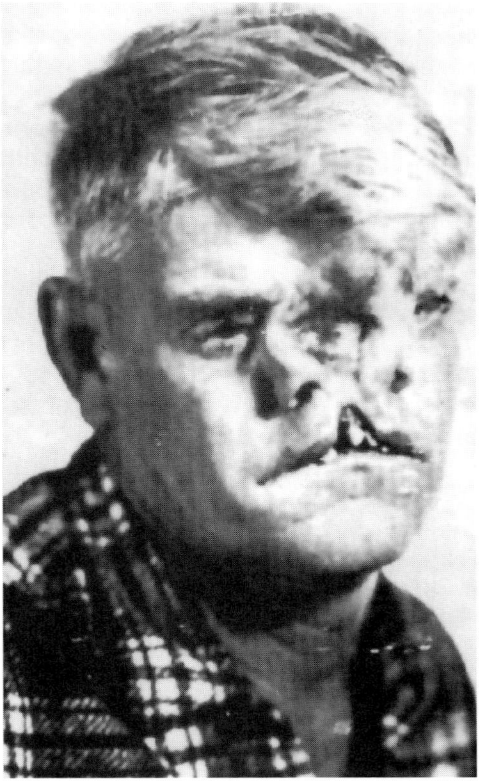

Bill Durks

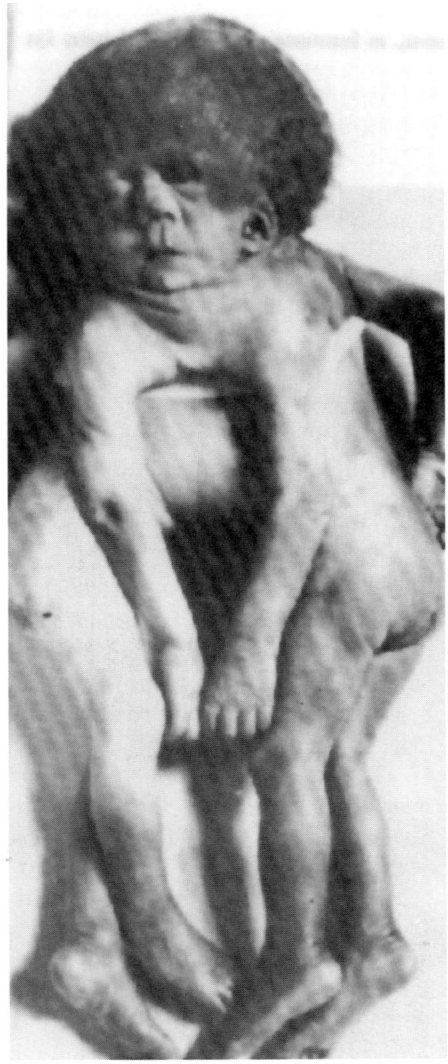

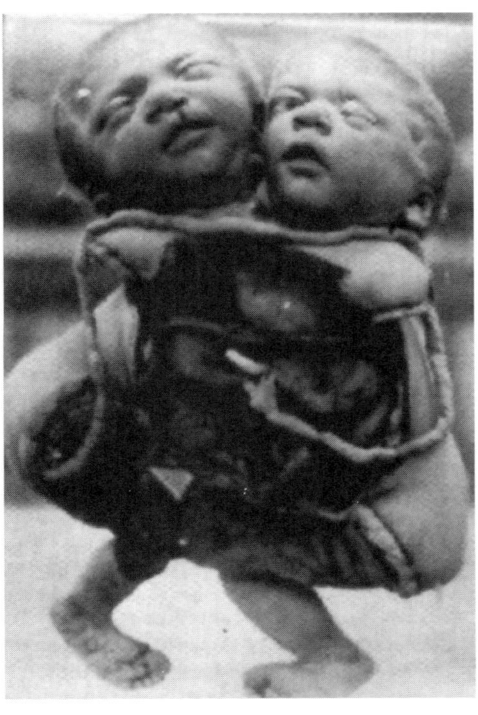

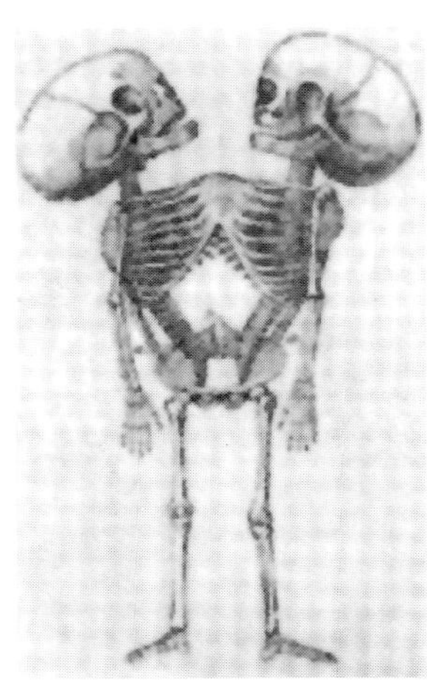

Symelians and Podurges, or 'half' monsters:
These are those born armless or legless, the completely limbless ("basket cases"), or those born with severely truncated limbs. Early examples include Thomas Schweiker (1541-1602), Catherina Mazzina (born 1577), Magdalena Emohne (born 1596), Matthias Buchinger (born 1674), Peter Stadelmann, Elisabeth Simson, Theodor Steib, Bartholomé, Philippe Ludovic Herr, Antonius Maria Reuter (born 1716), Johann Jacob Ewerth, the phocomelian ('seal-armed') Petit-Pépin (born Marco Catozze in 1741), scourge of the French court circa 1775, Louis César Joseph Ducornet (1806-56), and the peromelian Rosalie Fournier, born November 12th 1813 in Marseilles, described in her show advertisement as *"a living female without legs or thighs, with a woman's breast and nipple on the end of the left-hand stump, and a coral-shaped ear-ring of flesh on the right"*. In reality, her feet grew directly from her hips. Legend also tells of a sirenomelian, or mer-creature, born with both legs fused into a single limb, but there are no authenticated cases.

Armless notables include Ann Leak Thomson, saxophonist James Elroy, John Chambert (born 1854), Anton Pohl, Annie Lee, the Russian Rebecca Stromynka, Margarete Mariot, Luis Steinkogler, Gazay the Great, the Japanese Oguri Kiba, Tommy "Toes" Jacobsen, Frances O'Connor (born 1917, a regular with the Cole Brothers circus) and Martha Morris, who both appeared in *Freaks*, Canadian Charles Tripp (1855-1939), Freddie Esele ("The Armless Wonder"), and perhaps the greatest of them all, Carl Hermann Unthan. Born in 1848, Unthan became known as the 'armless violinist of Leipzig', and was also accomplished in many other activities. He went on to appear in the Danish film version of Gerhardt Hauptmann's novel *Atlantis* (August Blom, 1913), and in the German film *Der Mann Ohne Arme* (also 1913). His autobiography, *Das Pediskript*, was published in 1925. He died in 1929, in Berlin. Best-known of the show phocomelians were Andy, the "Sea-Lion", and Sealo, the "Seal Boy", a Ringling Bros. regular.

Tod Browning's *Freaks* brought notoriety to one Prince Randian, the Living Torso, born without limbs, but who nonetheless sired five children by his devoted wife. Though he could only move by wriggling along the ground like a worm, Randian could perform various tricks with his mouth including rolling and lighting a cigarette. He died in 1934, aged 63, after appearing at Sam Wagner's 14th Street Museum. One of the other most famous 'human trunks' was Kobelkoff, born in Siberia in 1851 with only a right shoulder-stump to speak of. Yet his show repertoire included tapestry-weaving, painting and rifle-shooting. He married one Anna Wilfert in 1876, giving her fifteen children and allegedly beating her with his stump when angry. He died in 1933. Other 'living torsos' have included the Englishman Thomas Goy, the American Emmett, the Frenchman Pierre Mahieux, and such women as Marie Bury, Marta, Annitta, Frieda Puschnik, and the celebrated Violetta.

Others born with little or nothing below the waist have included John Doogs (aka Nicodemus, born 1869), Princess Ida (born 1879), Sandu, Jeanie the half-girl (who married the giant, Al Tomaini in 1936), Tiny LaVonda, Lloyd Skelton, Lilli the Living Bust, and Eli Bowen (born 1844), who famously teamed up with the armless Charles Tripp to ride a special bicycle, with Tripp pedalling while Eli steered. Bowen, whose feet grew direct from his hips, was also an accomplished acrobat.

Perhaps the most famous half-boy of all time is Johnny Eck, another star of Tod Browning's *Freaks*; his remarkable and illuminating story is one of the most famous in carnival legend. Of all the human anomalies who appear in *Freaks*, none have caught the public's imagination so much as Eck, the 'most remarkable man alive', the self-styled 'King of the Freaks'. His life story, which begins one stormy August night in 1911, in Baltimore, is one of the most remarkable ever told and provides a telling complement to Browning's own black fable.

That summer night, a perfectly normal woman gave birth to twins; the first-born, Robert Eckhardt, weighed 6 pounds and was in fine health. Twenty minutes later the second child, who would be christened Johnny, emerged, and by the scant illumination of chain lightning the nurse and other attendants could see that he was somehow much smaller than his twin brother; in fact, Johnny Eckhardt had been born weighing just 2 pounds, a "broken doll" with virtually no body whatsoever beneath the bottom of his rib-cage. Miraculously, he survived.

Johnny's family, though they were poor, did not desert their half-formed child; he was perfectly intelligent, and he and Robert were brought up and educated with care. Johnny learnt to walk on his hands, and was extremely athletic. From a young age, he liked to entertain, and was naturally drawn towards the travelling carnivals which came to town. He later recalled: *"When I saw those tents, that was the end of sitting at a desk for me. God, how I loved to get out under those big tents. I loved the animals and I loved camping out. Rob and me, we'd go over to the horse barn and get the sweetest-smelling hay for a bed, and we'd sit up late and shoot the breeze with some of the most wonderful people in the world. I met hundreds and thousands of people, and none finer than the midgets and the Siamese twins and the caterpillar man and the bearded woman and the human seal with the little flippers for hands. I never asked them any embarrassing questions and they never asked me, and God, it was a great adventure."*

One of the biggest days of Johnny's young life came in December 1923, when he and Robert were taken to see a big magic show in the local church. The act came to a premature close when Johnny jumped up on stage to claim a prize; the audience went wild, and the magician was so dumb-struck he was lost for words. Finally, he summoned Johnny's mother and offered to make her rich by letting him put her half-boy on the stage. This was to be Johnny's first bitter lesson of the cruelties and trickery of the carnival world he loved so dearly.

The magician had soon persuaded his mother to sign a contract making him Johnny's manager for 1 year; a figure which was later blatantly altered to read "10 years". Johnny's last name was shortened to Eck, for the stage; it was not the only thing to be reduced. The high salary promised turned out to be $20 a week, while the manager was raking in over $100 per day through exhibiting the boy prodigy. Johnny refused to continue after the first 12 months and, despite threats of legal action, escaped the magician's clutches – for a while. Aged 14, Johnny and Robert went off to work with Captain Sheesley's circus in Plainfield NJ, a far happier experience. Johnny, who had been painting and making wooden models since the age of 8, had by now added juggling, tightrope-walking, conjuring, acrobatics, animal-training and sax-playing to his incredible repertoire.

Then came the Great Depression. With Bob and Johnny out of work and back in Baltimore, the Eckhardt family were down on their luck and in danger of losing their home. Out of the blue, a letter from Johnny's ex-manager arrived, inviting him to pay a visit to Maryland. There was nothing to lose, and so Johnny accepted. He had a great time, and it seemed like the manager was a reformed man; not long after he came through with a booking, and Bob and Johnny found themselves bound for Canada, to appear at the National Exposition. It so happened that two talent scouts from MGM were at the shows, and they got Johnny to take a screen test. Within 4 weeks, the Eckhardt brothers were bound for California, where the shooting for Tod Browning's *Freaks* was about to commence.

Johnny recalled how right from the start he became Browning's favourite; the director would address him as "Mr. Johnny", and have him sit next to him at all times. Indeed, the whole crew loved the half-boy, and it was to be one of the happiest times of his life. He was the star of the show, without doubt, and even had his own private dressing room, emblazoned with 'The Great Johnny Eck'. Inevitably, it was all too good to be true; it turned out that Johnny's manager, who had negotiated the MGM deal, had secured himself *over 90%* of the star's salary – and Johnny estimated that he was being paid around $1,000 a week. Once again he had fallen prey to the type of merciless exploitation which was, sadly, all too commonplace in the world of carnivals and sideshows.

After shooting, Johnny returned to Baltimore. He soon heard that Browning was planning another film, in which he wanted the half-boy to star. But again, MGM were negotiating with the crooked manager. Determined not be exploited again, Johnny wrote to both the studio and his manager, demanding a fee of $600 a week; as a result, the deal fell through, and although Johnny did suit up for MGM's *Tarzan The Ape Man* (as a bird-creature), his Hollywood career was effectively at an end.

Johnny continued to work in the carnivals and road shows, performing with Robert L. Ripley of *Believe It Or Not* fame in Chicago, Cleveland and Dallas, and also touring with various magic acts (he was made to be 'sawn in half'). His other exploits included conducting an orchestra in his home town, and driving a midget racing car in fairs throughout the south. But Johnny increasingly believed that this way of life was endangered, that his innocent form of entertainment was out of step with public taste. He retired in 1940, later reflecting that "people wanted sex from then on... now it's crime, dope and filth," poignantly adding: "If I want to see freaks, all I have to do is look out the window."

As if to confirm his worst fears, Johnny was assaulted during a burglary on his Baltimore home in 1988, and subsequently became withdrawn and reclusive. He died three years later.

During his career he had made thousands of friends, both carnival workers and public alike; people who saw Johnny Eck not as a freak, but as a great performer, a friendly and genuine person, and a truly unique human being.

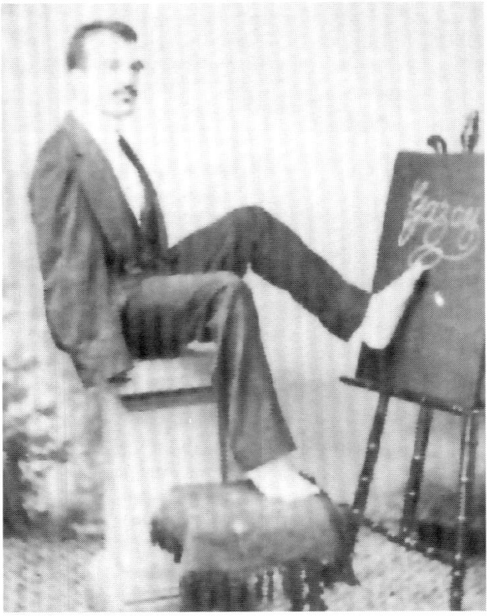

Gazay the Great

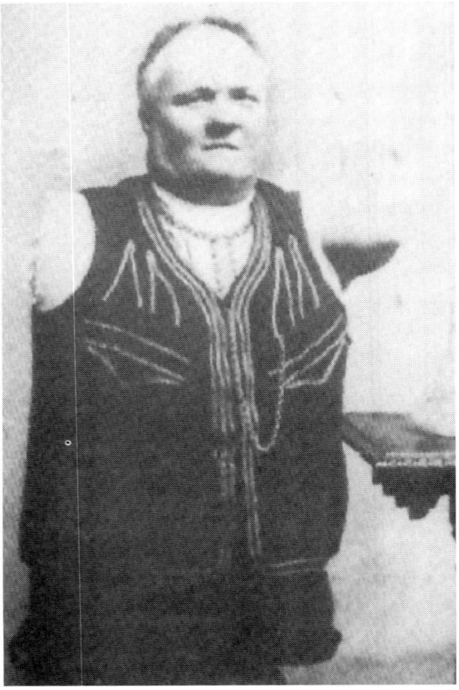

Kobelkoff

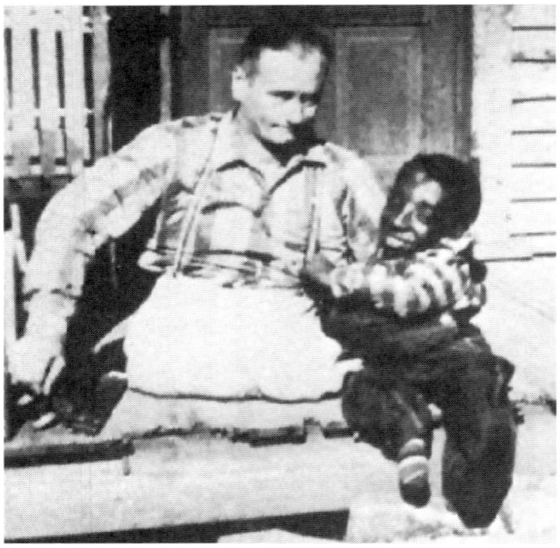

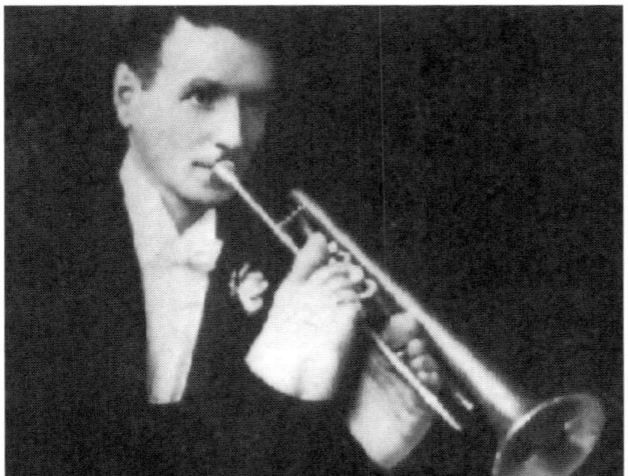

James Elroy

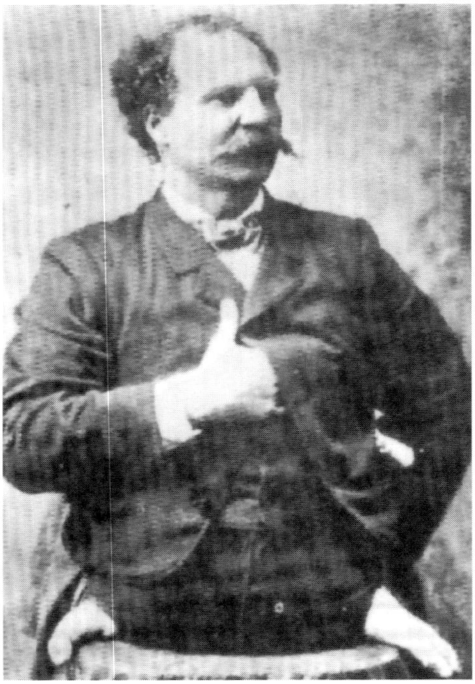

Eli Bowen

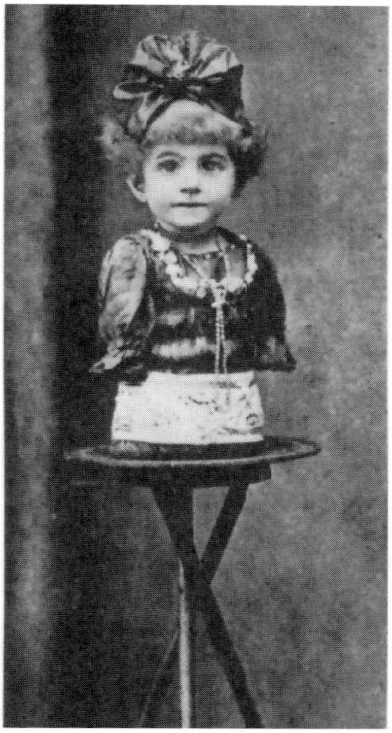

Miss Marta

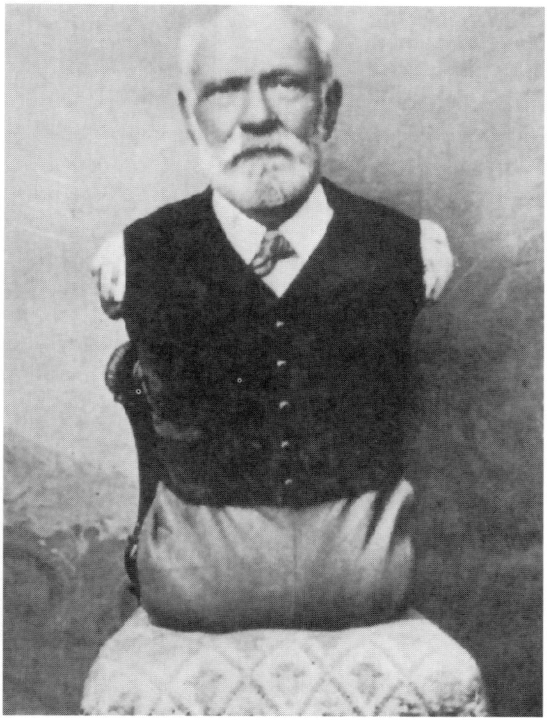

Thomas Goy

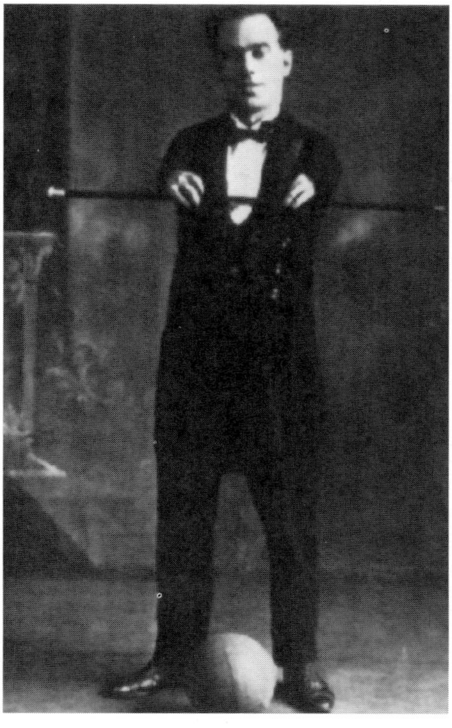

Andy

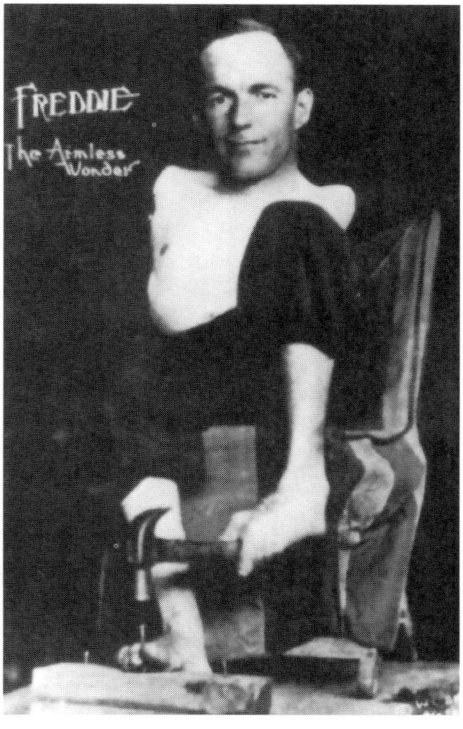

Freddie Esele

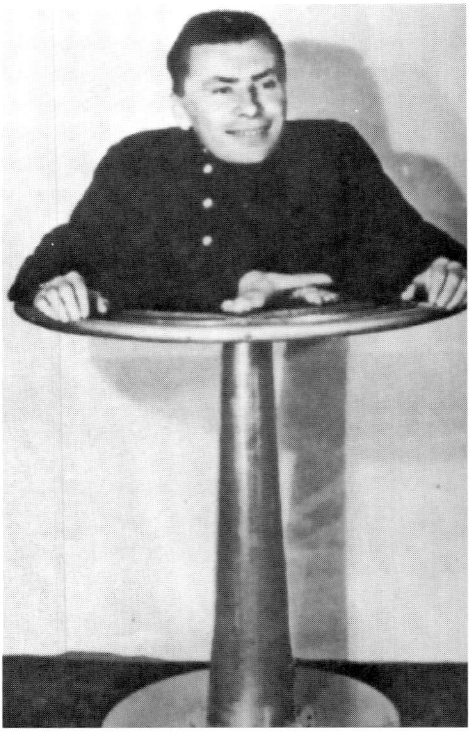

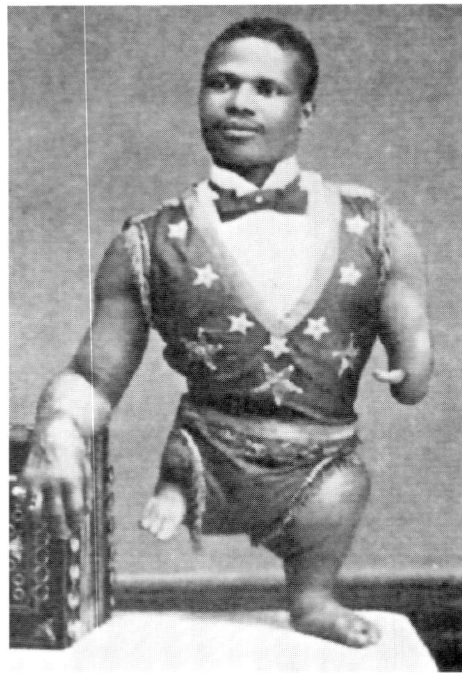

Nicodemus

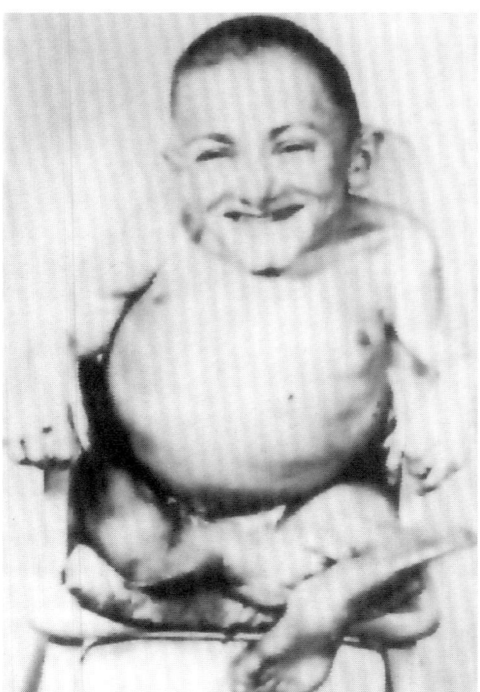

Lloyd Skelton

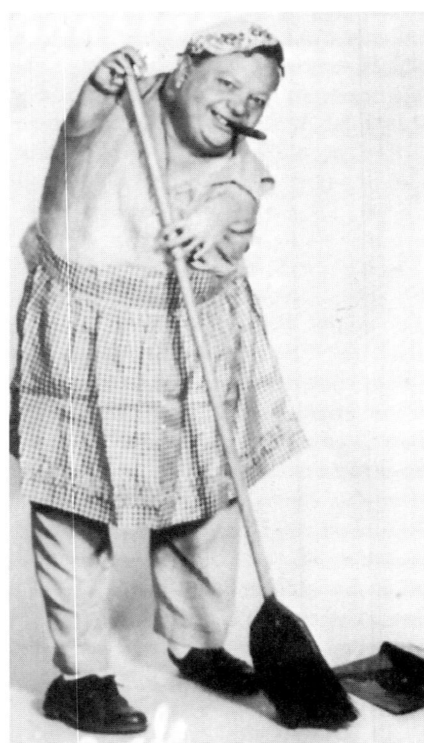

Sealo

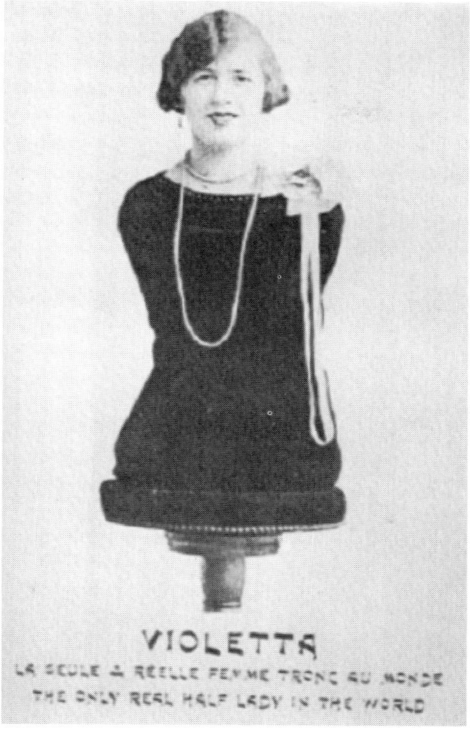
VIOLETTA
LA SEULE & REELLE FEMME TRONC AU MONDE
THE ONLY REAL HALF LADY IN THE WORLD

Violetta

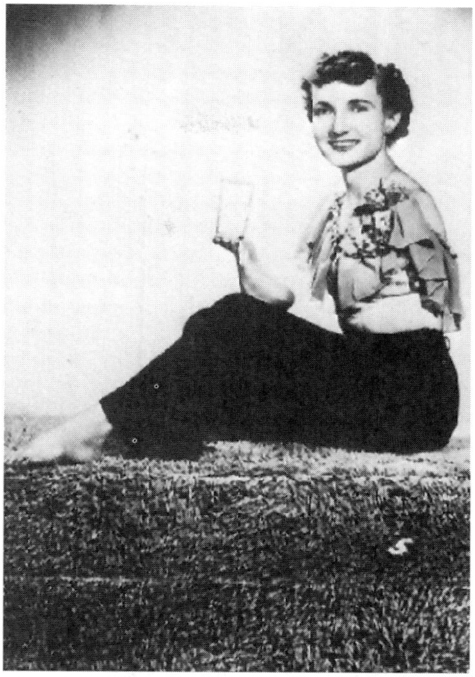

Frances O'Connor

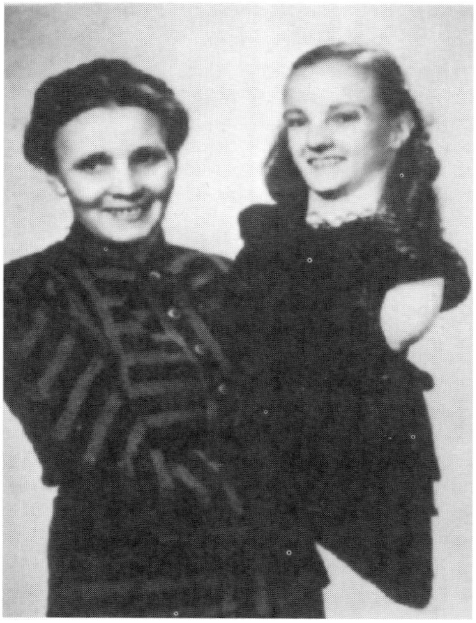

Frieda Pushnik

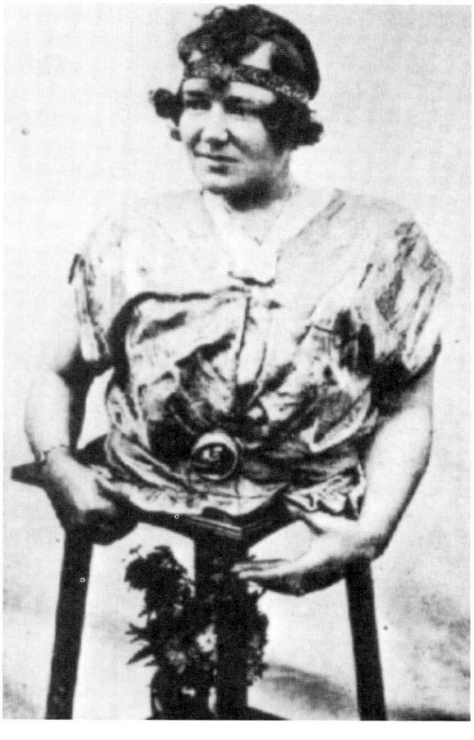

Lilli

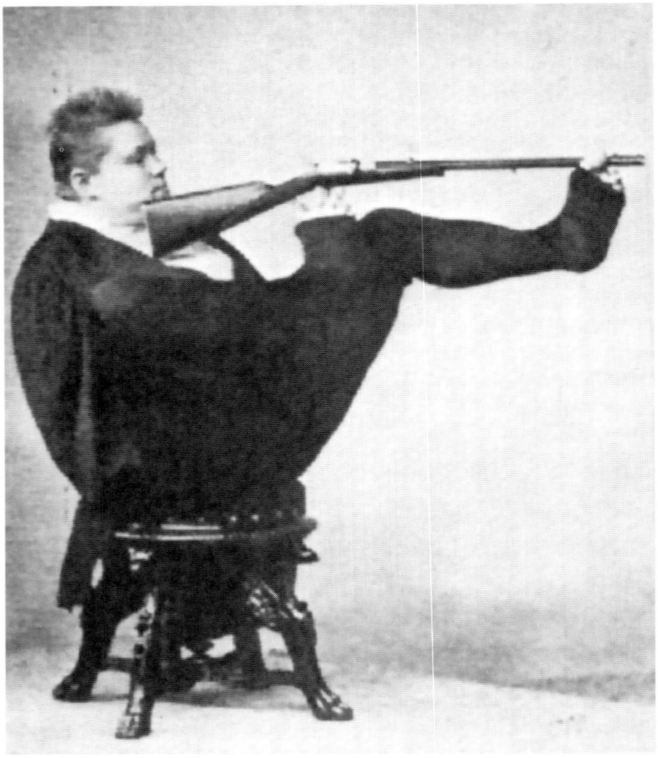

Unthan

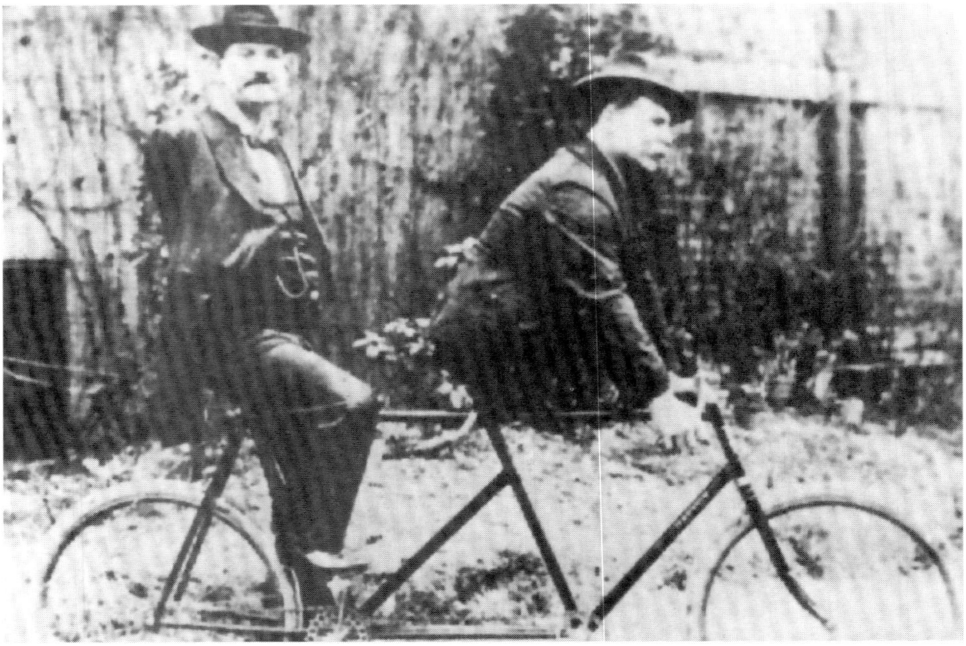

Charles Tripp and Eli Bowen

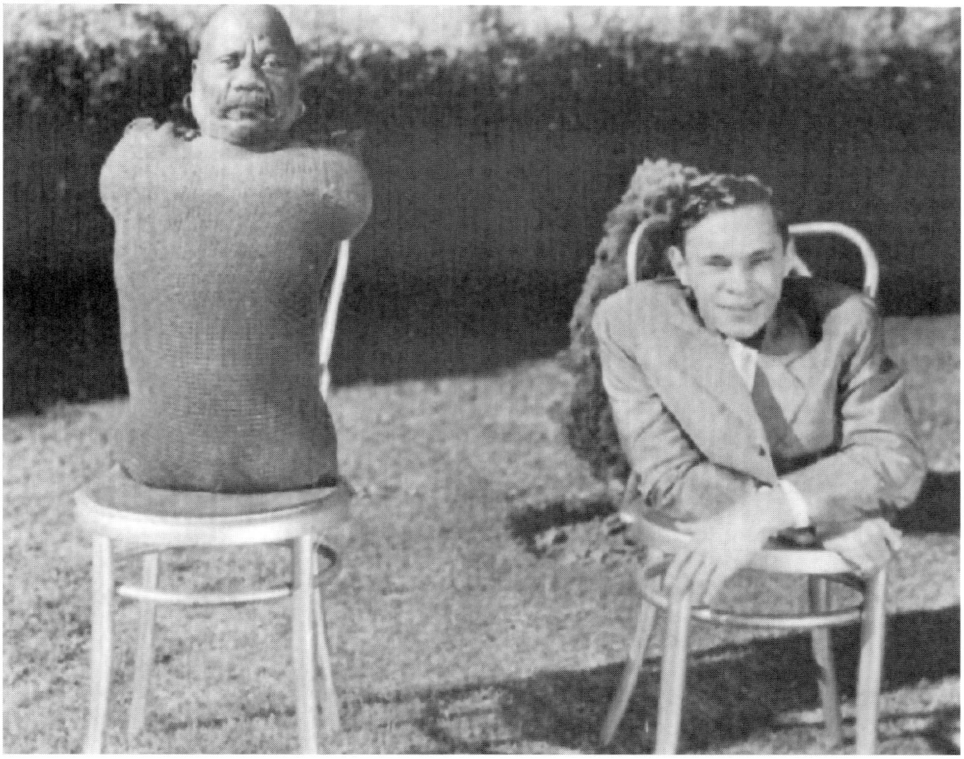

Randian, The Living Torso, and The Great Johnny Eck

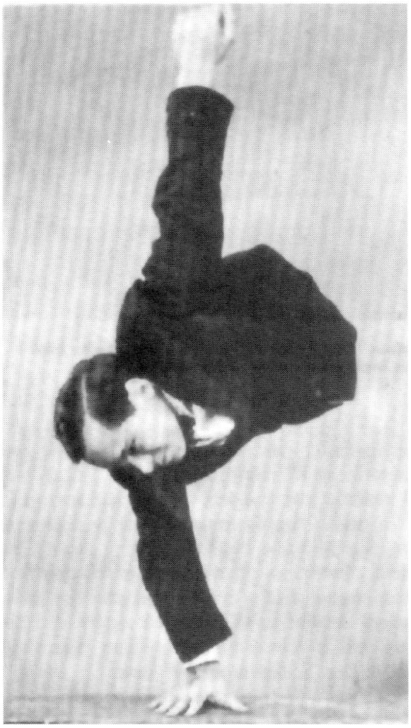

Mr Johnny

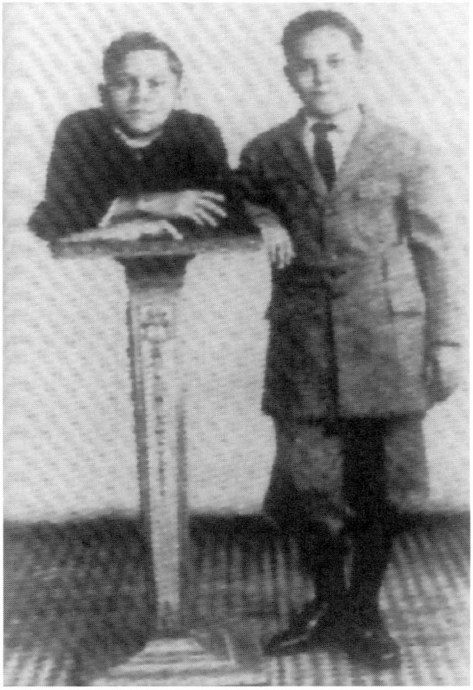

John and Robert Eckhardt

Dwarfs and Giants:
These are the most commonplace of human prodigies, with dwarfs in particular occurring in great number throughout the world even to this day. The most common kind are achondroplasic dwarfs, victims of a deforming, bone-truncating condition, while the name 'midget' is more usually given to those diminutive beings whose frames are in more harmonious proportion, resembling normal people in miniature. Other dwarfing conditions include spinal osteomyelitis (causing 'rachitics'), thyroid or ovarian deficiency, and metaphysical dysostosis. Dwarfs and midgets of renown have included: John Decker, Jimmy Camber (also notoriously fat), Hannah Warton, Jeffrey Hudson, Owen Farrel, Robert and Judith Skinner (1698-1763), John Coan (1728-64), Joseph Boruwlaski (1739-1837), Richebourg, Wybrand Lolkes, Hokins Hopkins (1736-54), Thomas Carter, Kelham Whitelamb, George Romondo, Nicolas Ferry, Catherina Helena Stoberin, Ignatz Ackenheil, Emma Leach, Calvin Philips, Nannette Stocker, Simon Paap (1789-1828), Tom Thumb (1838-83) and his wife Lavinia Warren, Thumb's love rival Commodore Nutt, Admiral Dot, Prince Nicholi (reputedly the smallest man ever, at 18" tall), Lucia Zarate (1864-1890, reputedly the smallest woman who ever lived), Count Magri, Major James Doyle, Carrie Akers (also obese), Mr. & Mrs. Mite, Smaun Sing Hpoo, Princess Pauline Masters (1876-95), Princess Elisabeth, Prince Puck, Princess Martha, the Speck Brothers, Franz and Carl Rossow, Princess Reta, Abdurrhama Pascha, Georg Theodor Ulpts, Prince Colibri (aka Dimitri Ossopoff), Millie Edwards, General Peanuts, Prince Mignon, Tiny Tim (aka Harold Pyott), Tom Sodrie, Fred "Pip" Aslett, Lia Graf (gassed by the Nazis), Walter Böning, Friedrich Hakl, Giuseppe Bignoli, Willy Rolle, Carl Norwood, Dolly Regan (the "ossified girl"), Caroline Cramachi, Charles Lockhart (three times Texas State Treasurer), Franz Ebert (who appeared on baby food labels), clowns Andrea Barnabé, Frankie Saluto, Jimmy Armstrong, Pooh-Bah (aka Pete Terhune), Buddie Thompson, Ferry and Gin, and Kiki (aka Otto Moskowitz), and such troupes as the Liliput Revue, the Singer Midgets, the Doll Family, and John Lester's Midget Ladies.

Giants, contrary to reputation, are seldom strong. Caused by pituitary deficiency, their condition very often renders them sluggish and clumsy. They are prone to acromegaly (a deforming skin condition) and kyphoscoliosis (crippling spinal curvature); poor circulation can often result in gangrene and limb amputation, and few specimens live to anything approaching old age. Giants and giantesses of renown have included: Anthony Payne, William Joyce, Anton Franck, Edmund Malone, Cornelius MacGrath (1736-52), Bernardo Gigli, Mrs. Gordon of Essex, Daniel Cajanus (a reputed, but unsubstantiated, 12' 1"), Charles Byrne, Edward Bamford, Basilio Huaylas, Thomas Bell, James Toller (1795-1819), Elizabeth Stock, Ann Hardy, Josef Behin, Louis Frenz, Joseph Brice, James Murphy, Amelia and Priscilla Weston, Martin Bates (1845-1919), Anna Swann (1846-88, who reputedly gave birth to a still-born child 24 inches long), Chang Yu-Sing (1840-93), Ella Ewing, Carl Brustad, Joseph Drasal (1841-86), Louis Wilkins, Emanuel Andersson, Oswald Balling, Trante Victor, Abomah, Jakob Murdel (1874-1904), the Russian Pisjakoff, Hugo, George Auger, Teddy Bobs, Waino Myllyrinne (1909-63), Angus McAskill, Dora Helms, Paul Herold,

Jan Van Albert, Jack Earl, Henry Hite, Max Palmer, Robert Wadlow (an authenticated 8′ 11″), Johann K. Petursson, Al Tomaini, Ted Evans, Eddie Carmel ("The Happy Giant"), Gabriel Munjane, and Dolores Pullard ("The Amazon Girl"). The American Eugene Berry (born 1872) was one of many stricken with elephantiasis, giving him giant and deformed appendages. The greatest authenticated height on record was achieved by the Russian Fédor Machnov (1881-1905), who measured in at an incredible 9′ 4″. His customary four meals a day consisted of two litres of tea, twenty eggs and eight buttered rolls for breakfast; two and a half kilos of meat, a kilo of potatoes and three litres of beer for lunch; a tureen of soup, another two and a half kilos of meat, three loaves of bread and two litres of tea for supper; and fifteen eggs with bread and a litre more of tea before bed.

Sharing the polar physical relationship of midgets to giants are the extremely thin and extremely fat people who have come to prominence throughout history. Famous thin men have included: Claude-Ambroise Seurat, the "Living Skeleton", who lived in early 19th century France and was reputedly 3 inches thick; Calvin Edson; Isaac Spragues, born 1841, who weighed 44 pounds; Harry V. Lewis; James Coffey; John Darrington; the Austrian Carl Noisée, born 1861; the Belgian Dominique Castagna, born 1907, who weighed 50 pounds; Eddie Masher, the "Skeleton Dude", who weighed 38 pounds; Harry Jones, born 1860, who weighed 49 pounds; Percy Pape, born 1932, who weighed 68 pounds and by 1960 had sustained over 75 limb fractures; Milton "Slim Jim" Malone (68 pounds); the negro, Seip, too weak to stand; Mac Intosh; Pete Robinson, weighing 64 pounds, who in 1933 married circus fat lady Bunny Smith (518 pounds); and Glen Pulley, weighing 72 pounds, who also married a fat lady weighing nearly 600 pounds. A rare example of a professional thin lady was Rosa Lee Plemons.

Famous fat ladies – much more traditional in show business than their male counterparts – have included: Miss Bertha (415 pounds), Olga, Anna (542 pounds aged 18), Victorine, Flossie, Marie Lill, Celeste Geyer (born 1901, better known as Dolly Dimples, who once weighed 500 pounds), Baby Ruth Pontico (1904-1941, said to weigh 814 pounds), Miss Susan Barton (Barnum's "Mammoth Lady"), Mademoiselle Rose (600 pounds), Jenny Letto, Teresina (star of the Gallery of Monsters at the Neuilly Fair, 583 pounds), Baby Irene, Baby Betty, Baby Thelma (655 pounds), Jolly Josephine, Alice From Dallas, the Canadian Miss Miranda, the Dutchwoman Juliana Voort, and the American negresses Lucy Morris, Flora Mae "Baby Flo" Jackson (840 pounds), "Captivatin'" Liza, and Miss Jean Hill (500-pound star of John Waters' *Desperate Living* [1977]).

Amongst the fattest men recorded in history have been: the Englishmen Nickolas Wood of Kent, Jack Biggers of Witney, Edward Bright of Maldon (584 pounds), and Daniel Lambert of Leicester (1770-1809, 739 pounds); the Americans Johnny Alee (an alleged 1,000 pounds) and Mills Darden (1799-1857, again an alleged 1,000 pounds); Emil Naucke (born 1855, 518 pounds), John Hanson Craig (1856-94, 745 pounds), Wilhelm Loter, the Cannon Colossus, William J. "Happy Humphrey" Cobb (802 pounds), William Campbell,

Leo Whitton, John McDonald, and "Happy" Jack Eckert (1877-1939, 739 pounds). The fattest man to have been medically authenticated remains the American Robert Earl Hughes (1926-58) of Fish Hook, Illinois. Some ten feet four inches around the waist, Hughes fell ill with measles at the age of 32. Too big for an ambulance, he was driven to hospital in a trailer and treated on the hospital forecourt. He died soon afterwards, and was buried in a piano-case. His weight at death was 1,069 pounds.

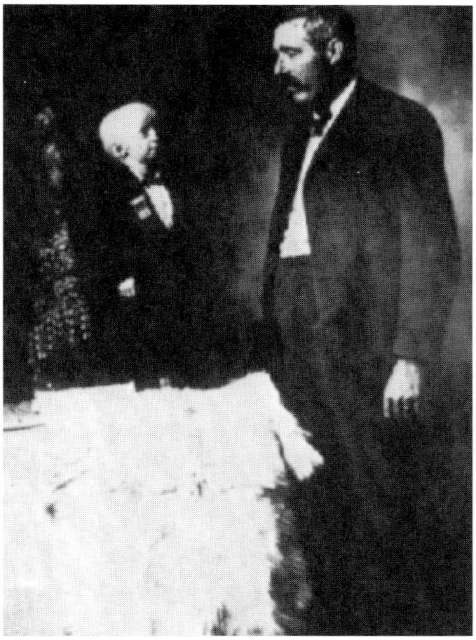

Prince Nicholi

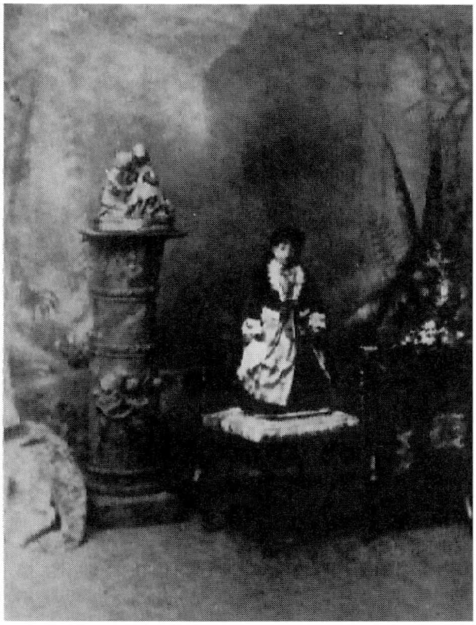

Lucia Zarate

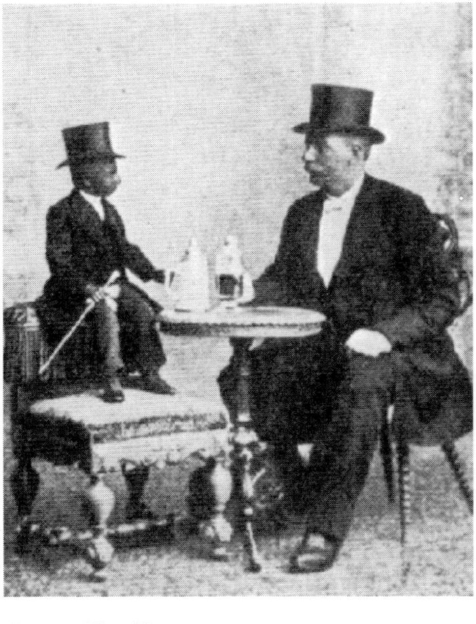

Smaun Sing Hpoo

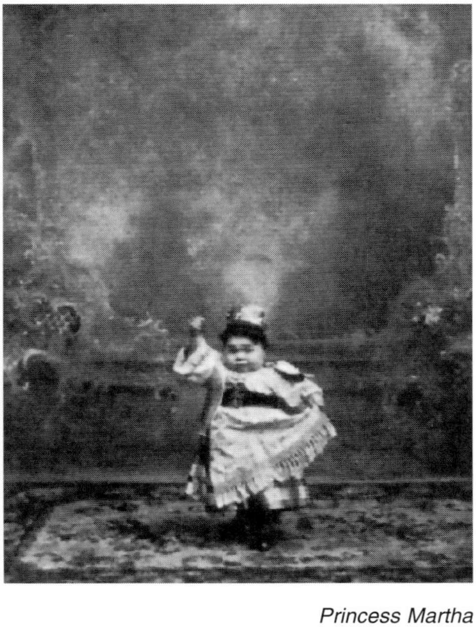

Princess Martha

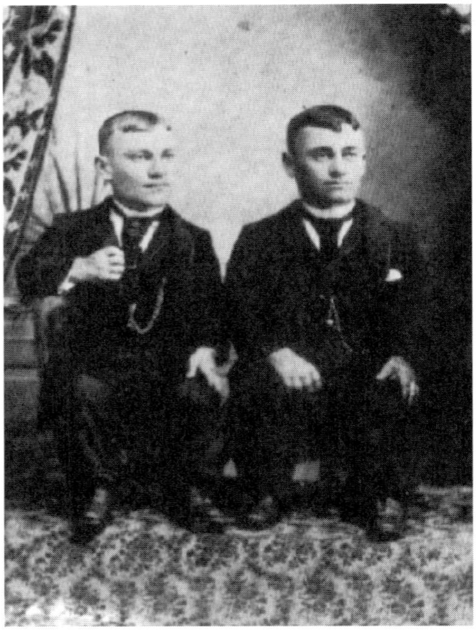

The Speck Brothers

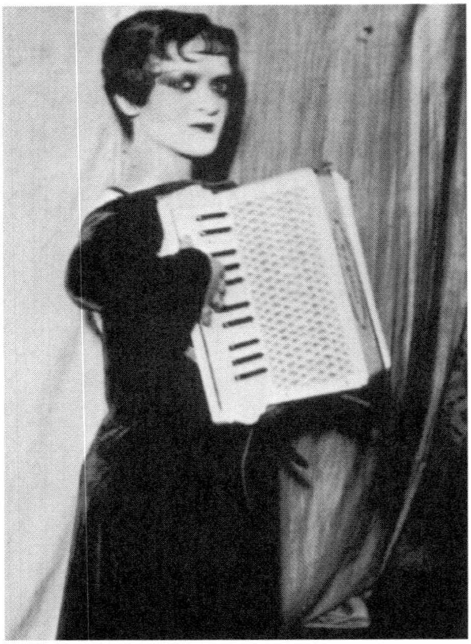

Princess Reta

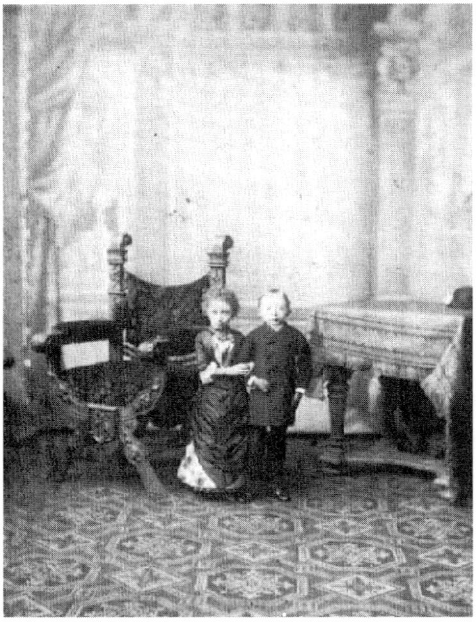

Mr and Mrs Mite

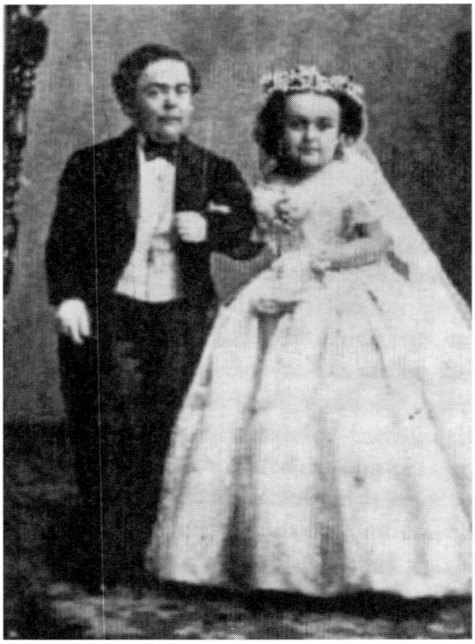

Tom Thumb and Lavinia Warren

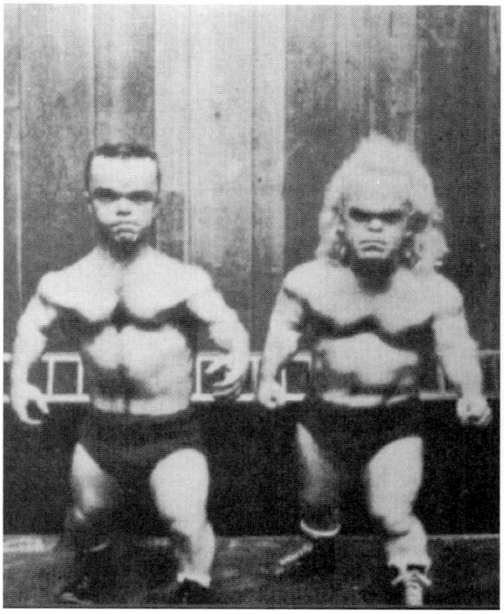

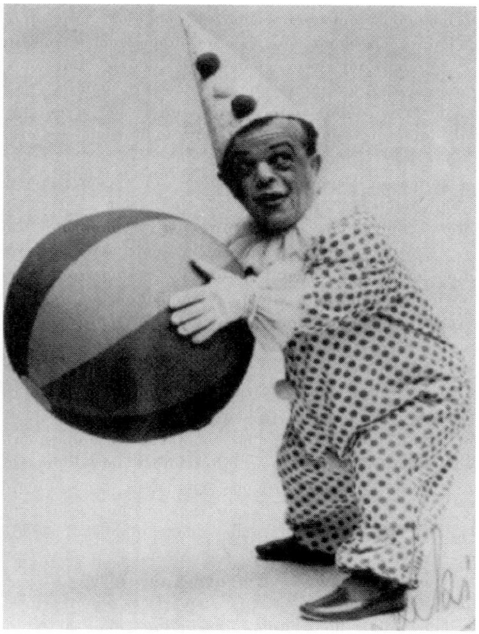

Kiki the Clown

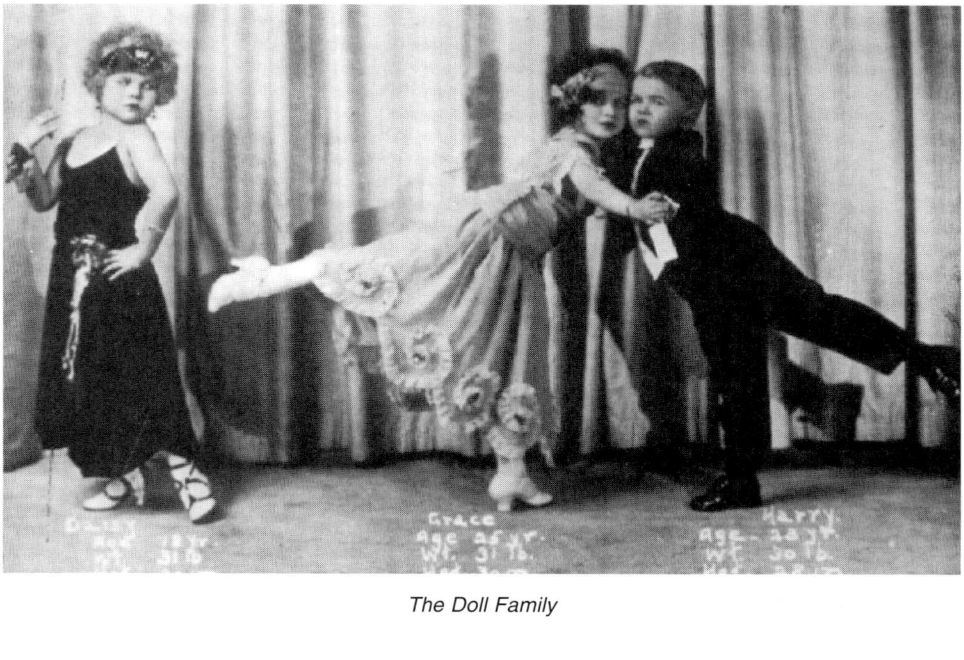

The Doll Family

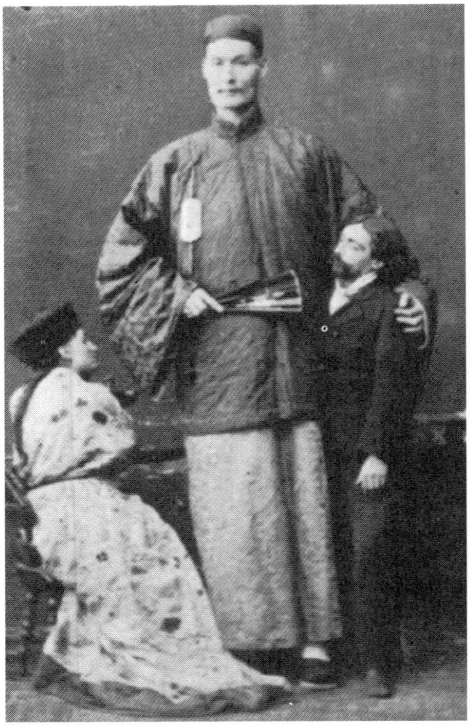

Chang Yu-Sing

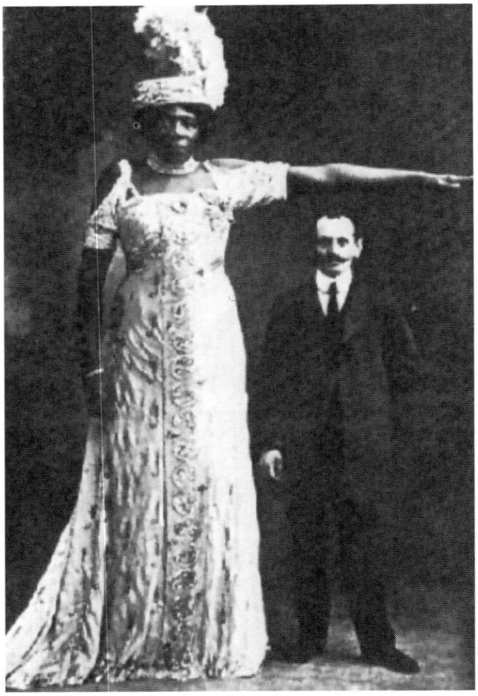

Abomah

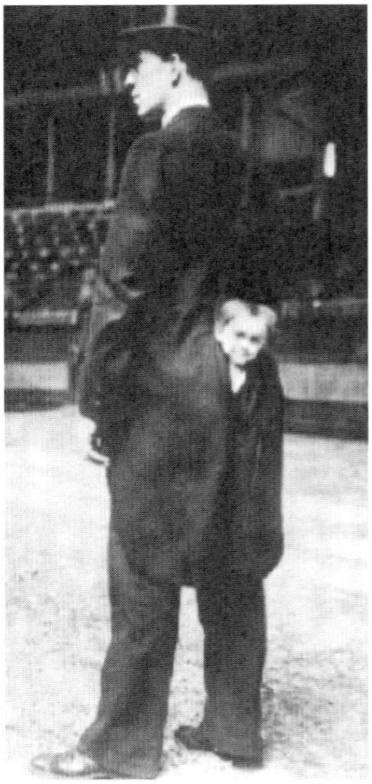

George Auger

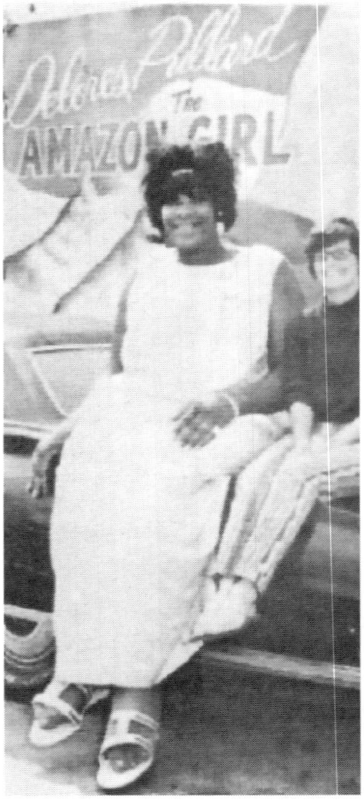

Dolores Pullard

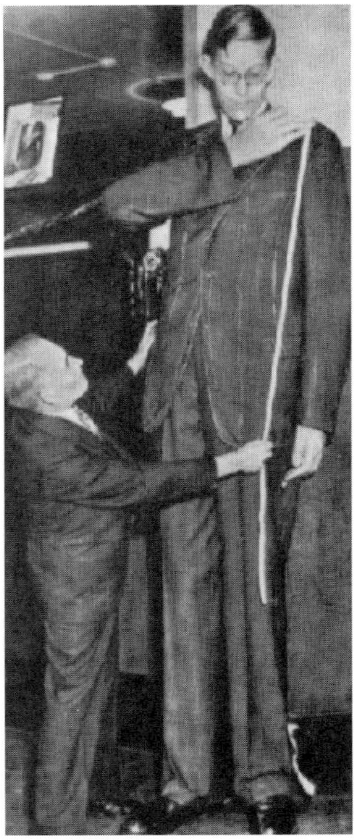

Robert Wadlow

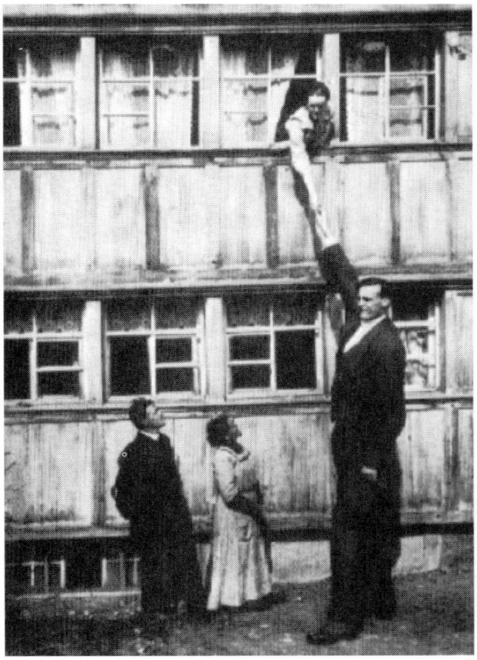

Van Albert

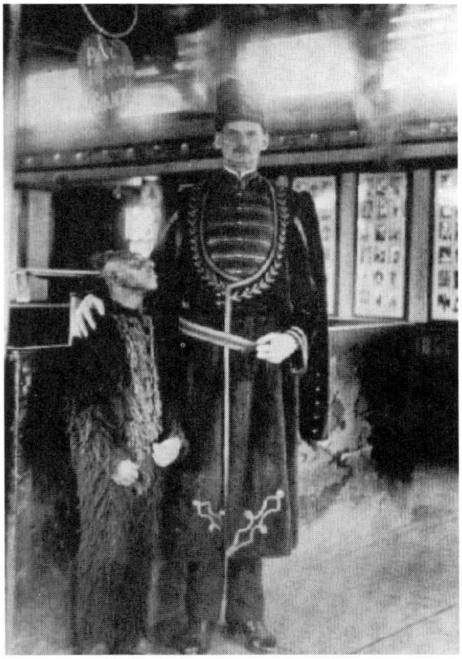

Paul Herold

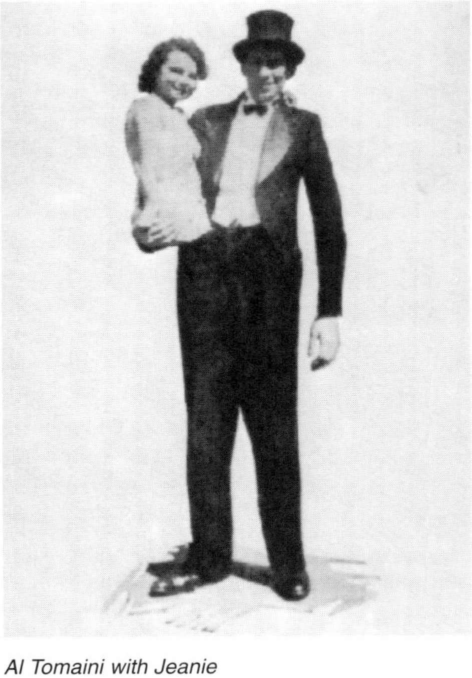

Al Tomaini with Jeanie

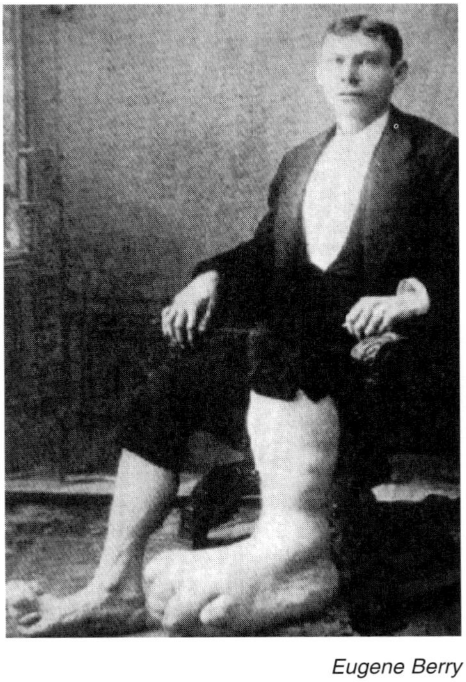

Eugene Berry

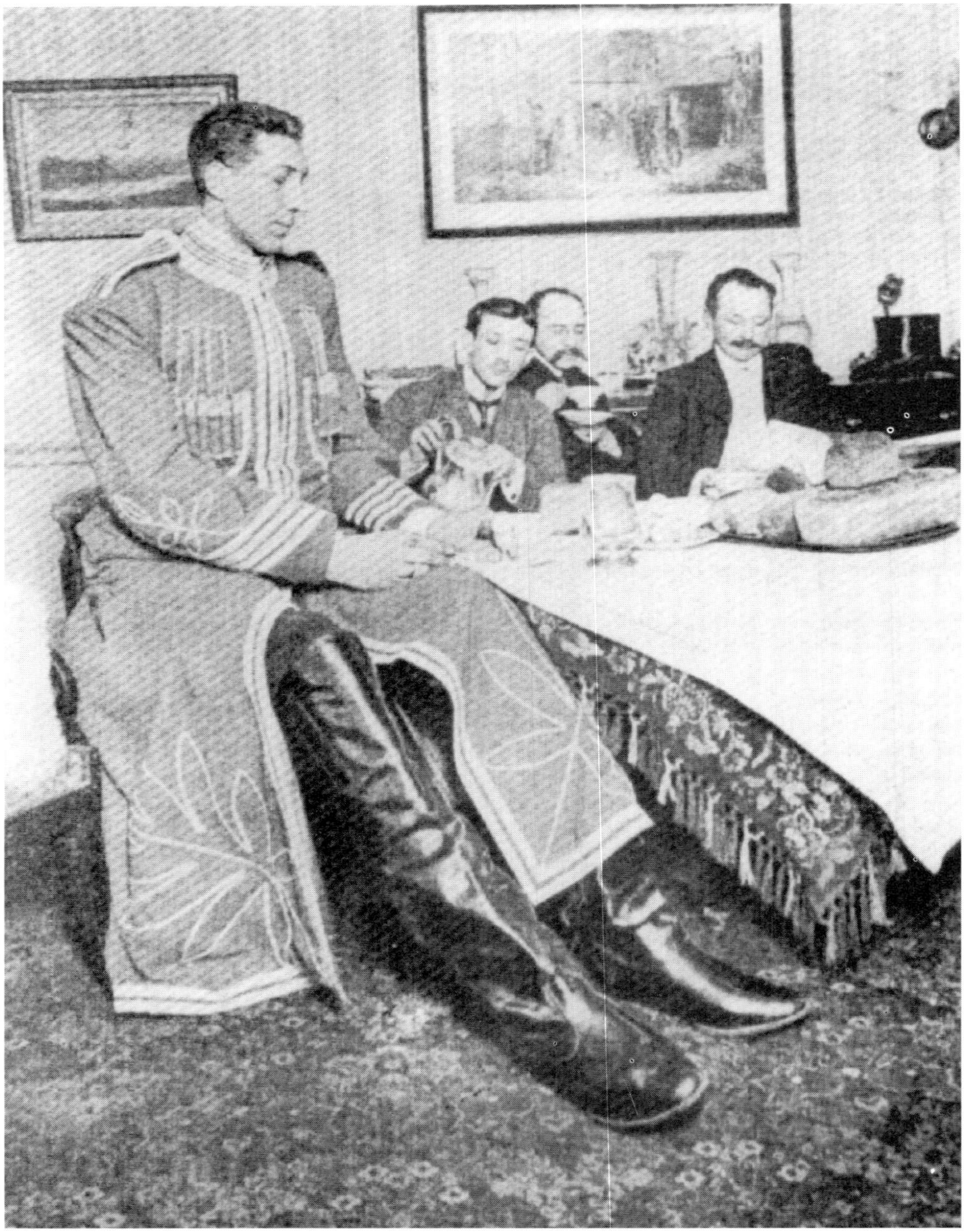

Machnov

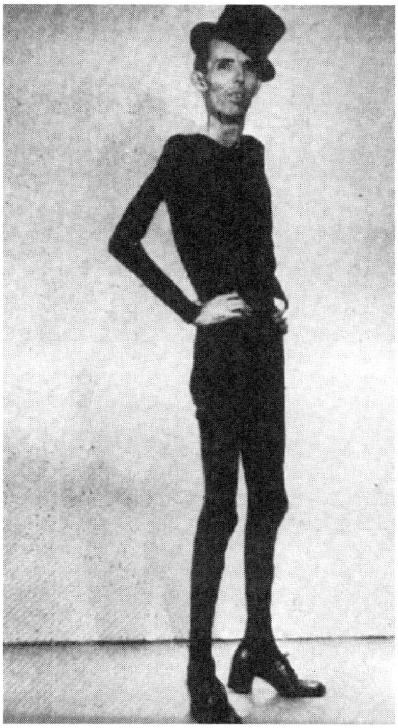

Glenn Pulley

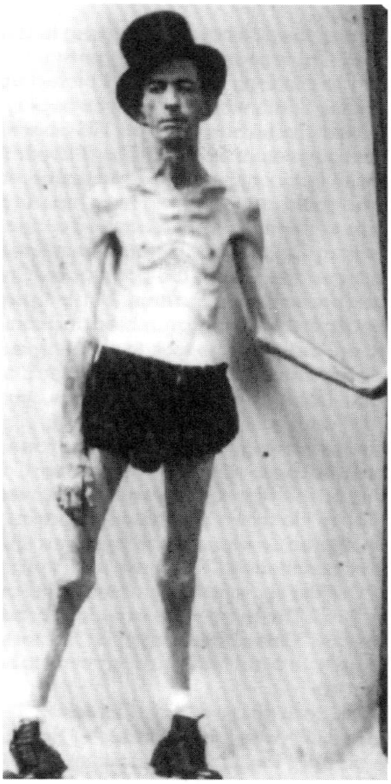

Slim Jim

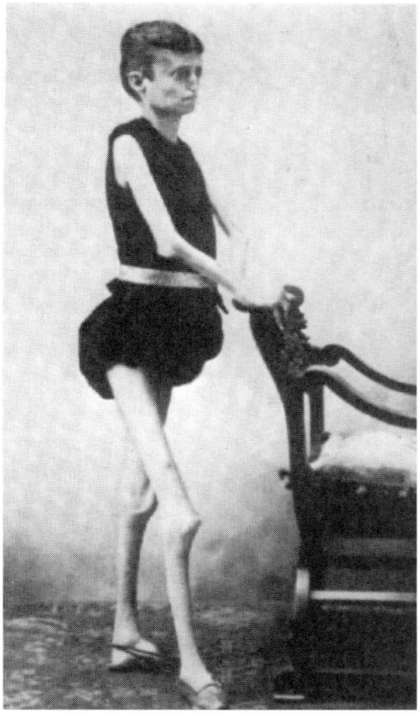

Dominique Castagna

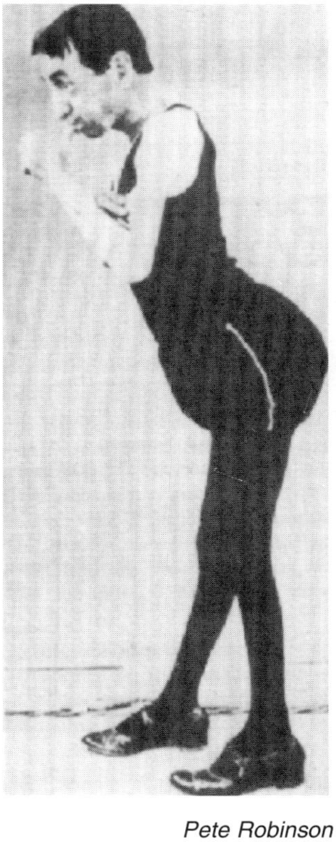

Pete Robinson

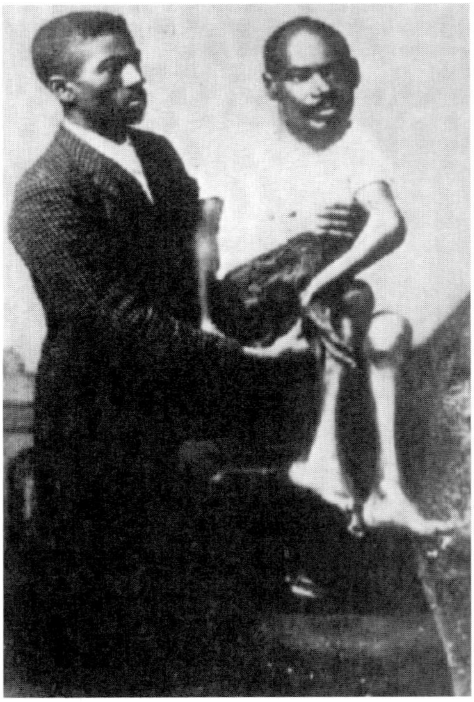

Seip

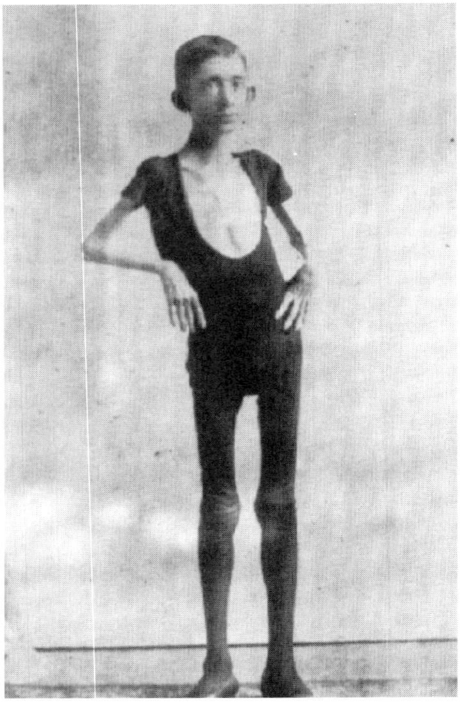

Harry Jones

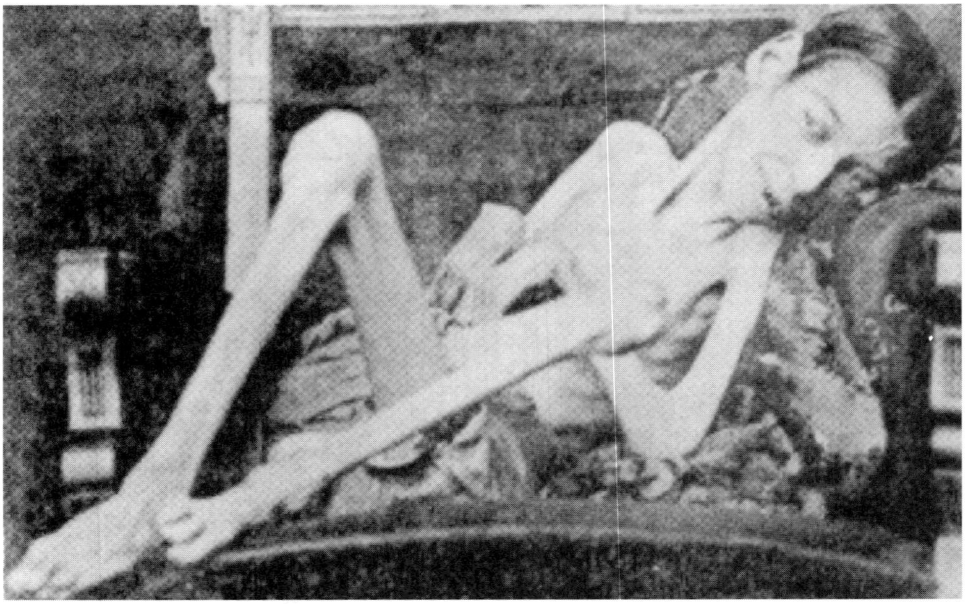

Rosa Lee Plemons

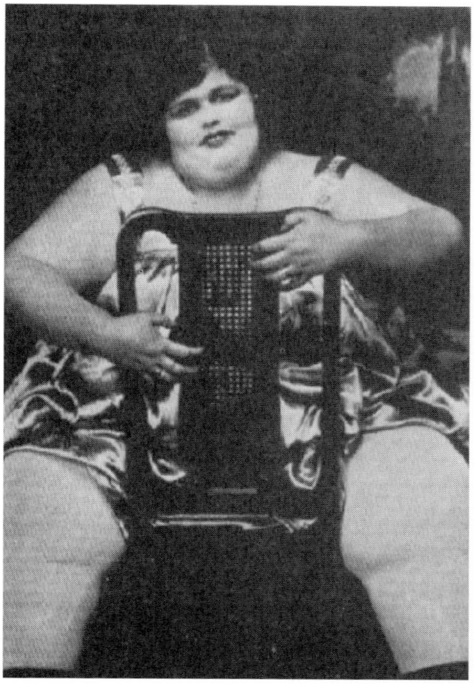

Alice from Dallas

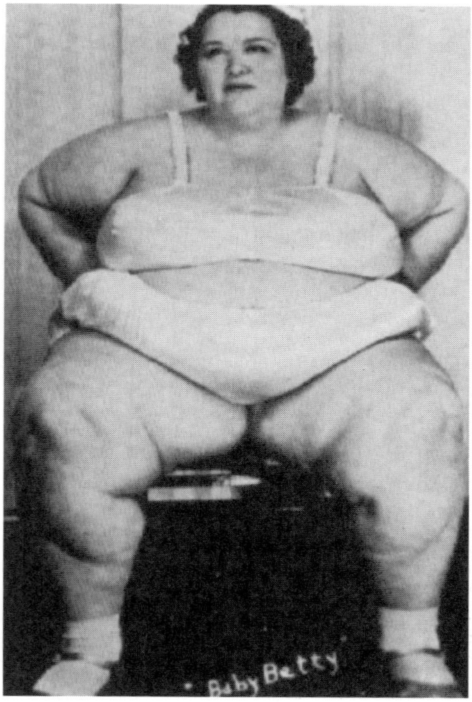

Baby Betty

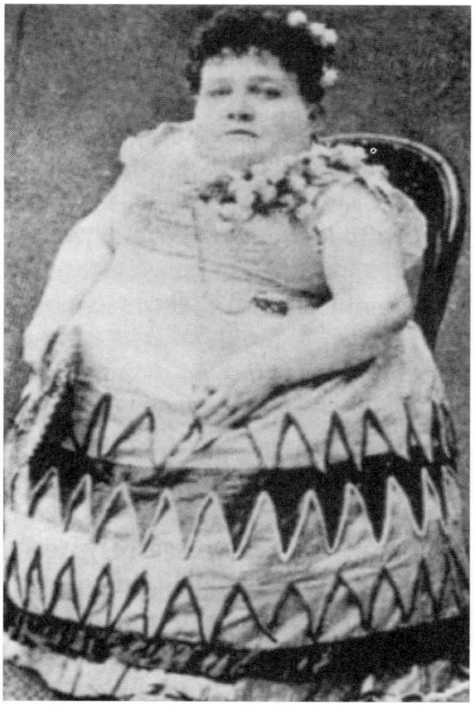

Carrie Akers

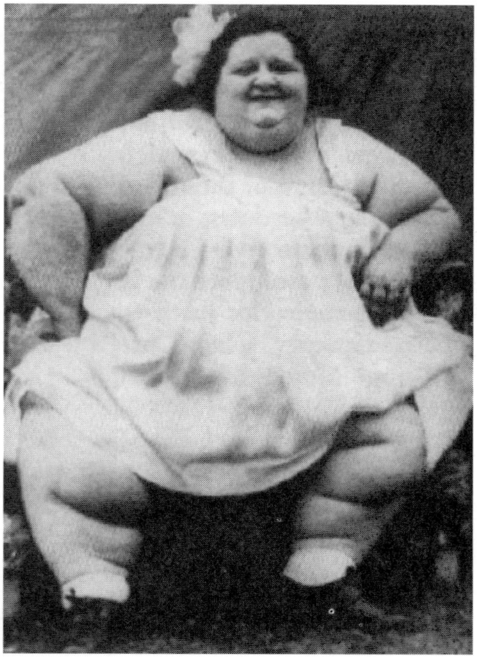

Baby Ruth Pontico

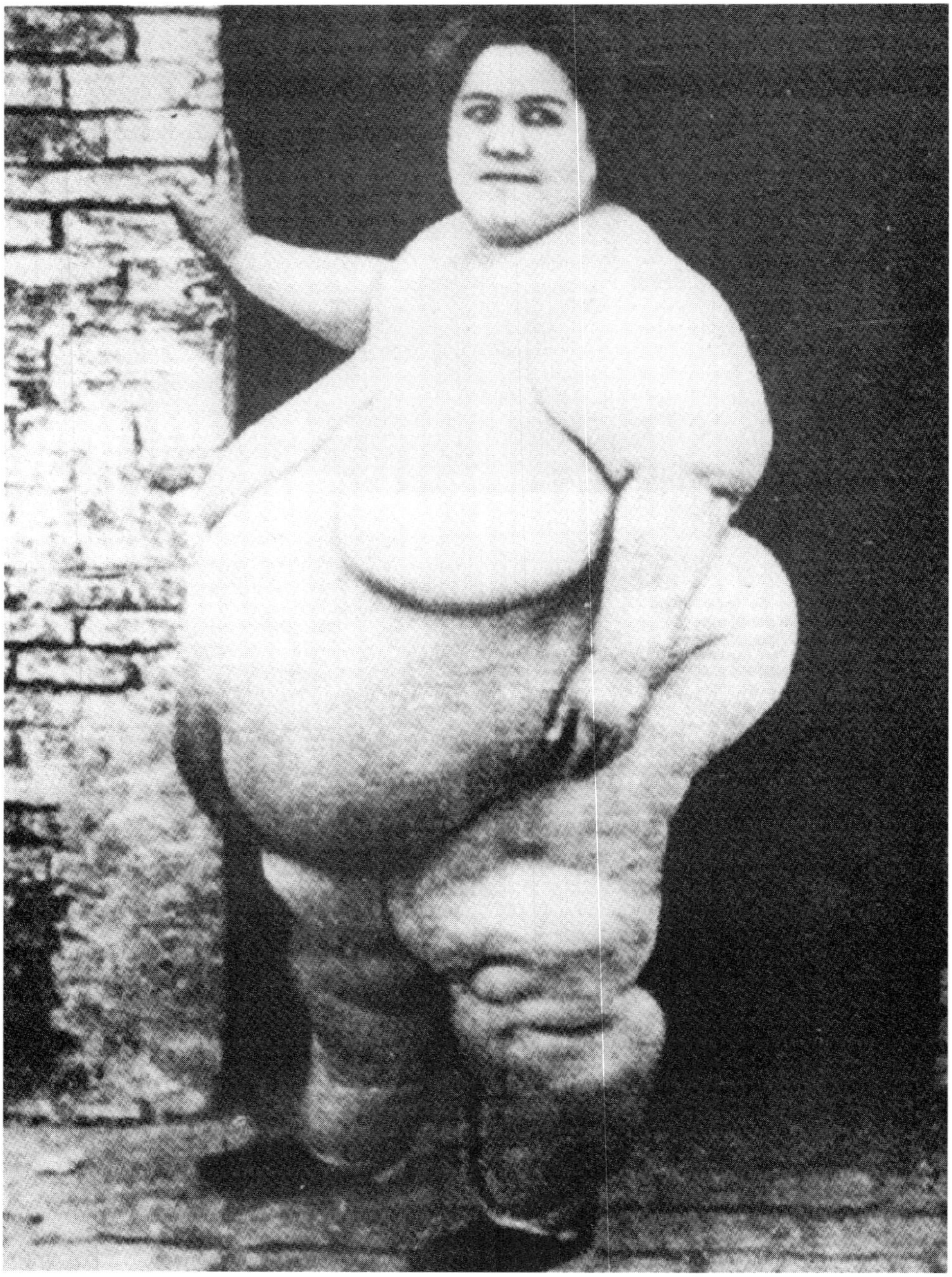

Dolly Dimples

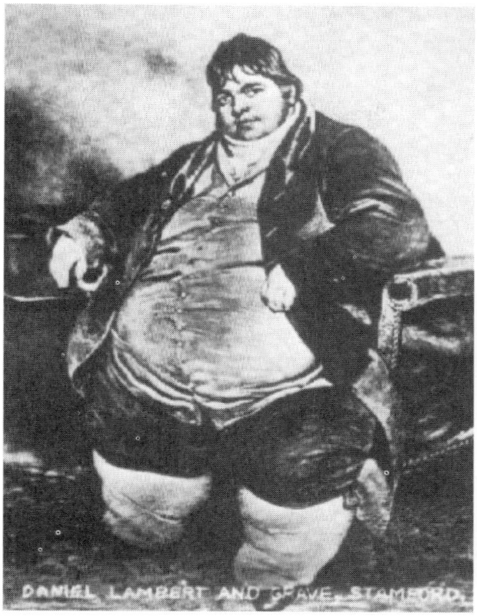

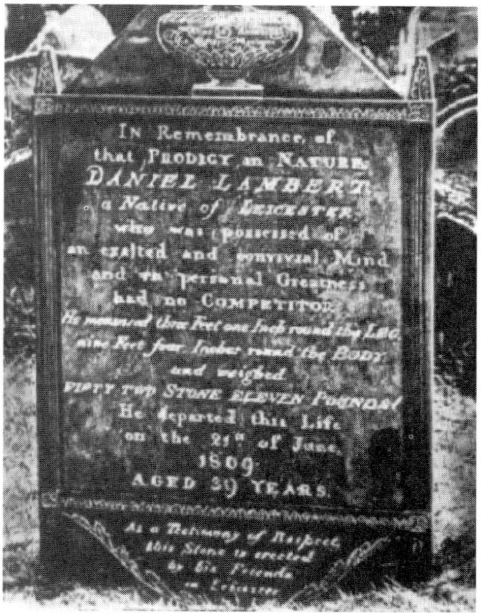

Daniel Lambert

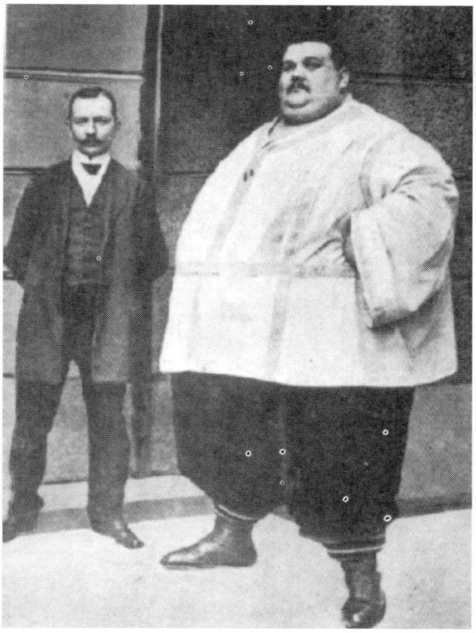

Cannon Colossus

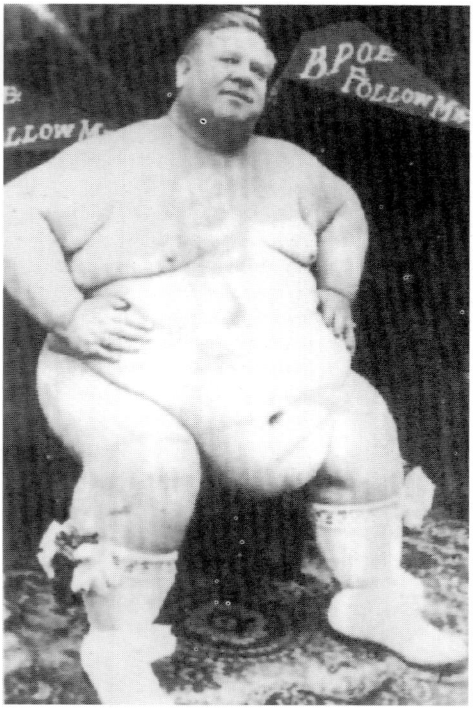

'Happy' Jack Eckhert

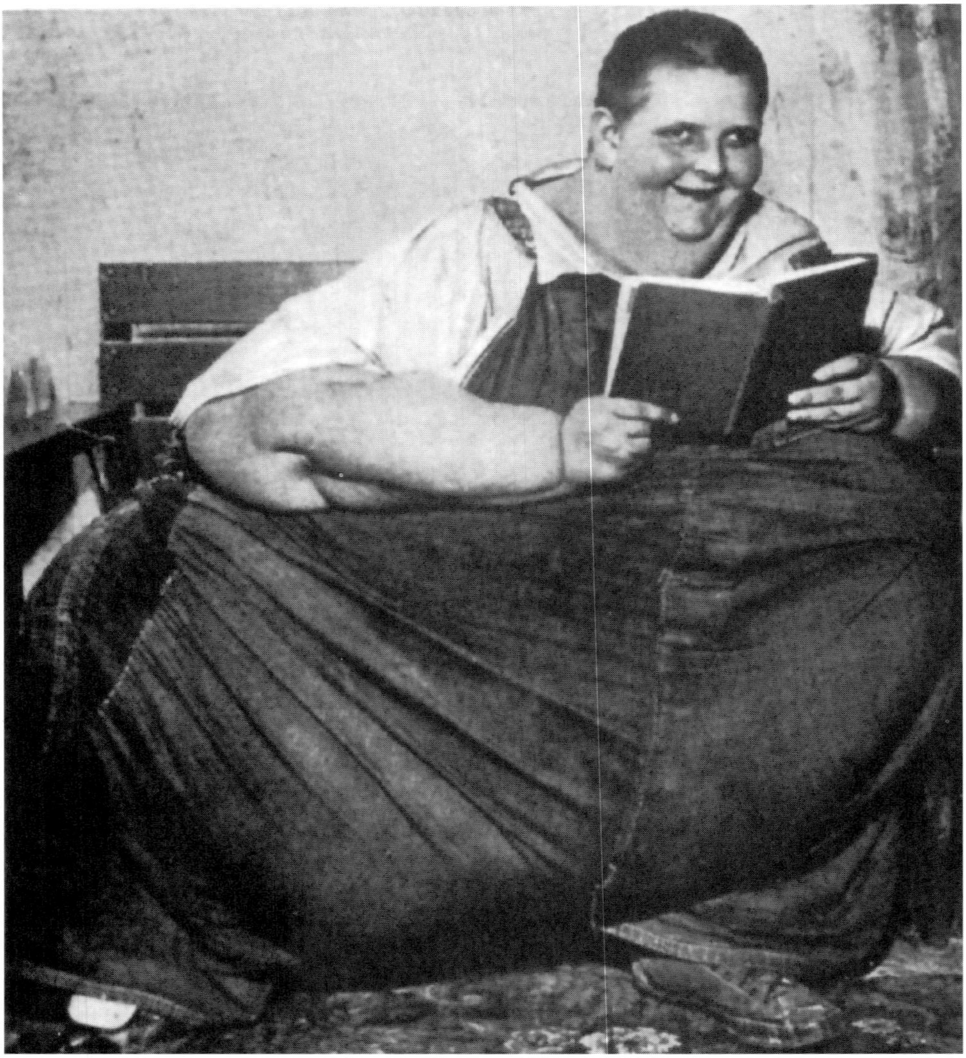

Robert Earl Hughes

Hermaphrodites, and other sexual anomalies

The most coveted, and covert, carnival attractions have always been so-called 'sexual freaks'.[5] Though transsexual surgery can now create hermaphrodites – a male and female in the same body – the authenticity of such 'natural-born' creatures remains in doubt. These androgynous marvels have always figured in classical mythology, but most carnival hermaphrodites ("half-and-halfs") are deemed to have been fakes, despite being perennial crowd-pullers. These 'morphodites' were usually divided laterally, such as Josephine-Joseph who appears in *Freaks*. Others have included Albert-Alberta (aka Bobby Kork from New Jersey), Mary Casey, Benny Rogers, and Donald-Diane.

Some women have been born with virtually no breasts and a clitoris so over-developed as to resemble a vestigial penis; others with neither ovaries nor testicles, but a sterile combination of the two. Neither can be classed as 'fully-functional' hermaphrodites. Nearer to true hermaphrodism are males with the chromosomal dysfunction Klinefelter's Syndrome (who display female breasts and small genitals); these correspond to females with Turner's Syndrome (web-necked, dwarfed, flat-chested). Other genital anomalies have included men with two penises or three testicles, less fortunates with only one testicle ('monorchids') or even none ('eunuchs'), and women with two vaginas. Hypospadias, a condition where the urethral opening is situated on the underside of the penis, can result in deformity of the glans. Related conditions include double or multiple urethral ducts, paired median raphe ducts (causing 'tunnels' in the skin), and even single dorsal ducts. Priapism – a psychotic disorder resulting in permanent erection – was once thought to indicate a boned penis.

Women have also been reported as possessing a third, or 'supernumerary' nipple – once regarded as the sign of a witch – a complete third breast, or a second or even third set of breasts. Anne Boleyn, besides having six fingers on each hand, is reputed to have had three breasts arranged in a triangle. In 1894, the case of a *man* with no less than six extra nipples was reported; men have also been said to give milk. Certain races of women, such as the Hottentots, are fabled not only for their hyper-extended buttocks, but for labia which dangle down between their thighs.

Finally, the most basic aberration – that of excessive size – made both overly buxotic women and exceptionally 'well-endowed' men much sought-after for an institution which went far beyond what the closely-monitored sideshows had to offer: the stag-movie (forerunner of today's hardcore porno flick). We will see that, since its inception, the moving film has always drawn on sideshow tradition in this way, only to eclipse and, ultimately, supersede it.

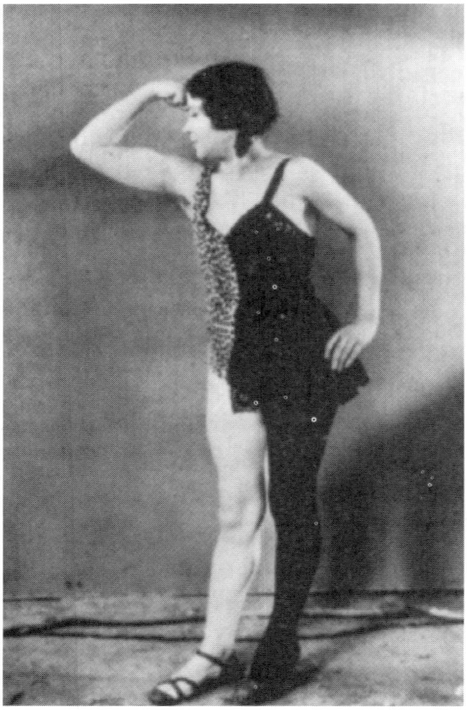

Josephine-Joseph

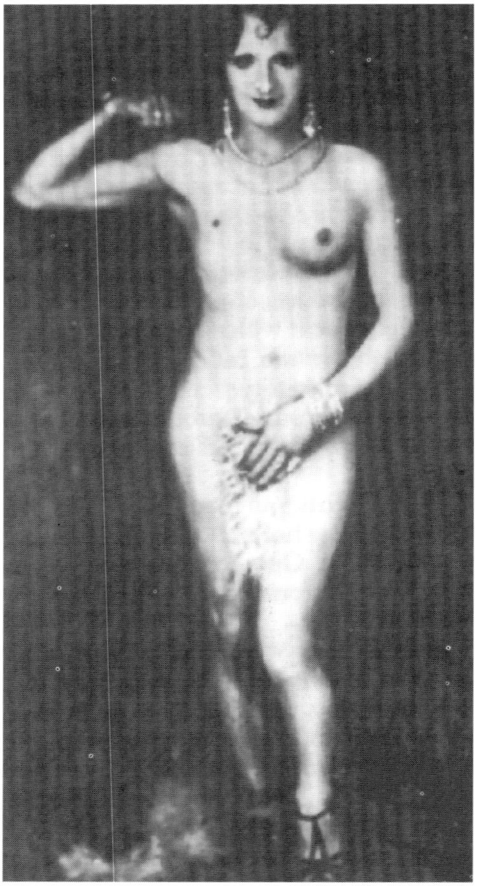

Bobby Kork

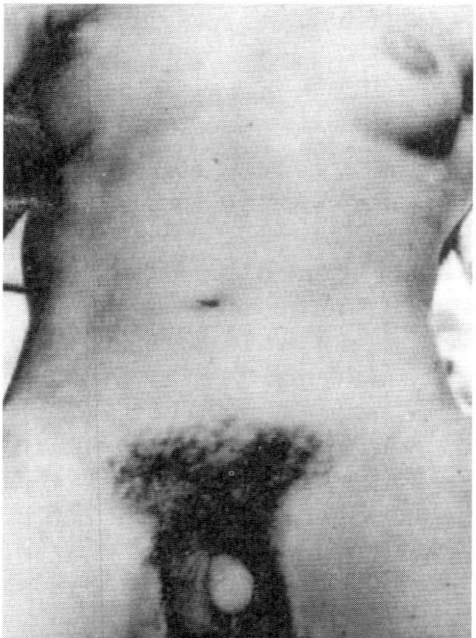

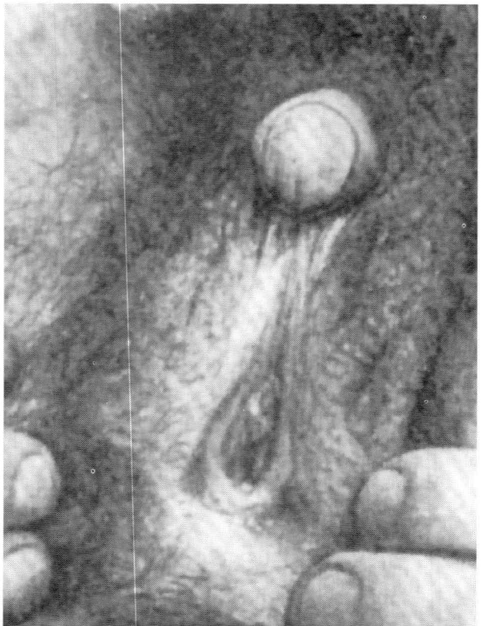

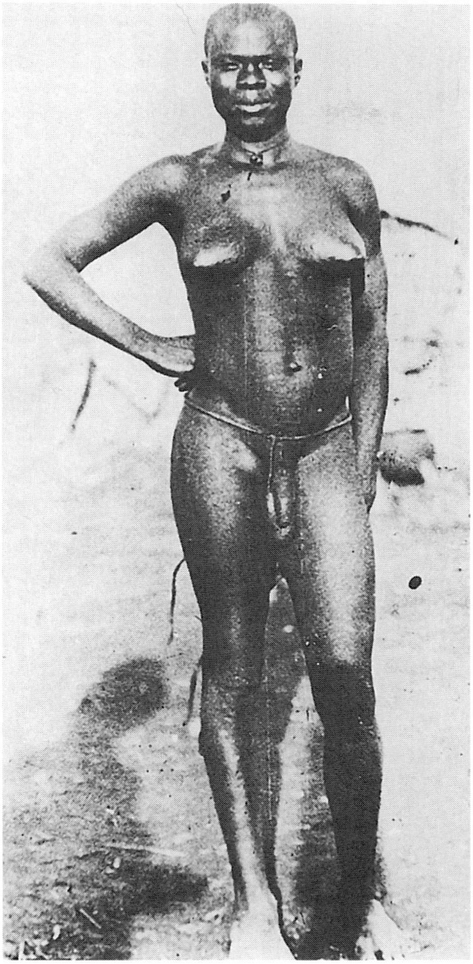

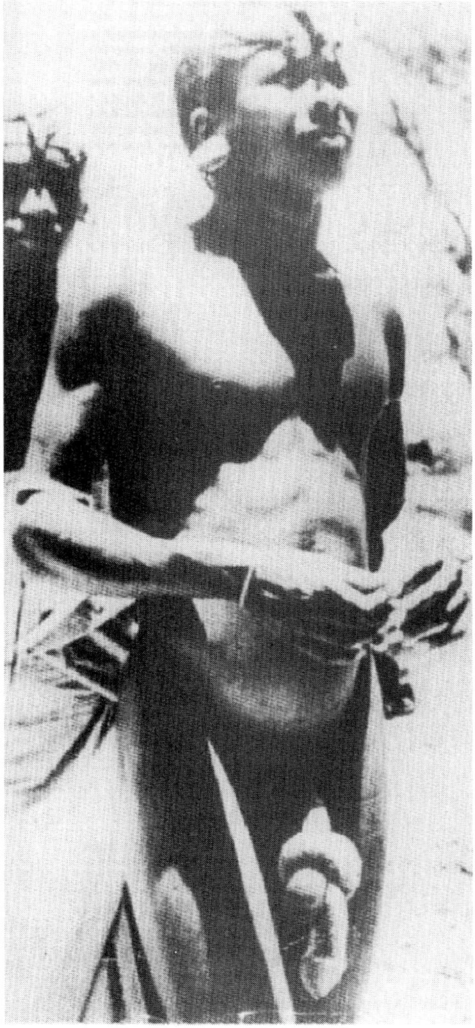

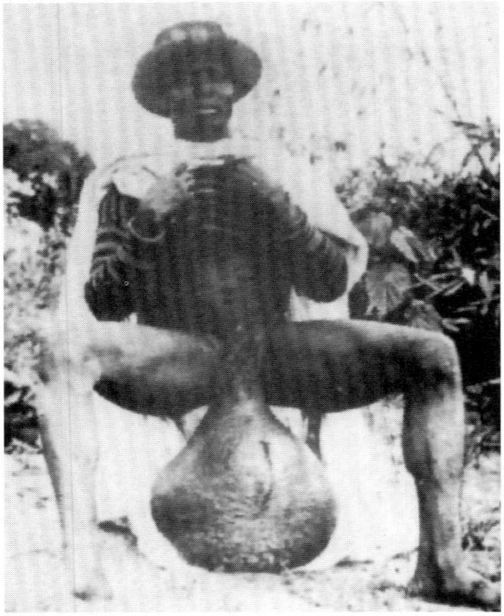

Elephantiasis of the scrotum

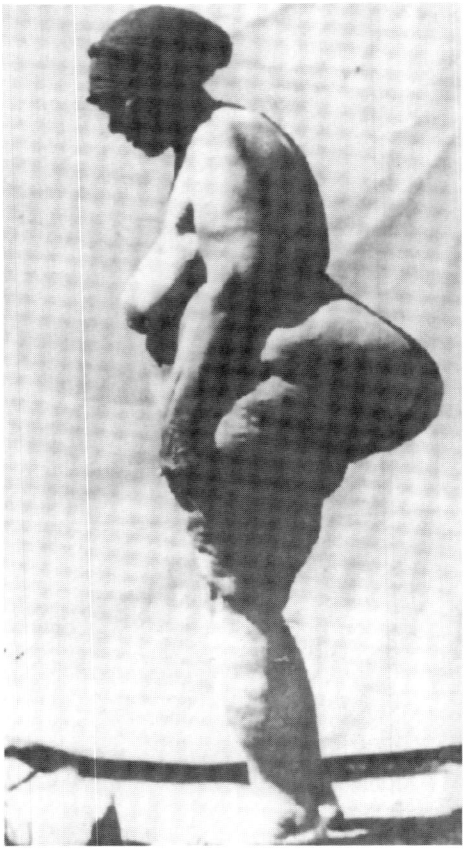

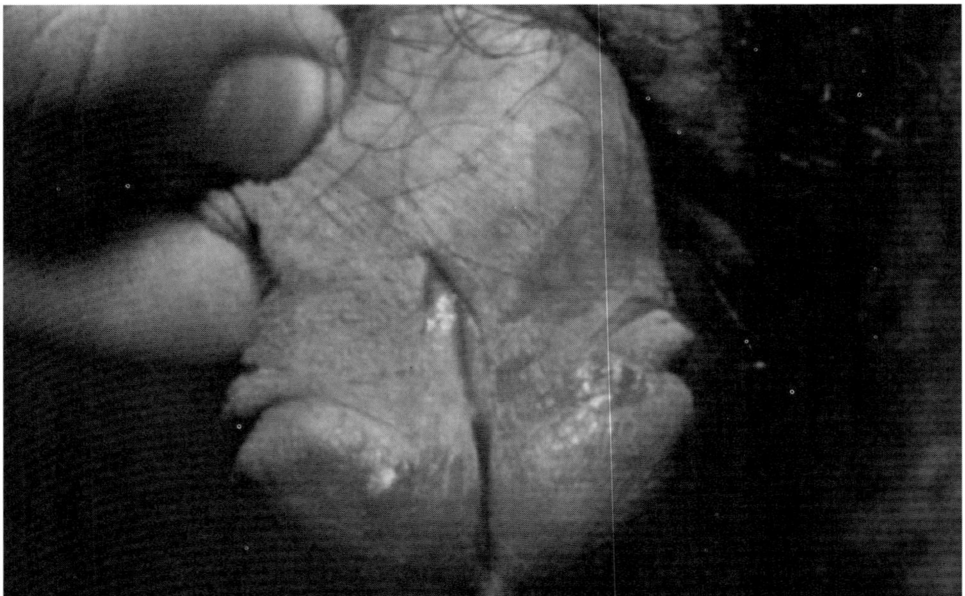

Hypospadias

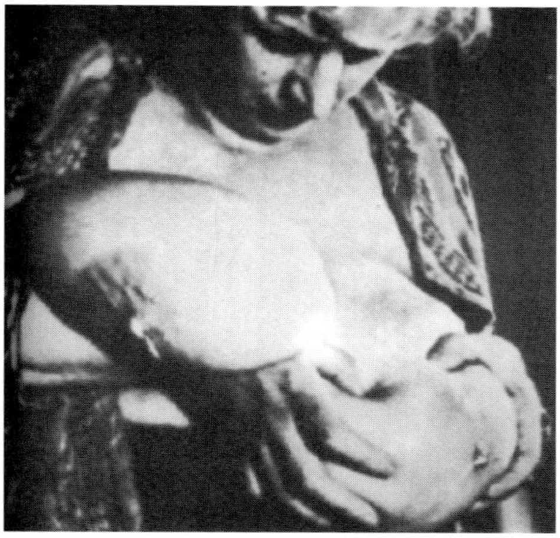

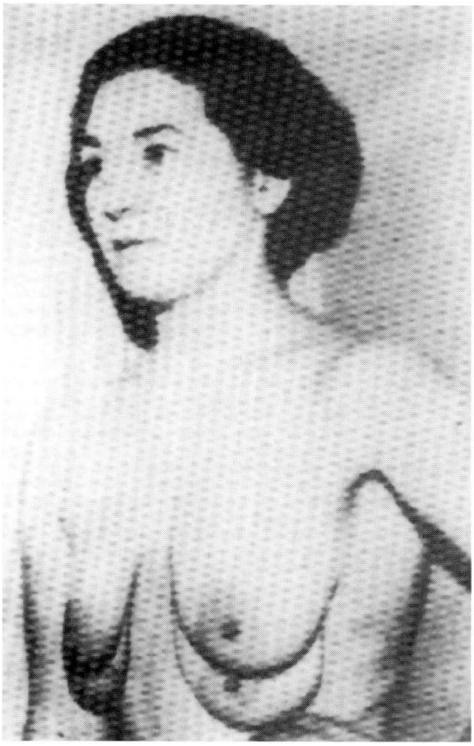

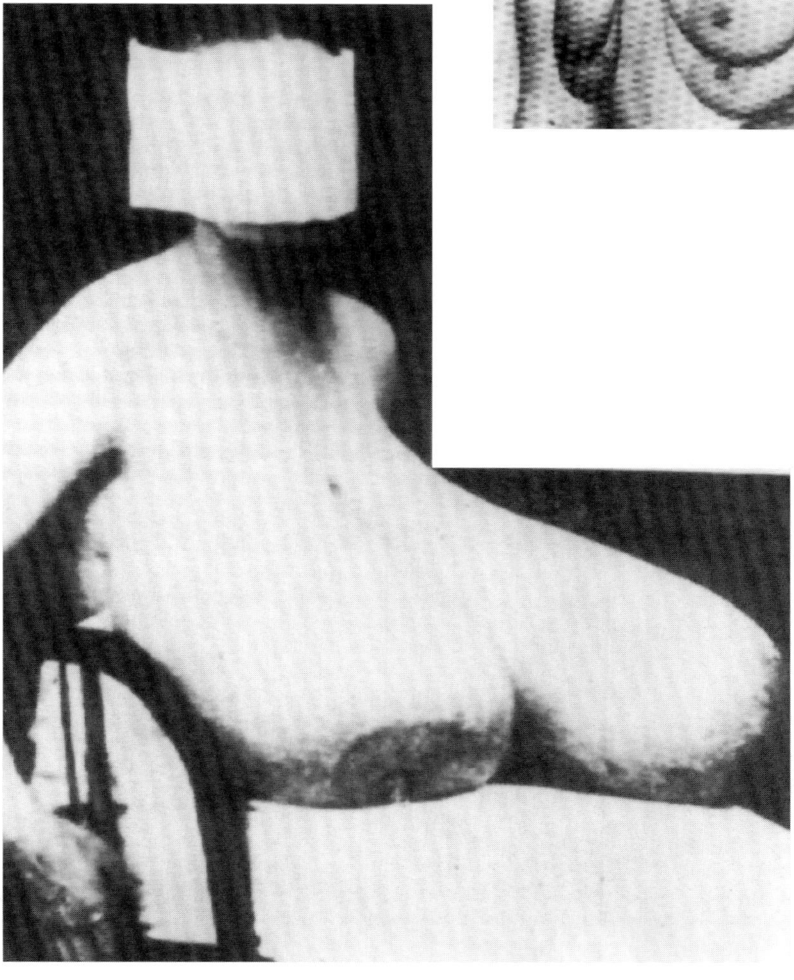

TARTARUS

After the war, interest in sideshows began to wane; this was due in part to the ascendence of cinema, both mainstream and underground, where darker and stranger marvels could be created for view. Advances in medicine were also reducing the number of 'freak' births, and the public's growing sophistication was leading them both to scorn the ever-increasing ratio of obvious self-mades and fakes ("grifts"), and to frown more and more upon the 'exploitation' of those unfortunate enough to have genuinely slipped through Nature's net. The freakshow was being marginalised. More crucially, a preponderance of global atrocities was accruing which would eventually outstrip even the worst horrors dreamt up by the cinema; through war, drugs, and radiation, man was about to supersede Nature once and for all in his seemingly limitless capacity for the twisting and destruction of human flesh.

The liberation of the Nazi death-camps finally revealed the true horrors of war; whereas the limbless, the faceless and the broken insane of World War I had been largely shielded from the world's gaze, the systematic extermination of not only the Jews but also the physically or mentally impaired in the ovens of Auschwitz, Belsen and the other death camps could not be ignored. Singling out such people, even if only to ogle at in sideshows, was nonetheless the first step necessary to eradicate them. In this sense, the carnivals – and their patrons – were as guilty of persecution as Hitler and his cohorts. The Nazis banned freakshows in 1937, thereby enabling 'freaks' to be arrested and incarcerated as 'useless people'; their 'Degenerate Art' exhibition damned most modern art, proclaiming it could only be the work of the mentally or physically retarded; while Hitler (whose favourite movie was reportedly Disney's *Snow White And The Seven Dwarfs*!) instigated the mass cremation of anyone and everyone displaying such aberrations. And then there were the experiments.

Dr Josef Mengele not only had the blessings of the Führer, but also found validation for his activities in the eugenics and cloning theories of Dr Etienne Wolff[6] of the University of Strasbourg, as well as other 'experimental teratologists'. Mengele's skin lampshades and curtains were merely the trimmings on an ongoing quest to hybridise and homogenise, his sadistic surgical practises – almost a real-life parody of '30s Hollywood SF/horror movies like *Frankenstein* or *Island Of Lost Souls*, with its House of Pain[7] – resulting in the most hellish atrocities. With Birkenau as his hermetic empire, Mengele had suddenly found himself with the absolute power over life and death; like the mad Romans, he also indulged himself by collecting human oddities. Dwarfs were his favourite, particularly hunchbacks, although he also favoured cretins and imbeciles. There was even a resident portrait artist at Auschwitz whose task was to preserve the features of dwarfs on canvas, before their inevitable trip to the ovens. But his greatest obsession was with twins, upon whom he conducted endless tests and experiments. These included inter-breeding projects, the making of monsters. Though twins were generally treated better than other prisoners for this reason, Mengele would often kill one of a pair on a whim for immediate autopsy; the simultaneous execution of twin siblings was another favourite pastime. One report has him killing and dissecting fourteen twins in one night. Arbitrary castrations and other mutilations were commonplace.

Mengele's other area of interest involved facial deformity and characteristics. As well as studying noma – a gangrenous condition of the face occurring frequently in Gypsy children – he conducted intense research into eye colour, especially heterochromia (where a person has one blue and one brown eye). He was especially outraged at those who had blond hair yet brown eyes, and would inject their eyeballs with searing chemicals in an attempt to turn them an Aryan blue. Jars of Gypsy eyeballs, rows of severed heads and other anatomical ephemera proliferated his laboratories.

In direct contrast to the crematorial pall over frozen Europe, yet equally maiming to the human spirit, came the blinding nova heat as Hiroshima burnt in a nuclear firestorm. It is difficult to speculate on the level of guilt felt by Americans on a conscious level over the thousands of Japanese men, women and children reduced to seared raw meat in burns units, or the mutant children which would issue from the irradiated genes of the survivors over the next generations,[8] but on a subconscious level at least it must have contributed to the post-atomic angst which epitomised American life – and by extension its pop/pulp cinema (*cf.* Robert Aldrich's *Kiss Me Deadly* [1955]) – over the ensuing decades.[9] Future events would only compound the constant feeling of futility and vague but omnipresent threat to 'normal' ways of life. The sideshow freaks, once primal ciphers reminding us of our darker nature, were no longer required; the true horrors of man's inhumanity to man were for evermore exposed for all to see.[10]

In 1957, one of the most grotesque and unsettling murder cases in American history came to light. Police investigating the disappearance of a woman from Plainfield, a small farming community in Wisconsin, came to the dilapidated farmhouse of one Edward Gein and uncovered a veritable charnel-house. After first finding the woman's body strung up on rafters where it had been beheaded, butchered and gutted like an animal, they uncovered a succession of grisly remains taken both from other murder victims and from corpses exhumed from the local cemetery – including a sack of severed heads, human hearts and hands, bone necklaces, and a whole suit made from human skin which, it transpired, Gein would wear about the house and yard. Stories of cannibalism and necrophilia stunned the nation. It was the pure stuff of horror films, and sure enough a young pulp horror writer called Robert Bloch was quick to bring out a (sanitized) novelisation of the case: *Psycho*. In many ways – with his lip light-switch, belt made of human nipples, his face-mask of genital skin, his personal collection of excised, rotting vulvas – Ed Gein echoed the predilections of Josef Mengele. But Gein went one better – he'd used his own mother's body.

Middle America's shock over Ed Gein's Oedipal necro-sarco-transvestism – distinctly anti-familial behaviour – had barely subsided when another, far greater tragedy struck their beleaguered ideal of wholesome family values. In 1961 a new, supposedly safe tranquillizer for the relief of morning sickness in pregnant women was made available – thalidomide. The drug affected fetal development, and in forty-six countries women who had trustingly taken this virulent teratogen gave birth to profoundly deformed babies. Babies without limbs, without eyes, without mouths, without anuses, without viscera, without *brains*. The phocomelians we have come to associate with the drug represent only the tip of the iceberg; they were the ones (un)lucky enough to survive, to be equipped for some form of life. Indeed, the following description of a typical thalidomide infant, taken from the book *Suffer The Children*, reads like nothing so much as a blueprint for the nightmare foetus/baby of David Lynch's *Eraserhead*: *"He had a deformed and shortened arm and a hand without a thumb. The other hand had one extra finger. His palate had a gaping hole in it. His face was paralyzed on one side. One ear was completely missing, the other grossly deformed. For the first eighteen months of his life, he vomited his food across the room with projectile-like force. It soon became clear that his brain was damaged, that he was deaf and dumb."*[11] Reports such as this filled the international press, replete with horrifying photographs. It was nothing less than a global freakshow, a fist in the face for the hallowed nuclear family, and its eventual repercussions could only serve to increase the demand for suppression of all such ungodly workings and displays.[12]

A few short years later, America compounded this earlier chemical infanticide by sacrificing thousands of its finest young men in a Hellish killing arena – Vietnam. The details of that conflict do not need repeating. A generation of wounded returned to their home country as virtual outsiders, shattered and maimed in both mind and body; the horrific, pointless war continues to inspire both 'serious' and 'fantasy' film-makers alike.[13] Meanwhile, the highly toxic US defoliant Agent Orange has permeated the entire water-table of Vietnam, resulting in two-headed babies and many other freak births even to this day.

By the time Tod Browning's *Freaks*, banned for many years, was (partially) rehabilitated in 1962 – ironically at the height of the thalidomide scandal – the sideshow life it depicted was vanishing to a large degree. Though a few die-hards, such as Ward Hall and Whitey Sutton, would persist to the bitter end, most were rolling over. When the shows closed down, the freaks had nowhere to turn, and many of them readily joined an organisation inaugurated by former showman Anton Szandor LaVey in San Francisco in the '60s – The Church of Satan. LaVey had many carnival friends, and knew show business intimately, but summed up the attraction of his sect to the freaks thus: "They feel that God has treated them unfairly by allowing them to be born deformed, and Satan, himself an outcast, has more sympathy for their plight." The Church, which thus heralded Satan as fallen angel rather than devil, a figurehead for rebels against unjust authority, started with few members but very soon grew to have several thousand, including the likes of Sammy Davis Jr, Jayne Mansfield and, latterly, rock band The Eagles (*Hotel California* being, it is said, a reference to the Church's first premises on California street, San Francisco). It still flourishes today, and LaVey's books, such as *The Satanic Bible* and *The Satanic Witch*, are perennial sellers among the disaffected of all classes and professions.[14]

One of the many people who turned on to the revival of *Freaks* was a young New York fashion photographer, Diane Arbus. She became instantly obsessed with the film, or more specifically with its gallery of fascinating human oddities, and went to see it over and over again. Arbus declared that from then on, she would devote herself to cataloguing these near-extinct marvels, to creating a permanent record of the darker, "evil mirror" side of human society and nature. She began seeking out live freaks of her own to capture on film, frequenting such shady haunts as Hubert's Museum on 42nd Street – one of the last existing residential freakshows in America – in her quest. Here she encountered all the traditional sideshow acts, including the famous phocomele Sealo, and the tattooed man Jack Dracula, who boasted no less than 306 illustrations from horror movies on his face, limbs and torso. Other anomalies she photographed regularly included a group of Russian midgets, a Jewish giant called Eddie Carmel, and a Mexican dwarf by name of Morales. Hubert's shut down in 1965; Arbus went after shots of other odd people, such as winos, hardcore Village lesbians, junkies, drag queens, nudists, even identical triplets and twins, but she would always return to her beloved freaks. As she later reflected:

"I just used to adore them. I still do adore some of them. I don't quite mean they're my best friends but they made me feel a mixture of shame and awe. There's a quality of legend about freaks. Like a person in a fairy tale who stops you and demands that you answer a riddle. Most people go through life dreading they'll have a traumatic experience. Freaks were born with their trauma. They've already passed their test in life. They're aristocrats."[15]

Diane Arbus committed suicide in 1972, by which time the sideshows were all but banished, generally regarded as disgusting anachronisms. This was underlined by a case in 1972, when the North Fair Show (featuring seasoned pros Sealo and dwarf Pete Terhune), tried to pitch in North Bay Village, Florida. Residents brought an injunction, citing an old law by which freakshows were explicitly equated with pornography. Although the case was finally overturned (in the interests of free enterprise), the message was clear: displaying deformed flesh was now deemed as obscene as showing hardcore sex; the Seal Boy's flippers as forbidden and unwelcome in town by decent folk as a spurting penis, gaping vulva or sodomised anus.

We now have special-effects cinema in place of live freak shows; and indeed, the mutations of John Carpenter's *The Thing*, David Cronenberg's *Videodrome* or Paul Verhoeven's *Total Recall* far surpass anything Mother Nature could ever have concocted. Likewise, the terrible results of years of chemical pollution and radiation leakage – our shameful 'fourth world' of man-made freaks – can never be admitted or revealed by the regimes and corporations responsible. In Brazil – where thalidomide and similar drugs are still prescribed to pregnant women – singer Nick Cave tells of freaks performing in local nightclubs; limbless beggars – usually crippled by their own parents – throng the sub-continent of India; but in the 'progressive' West, such sights are a thing of the past. Despite the homages paid to a nostalgic geek/amputee underworld by *manga* artist Maruo Suehiro in *Mr Arashi's Freak Show* and by American artist Joe Coleman in such exquisitely repulsive books as *The Mystery Of Wolverine Woo-Bait* (1982) and *Cosmic Retribution* (1992) [Coleman also had a stage act which in 1981 reportedly involved him biting the heads off live mice], and a vain bid by the Jim Rose Circus to reinstate geeking (of sorts) as a pastime fit for mass consumption, the only traces of the old sideshows are locked away in the deathly still of hospitals or museums, teratological refuges such as the Mütter Museum of Pathology, a collection donated to the College of Physicians of Philadelphia in 1858 and augmented ever since. Besides a post-autopsy plastercast of Chang and Eng and their joint liver, this reliquary houses the burnished bones of giants and dwarfs alongside club-footed, cretin and craniopagic skeleta, plus the only known remains of a sufferer from the rare crippling disease Fibrodysplasia Ossificans Progressiva, a condition where surplus bone forms and spreads at random over the normal skeleton, resembling a curtain of molten wax.

Inspired by such very collections is perhaps the only man still carrying on – and indeed far superseding – the darker photographic preoccupations of Diane Arbus. Joel-Peter Witkin's astonishing photographs have been published and exhibited worldwide. His is a body of work as extreme and taboo (and yet strangely erotic) as any in existence; lush, chemically-treated monochrome images of dwarfs, bearded women, amputees, hunchbacks, (especially) hermaphrodites, and any other human oddities that may fall beneath his lens, juxtaposed with props from a black carnival in which medical appliances and prostheses are melded with S/M accoutrements to form a startling atrocity zone. *Leda, Art Deco Lamp, Bacchus Amelus, Picasso En Los Disparates De Goya*: these are just a few dispatches from a catalogue unparalleled in its depictions of a lascivious living Hell.

Not content with these living wonders, Witkin has also transgressed further, working with dead flesh and bone, raiding the necropolis for the body parts used in the composition of such pictures as *Le Baiser* and *The Feast Of Fools*.

In this religious quest for the Freudian uncanny, Witkin is clearly a soul in the tradition of not only Diane Arbus, but *Freaks* director Tod Browning himself; in his volume of perversely beautiful portraits, *Gods Of Earth And Heaven*, he proclaims the following manifesto:

"I need physical marvels – a person, thing or act so extraordinary as to inspire wonder: someone with wings, horns, tails, fins, claws, reversed feet, head, hands. Anyone with additional arms, legs, eyes, breasts, genitals, ears, nose, lips, head. Anyone without a face. Pinheads, dwarfs, giants, Satyrs. A woman with one breast (center); a woman with breasts so large as to require Dalíesque supports; women whose faces are covered with hair or large skin lesions and willing to pose in evening gowns. Active and retired sideshow performers, contortionists (erotic), anyone with a parasitic twin, people who live as comic book heroes. Boot, corset and bondage fetishists, a beautiful woman with functional appendages in place of arms, anorexics (preferably bald), the romantic and criminally insane (nude only). All manner of extreme visual perversions. A young blonde girl with two faces. Hermaphrodites and taratoids (alive and dead). Beings from other planets. Anyone bearing the wounds of Christ. Anyone claiming to be God. God."[16]

The persistence of the art of Joel-Peter Witkin and like-minded others may be seen as indicating the presence of a growing underground resistance to the all-pervasive corporate body-imaging of the '90s, a rebel movement to reclaim the human form by its individual owners. Whereas the demand for real-life ("voyeuristic") freak shows began to decline steadily after the '40s and '50s, the passion for tattooing as a private adornment has grown with equal progress. A similar, more recent increase in body-piercing, not only of ears and noses but also of nipples, genitals and other erogenous areas, has given rise to a trend known as "modern primitivism", where Westerners are willingly undergoing tattooing, piercing, scarification and other body modifications normally thought to be the sole province of Eastern or African tribes, in order to assert an independent control over their personal and private lives. Male and female infibulation, once a punitive or feudal imposition, is now highly desirable. This new ideology is also indubitably reflected by the rising interest in sado-masochistic and fetishistic sex iconography and ritual. The live shows of Californian Ron Athey represent the apex of this new aesthetic. Athey is run through with sharp implements by his heavily tattooed and pierced assistants, his bald head transfixed by a crown of needles; genitals are sewn together, the stage awash with blood by the time the rites have ended.

Hermaphrodites are commonplace due to the wonders of modern surgery, while budding porno starlets have undergone massive silicon implants to augment their bust sizes to unheard-of dimensions in a bid to top the ratings. Penis enlargement is an escalating industry, and many other cosmetic operations – in spite of entailing cutting and slicing more graphic than anything inflicted by the 'psychos' of slasher movies – have become routine. Women are giving men licence to legally inflict upon them the kind of wounds usually perceived as the 'sick' dreams of misogynistic serial killers.

With the advancement of 'cyborg' technology in replacing soft body parts with machines, we are heading toward an era of a new kind of freak; not made by nature, or drugs, but by computer science. Not a freak of deformity, but of *con*formity. It remains to be seen whether this craving for physical perfection, epitomised by the cyborg aesthetic projected by Arnold Schwarzenegger in his *Terminator* movies, and by the current 'super-model' anorexic chic (callously glorified while in Bosnia thousands once more starved in death-camps), will yet come full circle and precipitate a millennial backlash that plunges us once more toward the Hellscapes and apocalyptic bestiaries of our unconscious.

In a world of perfect people, difference is the only mark of recognition.

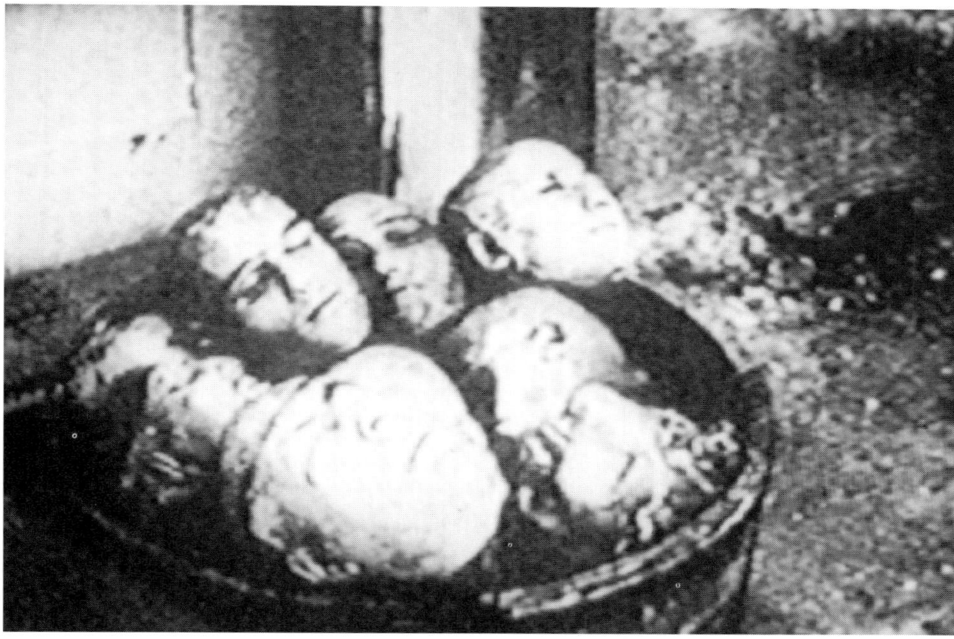

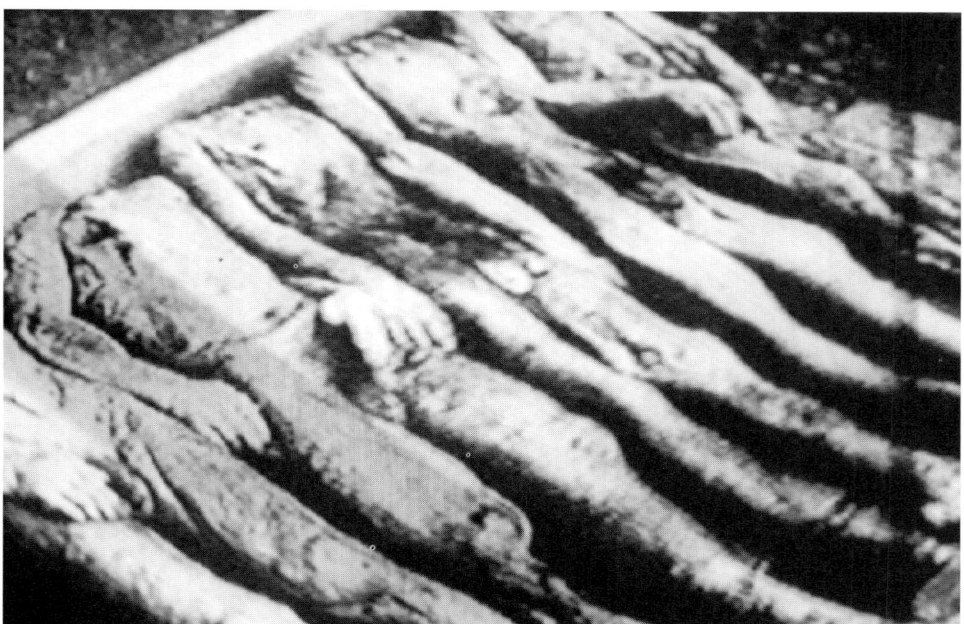

Holocaust

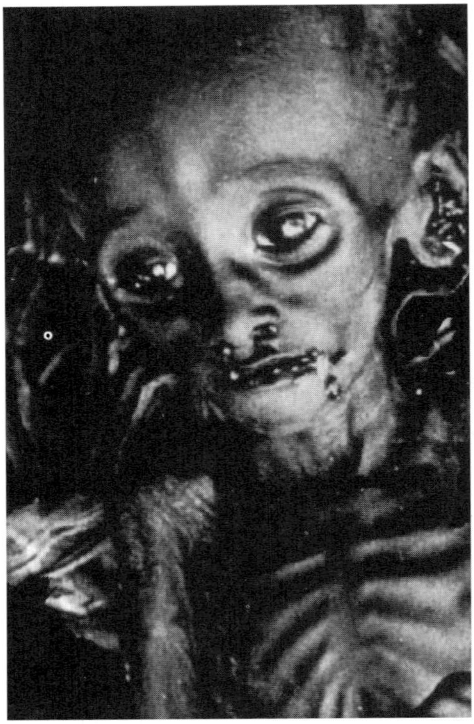

Famine

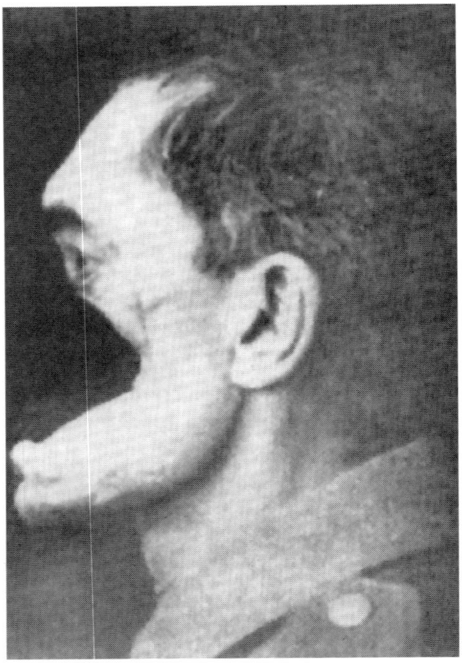

War

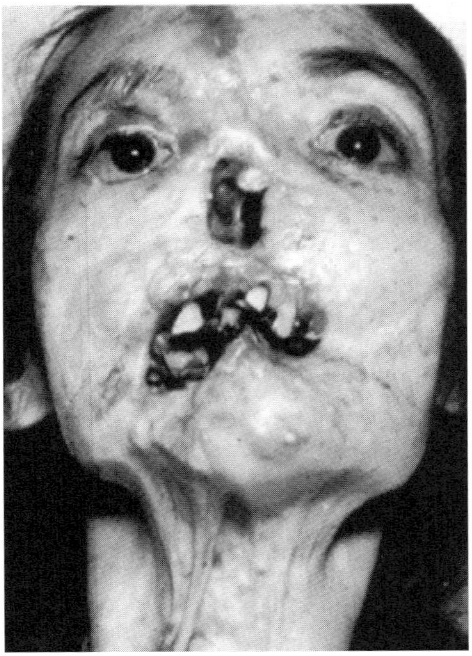

Plague

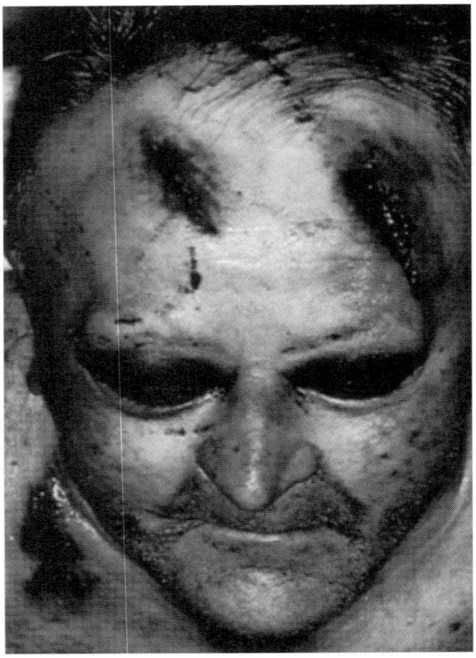

Death

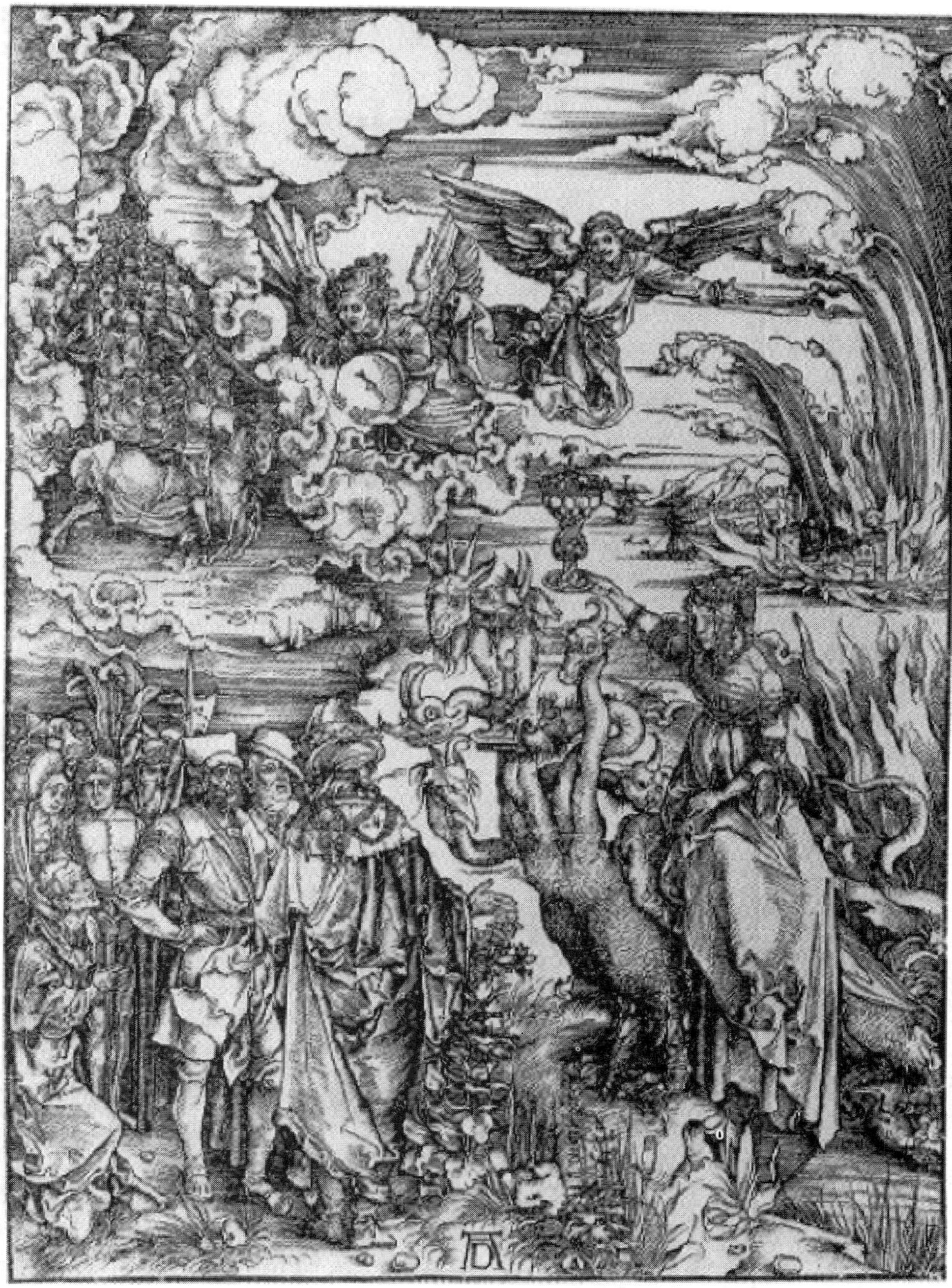

Albrecht Dürer, *Apocalypse* (1498)

NOTES

1 Deformed foetuses, usually preserved in formaldehyde – "pickled punks" in carnival terminology – have always been a mainstay of both teratological research and sideshows alike.

2 This mystical reverence towards the malformed typifies the shamanistic qualities consistently attributed to them throughout the ages. Actual shamans in various cultures have indeed used physical difference to accentuate their oracular status, hermaphrodism being particularly desirable. This is achieved through complete castration, or sometimes by slitting and inverting the penis to resemble an exposed vulva. Western culture typically twisted this, establishing the stereotypical ugly, hump-backed appearance of the witch as proof of malevolence. Even so, atavistic traces of this relationship reside in our fascination with freaks, a deep-seated notion that their difference somehow exposes them to arcane knowledge or power.

3 The legend of the feral child is closely linked to that of the "Missing Link", the creature who supposedly embodies the evolutionary stage between ape and man. Such 'human apes' have featured in many fantasy films, including Gordon Douglas' *Skullduggery* (1970). They have been shown as creations of science as early as 1908 (*The Doctor's Experiment*), and later in the likes of *Captive Wild Woman* (1943) and *Superbeast* (1972) [see also note 7]. One of the few serious film treatments of a feral child was François Truffaut's *L'Enfant Sauvage* (1970), inspired by Lucien Malson's *Wolf Children And The Problem Of Human Nature*, an account published in 1964 listing some 53 attested cases of this phenomenon.

4 Grady Stiles hit the headlines much more recently, when he was shot four times in the head on November 29, 1992 as he sat watching TV in his Gibsonton trailer. His wife, Mary Teresa Stiles, was later convicted of paying one Christopher Wyant $1,500 to kill Grady who had become a violent drunk prone to beating her savagely with his claws.

5 In Freudian terms, it is the onset of puberty, – the very sexualization of the child – with its physical distortions, which can first give rise to notions of the 'freakish'; while the increasingly obvious differences between male and female anatomy may instigate our permanent dread of (and fascination with) the 'other' (hence Freud's equivalence of notions of the 'uncanny' with castration/ lack).

6 Wolff's treatise *La Science Des Monstres* was eventually published by Gallimard (Paris, 1948).

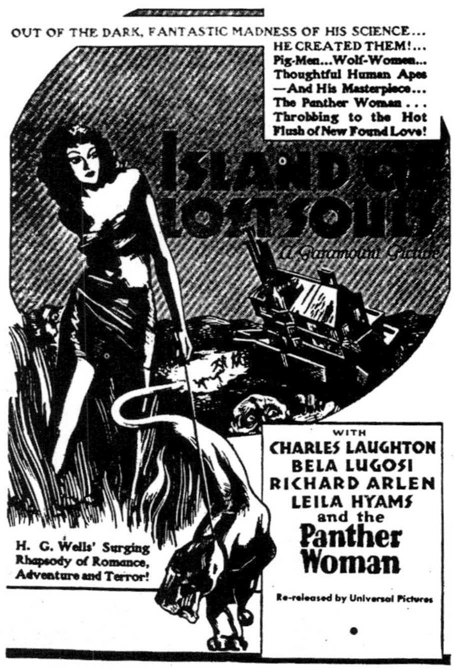
OUT OF THE DARK, FANTASTIC MADNESS OF HIS SCIENCE...
HE CREATED THEM!... Pig-Men...Wolf-Women... Thoughtful Human Apes —And His Masterpiece... The Panther Woman... Throbbing to the Hot Flush of New Found Love!
WITH
CHARLES LAUGHTON
BELA LUGOSI
RICHARD ARLEN
LEILA HYAMS
and the
Panther Woman
H. G. Wells' Surging Rhapsody of Romance, Adventure and Terror!
Re-released by Universal Pictures

7 These two films present a virtual blueprint for the huge body of fantasy film in which human monsters are forged by science fictional means (as opposed to the effects of nature, misfortune or common surgery). [At time of writing, it is still (officially) impossible to galvanize patchwork corpses into fresh life or hybridize living men with wild animals.] The sales pitch remained the same; the posters for *Island Of Lost Souls* (a film banned, like *Freaks*, for many years) in particular read like traditional, sleazy sideshow banners with their menagerie of zoomorphic oddities.

'Beast-people' have also been traditionally portrayed as victims of supernatural curses.

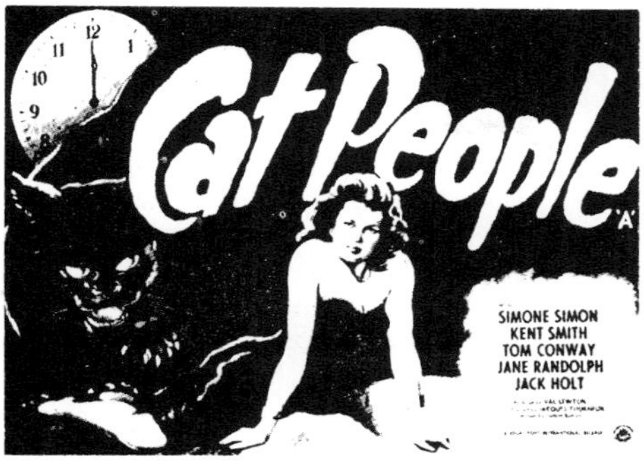
Cat People
SIMONE SIMON
KENT SMITH
TOM CONWAY
JANE RANDOLPH
JACK HOLT

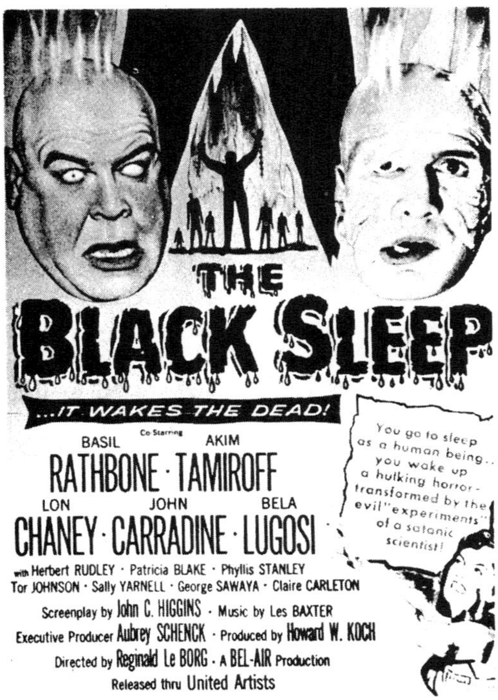
THE BLACK SLEEP
...IT WAKES THE DEAD!
You go to sleep as a human being.. you wake up a hulking horror-transformed by the evil "experiments" of a satanic scientist!
BASIL Co-Starring AKIM
RATHBONE · TAMIROFF
LON JOHN BELA
CHANEY · CARRADINE · LUGOSI
with Herbert RUDLEY · Patricia BLAKE · Phyllis STANLEY
Tor JOHNSON · Sally YARNELL · George SAWAYA · Claire CARLETON
Screenplay by John C. HIGGINS · Music by Les BAXTER
Executive Producer Aubrey SCHENCK · Produced by Howard W. KOCH
Directed by Reginald Le BORG · A BEL-AIR Production
Released thru United Artists

Werewolf films have thrived, from *The Werewolf Of London* (1935) through to *The Howling* (1981) and beyond, encompassing such kindred spirits as *The Cat People* (1942) and *The Reptile* (1966) along the way.

The intake of weird drugs provided film-makers with a third strand of metamorphic fantasy. Freaks and human monsters produced this way have included the many versions of Mr Hyde in *Dr Jekyll And Mr Hyde* (man into hypertrichotic savage), the mutant somnambulists of *The Black Sleep* (1956), and the likes of *The Alligator People* (1959). Ken Russell's *Altered States* (1980) is a notable post-psychedelic version [see also note 12]. [Russell's *Gothic* (1987) incidentally includes a laudanum-induced vision of a unique freak condition – a woman with eyeballs in her nipples.]

8 One report in *Medical News* stated that: *"Examination of children born in Nagasaki since 1945 reveals an enormous increase in deformities. The damage is lasting, because the origin of the defects is a change in the reproductive cells of all the inhabitants affected by radiation, a change that is inherited and cannot be reversed. Of 30,150 children examined, 3,630 have serious defects, which may be classified as follows:— 1,046 children: degeneration of the bones, muscles, skin, and nervous system; 429: deformities of the organs of sight or hearing; 254: hare-lips or tongue deformities; 59: lung deformities; 47: jaw deformities; 25: born without brains; 8: born without eyes or eye-sockets."*

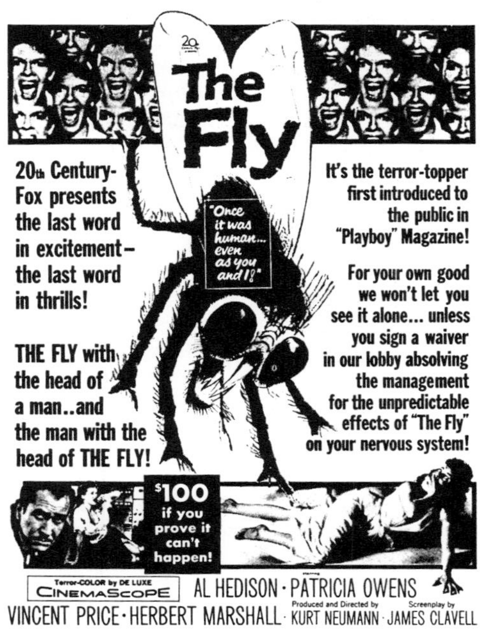
The Fly
20th Century-Fox presents the last word in excitement – the last word in thrills!
"Once it was human... even as you and I!"
It's the terror-topper first introduced to the public in "Playboy" Magazine!
For your own good we won't let you see it alone... unless you sign a waiver in our lobby absolving the management for the unpredictable effects of "The Fly" on your nervous system!
THE FLY with the head of a man..and the man with the head of THE FLY!
$100 if you prove it can't happen!
CinemaScope
AL HEDISON · PATRICIA OWENS
VINCENT PRICE · HERBERT MARSHALL · Produced and Directed by KURT NEUMANN · Screenplay by JAMES CLAVELL

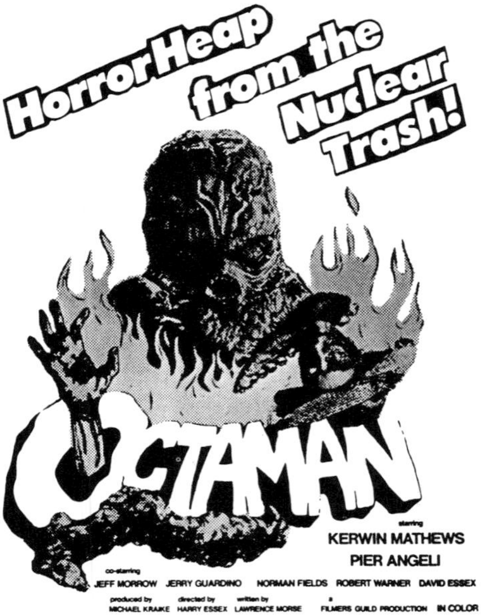

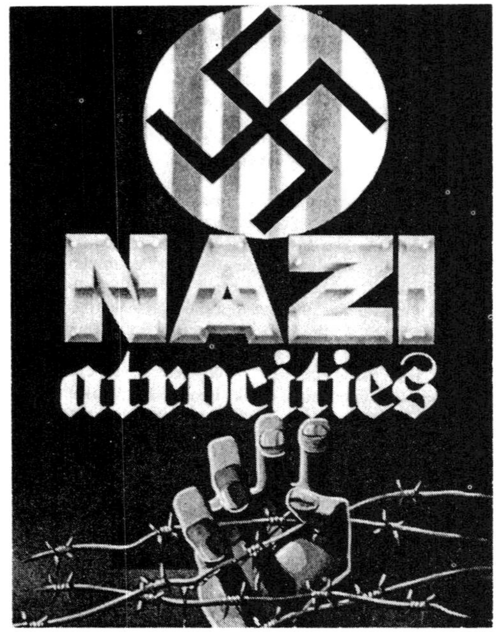

9 The advent of the nuclear and space ages also provided fantasy film-makers with a new excuse for dreaming up human monsters – radiation mutation. From *The Incredible Shrinking Man* (1957) and *The Amazing Colossal Man* (1957) to *The Fly* (1958), from *Atom Age Vampire* (1961) and *The Most Dangerous Man Alive* (1961) to *Octaman* (1971) and *The Bat People* (1974), all manner of freaks have been conveniently blamed on post-Atomic science.

A virus imported from outer space is culpable for the ghastly metamorphoses of *The Quatermass Xperiment* (1955) and *The Incredible Melting Man* (1977), while the alien itself in John Carpenter's version of *The Thing* (1981) is shown as an HIV-type, blood-borne virus causing terrible mutations in its host. Larry Cohen duly provided us with the first alien half-breed hermaphrodite in *God Told Me To* (aka *Demon*, 1976).

10 Documentary footage of the Allied forces liberating the concentration camps is included in such films as *Nazi Atrocities* and *Highway To Hell*; showing the piles of bones and corpses, ovens brimming with ashes, medical 'research' victims, collections of tattooed skin and severed heads arrayed on tables. The most notorious use of these real-life images in the context of a feature film was Alain Resnais' *Nuit Et Brouillard/Night And Fog* (1958).

Harrowing footage of the aftermath of nuclear attack, shot by the Japanese but confiscated and classified by the US army, was finally released in 1970 under the title *Hiroshima-Nagasaki: August, 1945*.

In the 1970s a counter-balancing film emerged from China. *Man Behind The Sun*, directed by one F. T. Mous, is a faked – though hideously realistic – documentary account of true war and experimental atrocities perpetrated by the Japanese *Kempei Tai* in Manchuria.

11 The Insight Team of *The Times* of London; *Suffer The Children: The Story Of Thalidomide* (New York: The Viking Press, 1979), p.112.

12 Drugs of a different nature – chiefly psychedelic – were to be a major catalyst in the further erosion of traditional family values in the '60s. The kids who tuned in, turned on and dropped out to live in communes also became dubbed 'freaks' by the establishment. This new kind of freak – stigmatized not by physical deformity but by a more superficial difference (clothes, hair) and by a profound spiritual alienation from convention – was duly documented in such films as *The Wild Angels* (1966), *The Trip* (1967), and *Psych-Out* (1968, all precursors of the Manson-type movie); it was

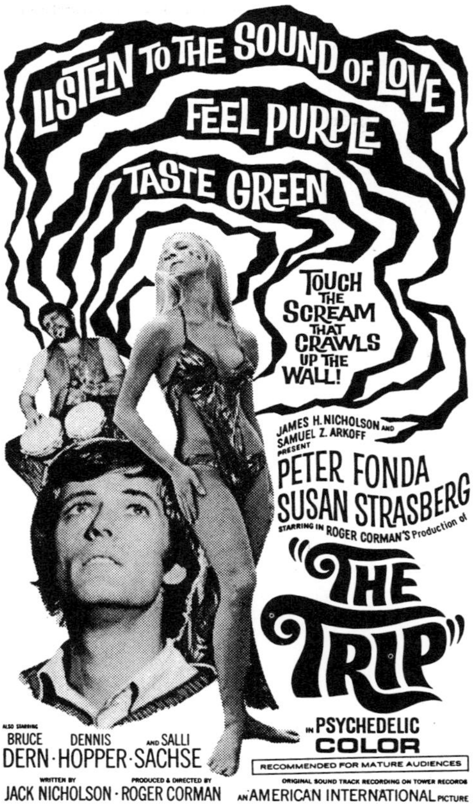

finally left to Jeff Lieberman in his *Blue Sunshine* (1978) to make these rebels into 'real' freaks (a group of straight citizens pay for their former rebellion when some bad acid they ingested as students ten years previously provides the ultimate flashback, turning them into bald, psychotic killers). A similar theme was explored by Adrian Lyne in *Jacob's Ladder* (1990), in which a Vietnam vet once subjected to experimental doses of a deadly hallucinogen is tormented by Baconesque visions of Hell as a basement littered with human limbs and viscera, peopled by legless, eyeless thalidomidic freaks and the crawling insane.

13 'Vietnam films' range from the sublime (*Apocalypse Now*) to the ridiculous (*Cannibal Apocalypse*) to the totally gratuitous (*Forced Entry*). Among the best are *Jacob's Ladder* [see note 12 above], and Bob Clark's allegorical psychodrama *Deathdream* (1972), in which a dead GI returns home as a murderous zombie.

The *true* horror of the war may be seen in *Army Medicine In Vietnam*, sickening documentary footage of field surgery on appallingly-wounded young GIs.

14 *Satanis*, a full-length documentary on the Church of Satan, was made in 1970 by Ray Laurent. Nick Bougas' later film *Speak Of The Devil* examines LaVey's rituals, philosophies and lifestyle even more closely.

15 Arbus, Diane; *Photographs* (New York: Aperture Books, 1972).

16 Witkin, Joel-Peter; *Gods Of Earth And Heaven* (California: Twelve Trees Press, 1989).

PART TWO:

MEAT BABYLON

Freak Film — Cinema Of The Bizarre

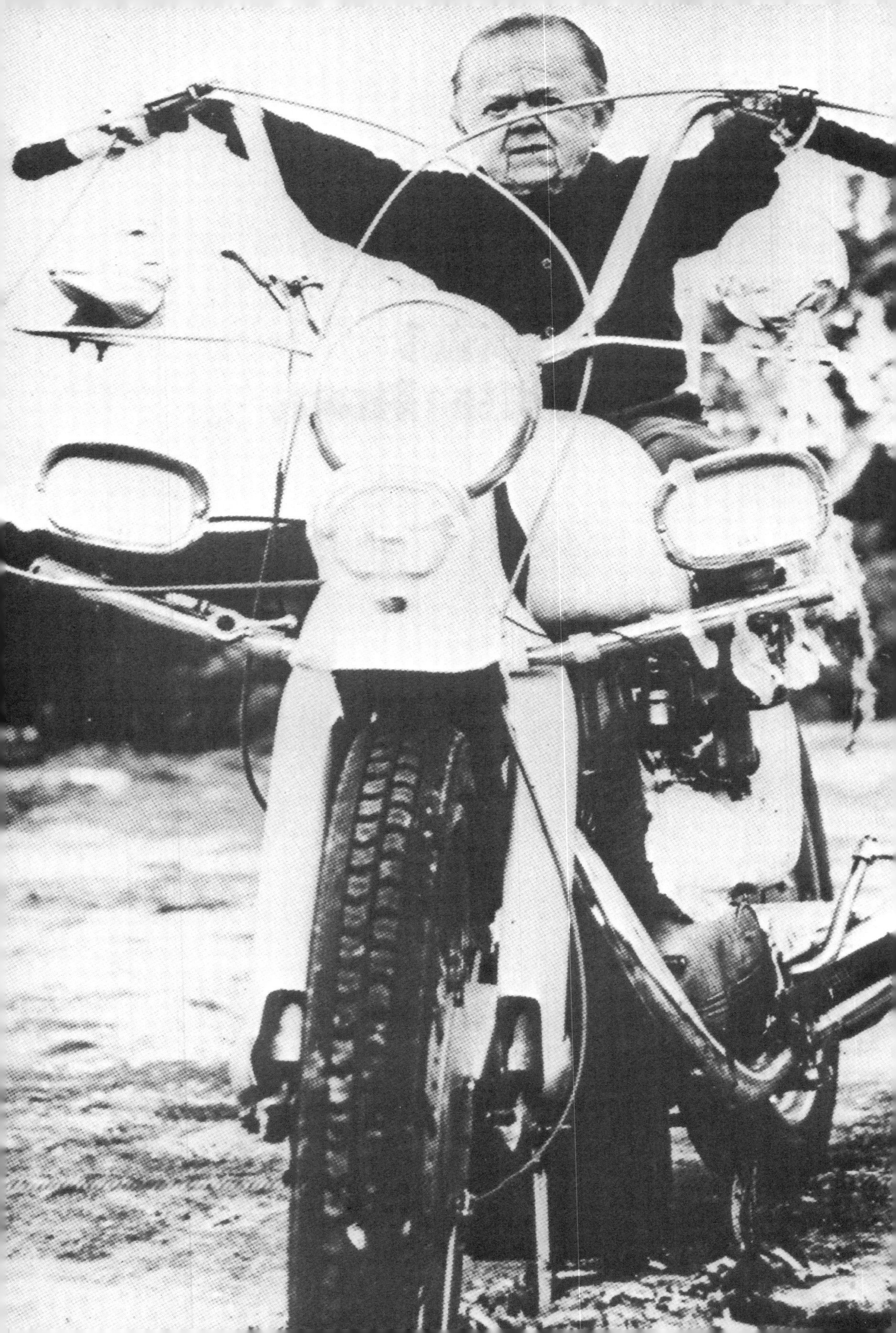

Chapter One:

BLACK CARNIVAL

(From Circus To Cinema)

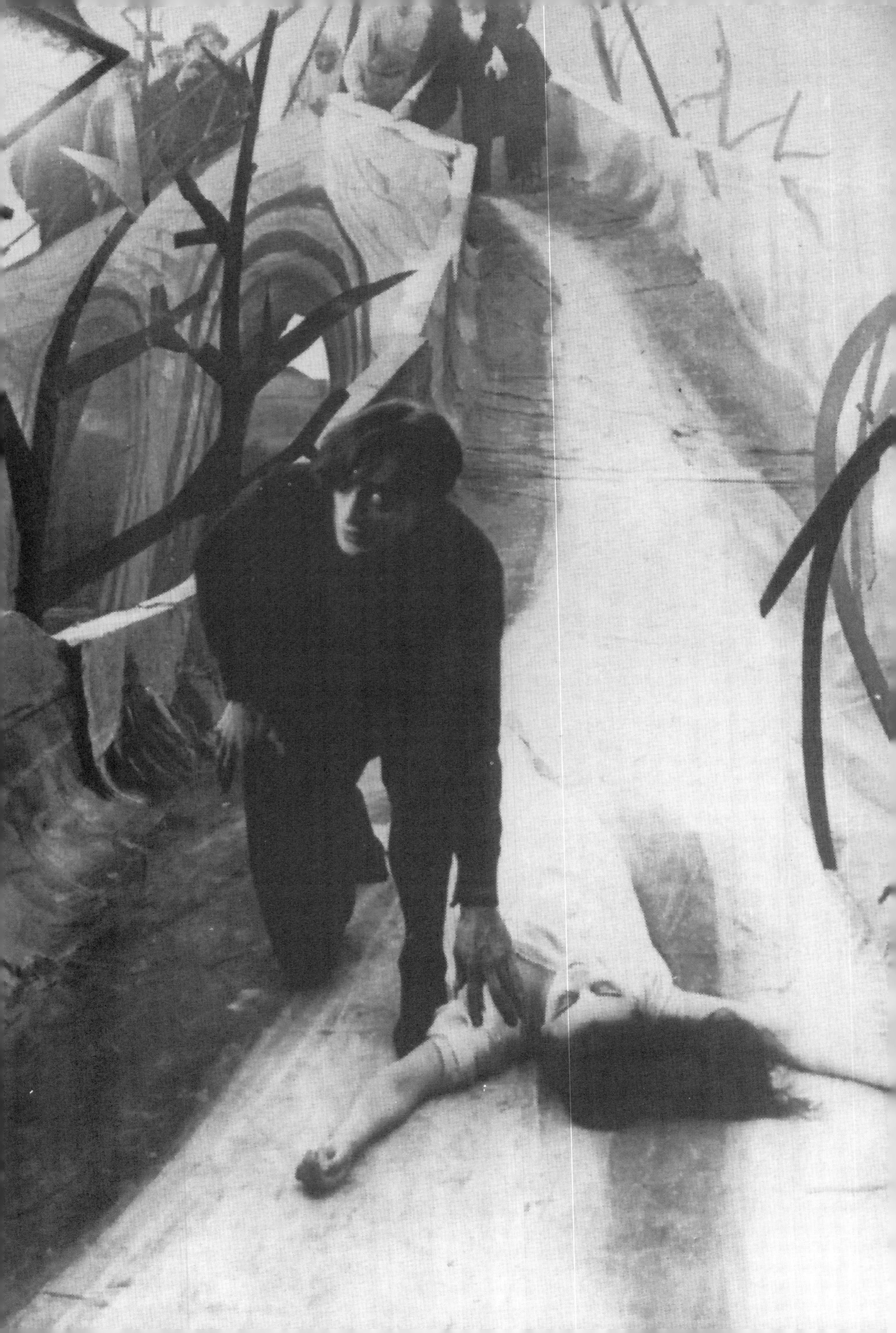

THE HAUNTED PALACE

Even before the great Barnum show of 1901, Paris in the 1890s had been gripped by a passion for extravagant theatre; the Grand Guignol, which opened in 1897, live beasts and, indeed, circus freaks were the vogue. At the *Théâtre de la Gaité* or the *Varietés* of the time, for instance, the crowds could marvel at the naked dancing girl Bob Walter gyrating behind a mass of snarling beasts, see the deadly Spider-Woman, Mlle Fougère, or witness the most famous Siamese twins in all the world, Rosa-Josepha Blazek. Paris even had its very own "Giants' Restaurant", where visiting goliaths were exhibited while prostitutes plied their trade.

At the same time, another burgeoning branch of the spectacular was about to reach fruition. Throughout the century, various experimenters had been investigating the phenomenon of the persistence of vision, developing ways to give the illusion of moving images either in the name of science, or in order to even further enhance their shows: Dr. John Ayrton Paris' Thaumatrope (1826), Joseph Plateau's Phenakistiscope and Simon Stampfer's Stroboscope (1833), William George Horner's Zoetrope (1834), Henry R. Heyl's Phasmatrope (1870), Emile Reynaud's Praxinoscope (1877) and his subsequent *Pantomimes Lumineuses*, Eadward Muybridge's Zoopraxiscope (1881), and finally Robert W. Paul's Theatrograph, Thomas Edison's Vitascope, Emil Skladanowsky's Bioscop, and the Lumière Brothers' Cinématographe (1895); all had their place in the development of moving pictures. It was this progression of invention which eventually gave birth to the cinematic arts in the mid-1890s. And it was during the formative years that followed, at the height of the carnival craze, that a certain Georges Méliès, not content with producing mere documentary footage, was busily developing his pioneering "cinema of magic and illusion".

Méliès was himself originally a magician in the music-halls and fairgrounds. In 1887, aged 26, he purchased the legendary *Théâtre Robert-Houdin*, where he had served his sorcerer's apprenticeship. For 8 years he ran the theatre, presenting breath-taking spectacles of sensational trickery; and then he discovered the camera. The Lumière Brothers, operating the first screening-room beneath the Grand Café, were already drawing over two thousand people a day to view their short, documentary-type films. When Méliès began to make films in 1895 (having customised his own camera and projector), he soon grew bored with 'real-life' subjects, and realized that the best effects could be achieved *within* the camera, rather than in the events being filmed; over the next few years his magician's mind would lead him to investigate every conceivable manner of trick photography, single-handedly pioneering the fantasy film.

Distortion of the human body was naturally one of the first tricks he developed; in one famous sequence from *The India Rubber Head* (1902), his own head was enlarged to a gigantic size – then exploded. His many other films of illusion and thrills, ranging from *The Laboratory Of Mephistopheles* (1897) and *Après Le Bal – Le Tub* (1897, often cited as the first 'nudie' film) to *A Trip To The Moon* (1902), *Le Monstre* (1903) and *An Impossible Voyage* (1904), were chiefly exhibited by his friends and associates, the fairground showmen. While his competitors, the Lumière Brothers and Edison and Pathé and Eclair, used theatrical outlets, Méliès trusted to the oldest exhibition pitch of all – the booth in a circus or fair.

The very origins of the cinema of imagination are thus intertwined with the tradition of using a sideshow to exhibit freaks and other wonders. And not only were the first films shown in the fairs, but one of the first genuine film classics chose the fairground as its sinister *mise-en-scène*. Robert Wiene's *The Cabinet Of Dr. Caligari* (1919) is regarded as the highpoint of German Expressionism, a movement which made many contributions to bizarre cinema. The shuffling, seemingly crippled Dr. Caligari (played by Werner Krauss) is a sideshow hypnotist who displays his somnambulist Cesare (Conrad Veidt), an emaciated figure who sleeps in a coffin-like box. Caligari is accused of using Cesare to commit a number of murders in the small-town community they have infiltrated. The 'hero' of the film is finally revealed to be a lunatic, telling this tale about the head of the asylum in which he is incarcerated. Remembered chiefly for its grotesquely-angled sets (designed by members of the Berlin *Stürm* group), and Veidt's striking, ambivalent portrayal of the doomed sleep-walker, *Caligari* may also be seen to pre-figure many themes which would later become 'horror-movie' standards: a small community penetrated or 'infected' by an unknown evil; the 'mad scientist' and his murderous creation; the gaunt, nocturnal shambler, risen from the oblong box, e.g. a vampire or zombie; possession (Dr. Caligari imagines himself the re-incarnation of a former mystic); the 'Jekyll & Hyde'-type duality of Caligari as both madman and scientist; the framing device of the lunatic telling the tale, plus the further suggestion that even this may be a dream (*cf. Dead Of Night* [1945]); differing perceptions of 'madness' and 'sanity'; and, not least, the carnival setting itself, with its voyeuristic ramifications reminding the viewer of his own participation in the whole cinematic process – a key element in all 'freakshow' films.

Conrad Veidt and Werner Krauss also appear in Robert Wiene's *Orlacs Hände* (1924, an early example of the 'surgical' strain of bizarre cinema), and in Paul Leni's highly expressionistic *Das Wachsfigurenkabinett/Waxworks* (also 1924). In the latter, a poet visits the wax museum at a sinister fairground; in the most frightening of three episodes, remarkable for their outlandish architecture, the figure of Jack the Ripper (Krauss) comes to life and pursues the man and his girlfriend through the night. Veidt appears as Ivan the

Terrible. [Probably the earliest 'waxworks' film was Maurice Tourneur's *L'Homme Aux Figures De Cire* (1913).] Arthur Robison's *Schatten/Warning Shadows* (1924) is also of interest: an atmospheric arabesque of macabre shadows, mirrors and reflections, telling of people driven to act out their own secret desires by a stage illusionist.

Mainly due to the influx of imported talent from Germany, the Hollywood horror films of the 1930s markedly displayed the direct influence of expressionism, particularly in the work of directors such as James Whale, Robert Florey and former cinematographer Karl Freund. Michael Curtiz' *Mystery Of The Wax Museum* (1933) drew on Paul Leni's previous scenario in telling the lurid tale of a deranged sculptor (Lionel Atwill) bent on repopulating his decimated mannequin collection with the wax-coated bodies of real people after his business partner has torched their museum. Heroine Fay Wray, ear-marked as a future Marie Antoinette, eventually cracks apart the maniac's artificial face, revealing his hideously burned and distorted features in the scariest unmasking since Lon Chaney in Rupert Julien's *Phantom Of The Opera* (1925). The film was shot in an early, primitive two-colour version of Technicolor, which lends the proceedings a uniquely eerie aspect and contributes much to this work's status as an early horror classic. Apart from the sideshow connection, it also relies heavily on a staple ingredient of bizarre/freak cinema: disfigurement (= derangement).

Mystery Of The Wax Museum was remade in 1953 as *House Of Wax*, an early 3-D feature directed by André de Toth and starring Vincent Price in his first major horror role. Although this version adds nothing new, Price is typically effective; Charles Bronson plays Igor, his mute assistant. The story was taken to new extremes by Bud Townsend's *Nightmare In Wax* (1966), starring Cameron Mitchell as the disfigured museum owner who lures his victims with a frenetic go-go dancer (Victoria Carroll) as bait.[2]

Of all directors working in Hollywood during the '20s and '30s, one in particular will always be associated with the fairground or travelling carnival and its darker aspects. Although best known for *Freaks* (1932), which would prove to be the thematic and artistic summation – and financial and critical ruin – of his career, Tod Browning left a remarkable legacy of films set in a similar, dark milieu. The carnival was in Browning's blood from an early age; he ran away from home in his teens and joined a travelling show, performing as half of acts called "The Lizard and the Crow", and the "Hypnotic Living Corpse". His Hollywood apprenticeship began with serving as D.W. Griffith's assistant on *Intolerance* (1916), after which he graduated to direct a string of undistinguished comedies and thrillers before meeting up with the actor who would help shape the darker visions to come – the 'man of a thousand faces', Lon Chaney. Chaney, who would make his name by playing characters of extreme ugliness or physical impairment, had a remarkable background which might even have provided a storyline for one of Tod Browning's films. He was raised by deaf-mute parents; his first wife became alcoholic and burned out her own vocal chords with poison; he then left her for a chorus-girl who was already married to a man with no legs.

Chaney very quickly made a reputation for himself playing grotesque, contorted characters, such as the feral, half-simian freak in *A Blind Bargain*

(1922). His first two films with Browning were mediocre, but after Chaney had accomplished his first major screen portrayal of deformity in *The Hunchback Of Notre Dame* (1923), the pair made *The Unholy Three* (1925), a sideshow tale based on the novel *Three Freaks* by Tod Robbins.

Chaney plays Echo, a larcenous ventriloquist who, bored by the carnival and its paltry rewards, devises a scheme with two of his circus cohorts. Echo dresses up as an old lady to sell 'talking' parrots, fooling customers by throwing his voice into their beaks. Any who complain about their silent purchase are visited in person by the 'old lady', pushing her baby in a pram before her. Anticipating later uses of freaks or the freakish to parody the nuclear family, this 'baby' is in fact a midget (played by Harry Earles), who takes the first opportunity to rob the hapless customers' homes. The third gang member, a strongman, provides muscle in case anything goes wrong. In the end, this unholy trinity of circus refugees are strangled by an escaped gorilla. With its use of real-life midget Earles, carnival connections and grotesque moments, *The Unholy Three* was very much a warm-up for Browning's later, more *outré* works in that area.

That same year, Lon Chaney would star as the hideously disfigured madman in another horror classic: *The Phantom Of The Opera*. Next came two more films with Browning, including *The Blackbird* (1926), in which Chaney once more played a fake cripple; the pair then produced their most extreme entry together yet: *The Unknown* (1927). For this story, Browning devised for Chaney his most freakish role to date; as he himself said of the film: "When I work on a story for Chaney, I never think of the plot. That writes itself when I know the characters. *The Unknown* comes simply from the fact that I had an idea about an armless man. So I asked myself what were the most surprising situations and acts which a man as mutilated as that could be involved in. A circus artist who used his feet just as well as his hands, who lost the woman he loved and tried to commit a terrible murder with his toes, that was the result of my speculations."

It was just so. *The Unknown* begins with a circus girl (Joan Crawford), whose act is to spin on a revolving wheel while a knife-thrower hurls his blades around her. The knives are thrown by Chaney, with his feet; he appears to be without arms. We then discover that the girl's father was murdered, killed by a man with two thumbs on one hand. Chaney is later shown removing his costume; a straitjacket has hidden his arms and hands, and we see with horror that one of his hands has two thumbs. The plot progresses, and it becomes apparent that Chaney is infatuated with the girl (not realising that her affection for him is more innocent). Yet he dare not ask her to marry him, as she would then discover he is her father's murderer.

One evening, after his act, he is relaxing in a chair and idly lights up a cigarette. When he realises that he is automatically using his toes, although his arms are free, a deadly train of thought is instigated. If he really were without arms, he could marry the girl with impunity; none would see his two-thumbed hand and suspect him of homicide. Obsession proves stronger than sanity, and he eventually goes ahead with the double amputation.

Returning to the circus, the learns the hideous truth: the girl never loved him, and has now given her heart to the strongman, Hercules. Insane with jealousy, Chaney plots his revenge. The strongman has a stunt, by which he seems to keep two galloping horses from tearing him apart merely with his own strength. In fact, the wild horses are galloping on revolving drums, so there is no pressure on his arms. The next night, Chaney uses his feet to jam the mechanism of the drums, and the horses begin to gallop apart, threatening to really tear off Hercules' limbs. Stage-hands finally rein the beasts in, but one breaks loose and, still frenzied, tramples Chaney to death.

This was the wild plot to result from Browning's speculations, a sado-masochistic tale of *amour fou* which André Breton himself might have written (the Surrealists reputedly worshipped Browning); the fact that it proved successful – despite being described by one outraged reviewer as *"a fiendish mingling of bloodlust, cruelty and horrors"* – was both a tribute to the sympathy Chaney could invoke from an audience, and to the ready familiarity of the public with such people and events in fairgrounds and carnivals. And while circus freaks could be glimpsed in various other films of the genre such as *Wheel Of Destiny* (1927), *The Sideshow* (1928), and *The Barker* (also 1928), none of these works approached the lurid perversity purveyed by Browning.

Chaney followed up *The Unknown* with a double role, again in excruciating make-up, in Browning's *London After Midnight* (also 1927), a pseudo-vampire tale (which the director remade in sound in 1935 with Bela Lugosi, as *Mark Of The Vampire*); and in Browning's *West Of Zanzibar* (1928) he played a sadistic, wheelchair-bound magician. Their remaining projects together, save for a sound remake of *The Unholy Three* in 1930, are less remarkable; Chaney died of throat cancer just after this last film was completed. Browning went on to make his most successful film, Universal's *Dracula* (1931) with Bela Lugosi, but not before he had presented yet another tribute to carnival life in *The Show* (1927). Centred around a Palace of Illusions sideshow, this film featured John Gilbert as a John the Baptist who is 'decapitated' nightly on stage after the dance of Salome (Renée Adorée). A jealous rival attempts to cut off Gilbert's head for real, while the entrance money of the Palace's patrons is seemingly collected by Cleopatra'a severed hand – another recurring and powerful 'horror' film icon. The potency of this disembodied appendage, its ability to breed anxiety, is as harbinger of an amputee zone, the negative space surrounding a bleeding stump. *"Dismembered limbs, a severed head, a hand cut off at the wrist... all of these have something particularly uncanny about them,"* says Freud in his essay *The 'Uncanny'*, going on to indeed specify that uncanniness is a feeling closely linked to fear of castration. It certainly appears to have been the driving force behind the pathological morbidity of Browning's cinematic visions. The presence of a legless 'half-girl' further underscores his obsession (fetish?) with amputation and loss (phallic or otherwise), while the film almost incidentally demonstrates the circular links between cinema, theatre and fairground.[1]

Browning's other films concerning the tricks and illusions of the sideshow included *The Mystic* (1925) and *The Thirteenth Chair* (1929), but it was not until the phenomenal success of *Dracula* that he found himself in a strong enough position to make the ultimate carnival/deformity film: *Freaks*, a true masterpiece of bizarre cinema.

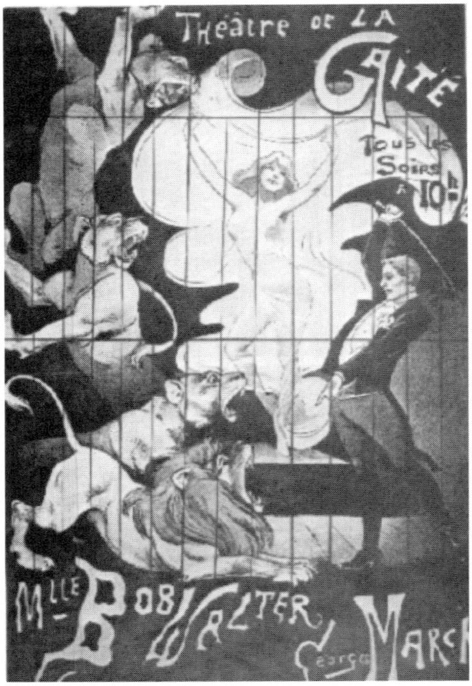

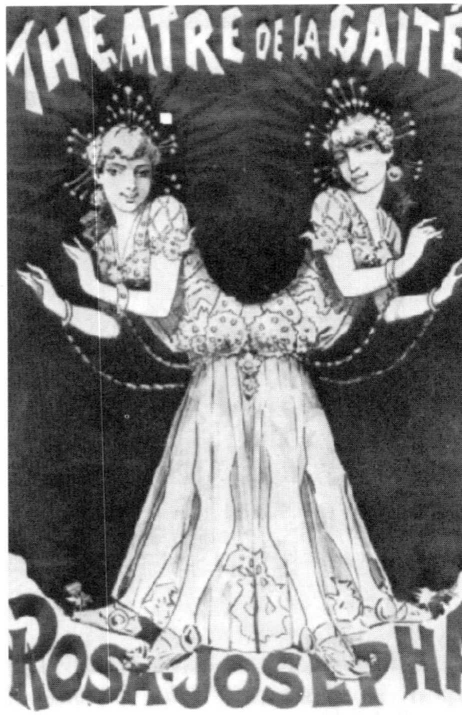

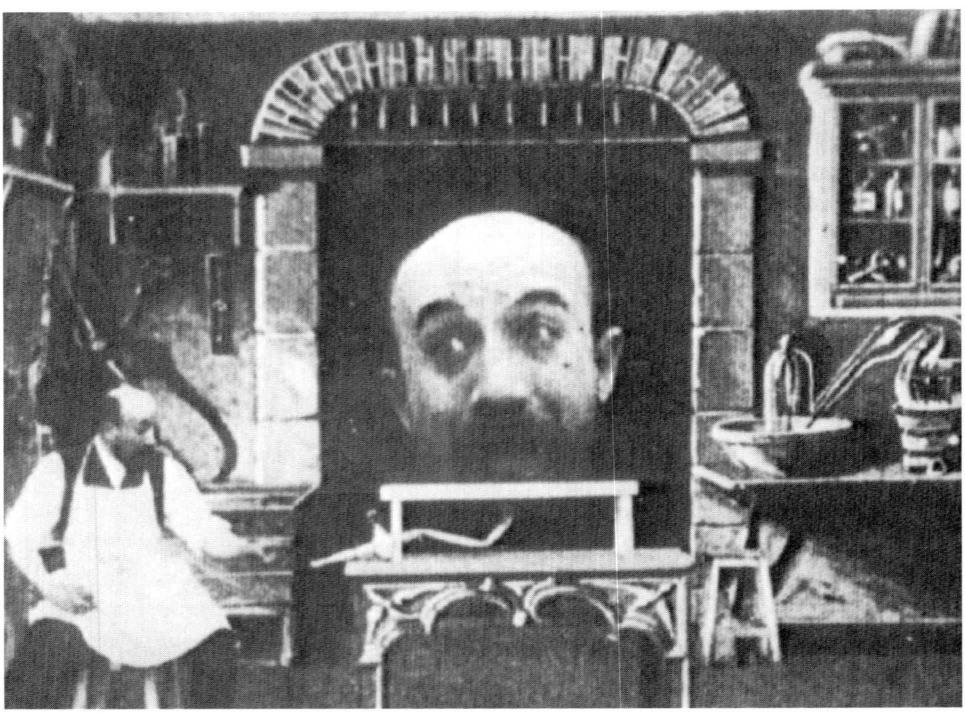

The India Rubber Head

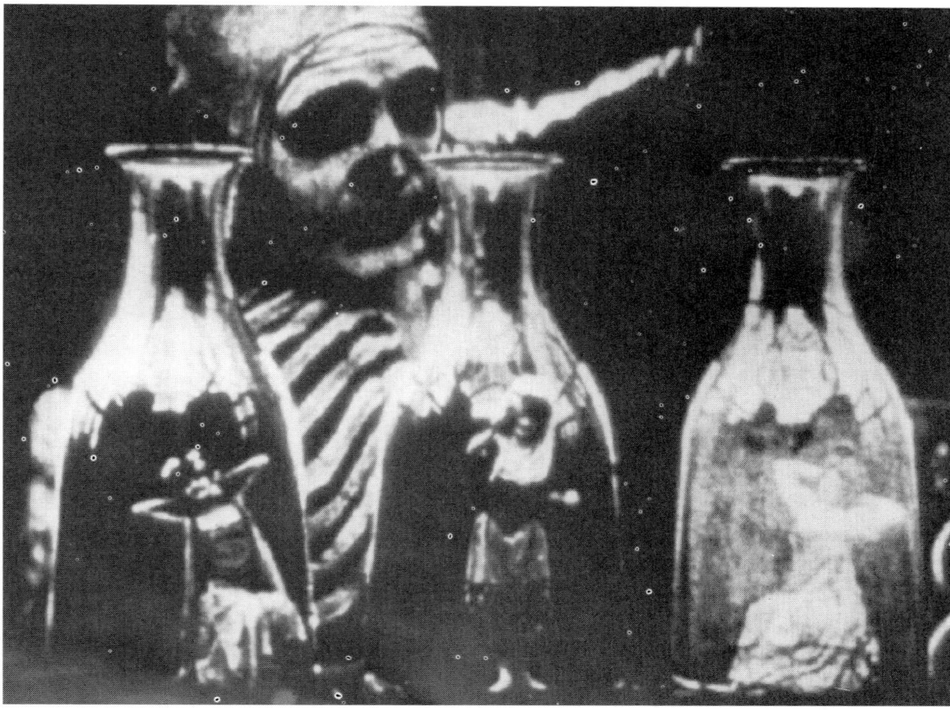

The Laboratory Of Mephistopheles

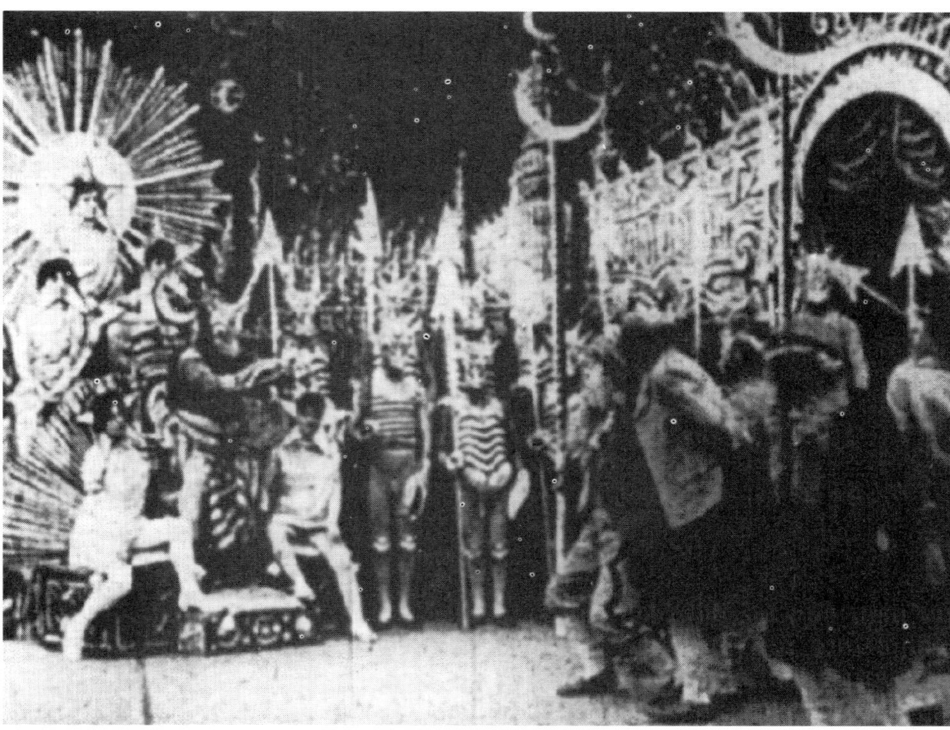

A Trip To The Moon

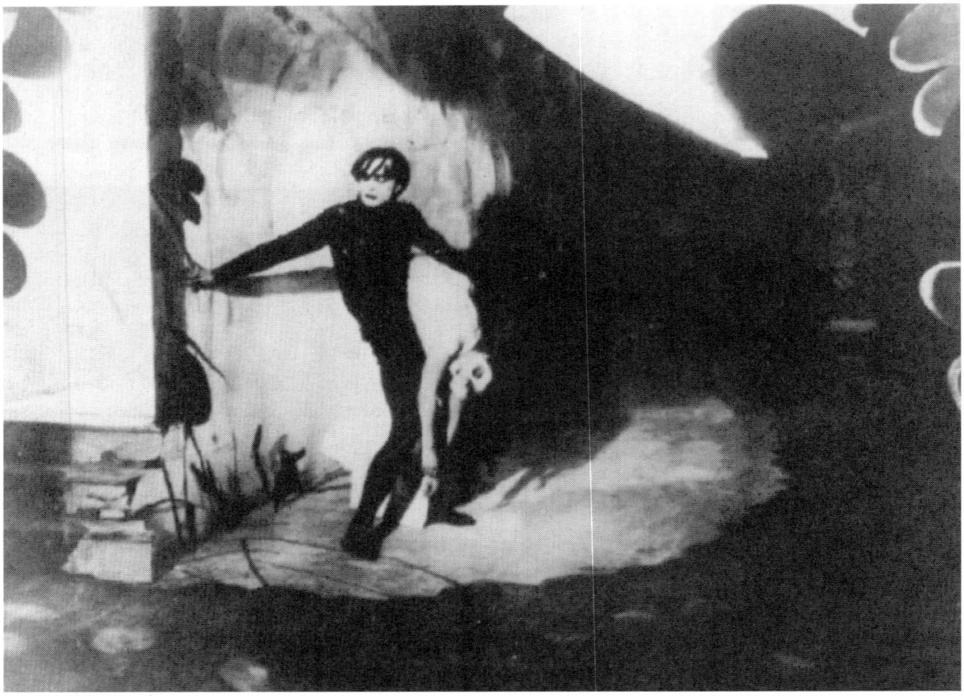

The Cabinet Of Dr Caligari

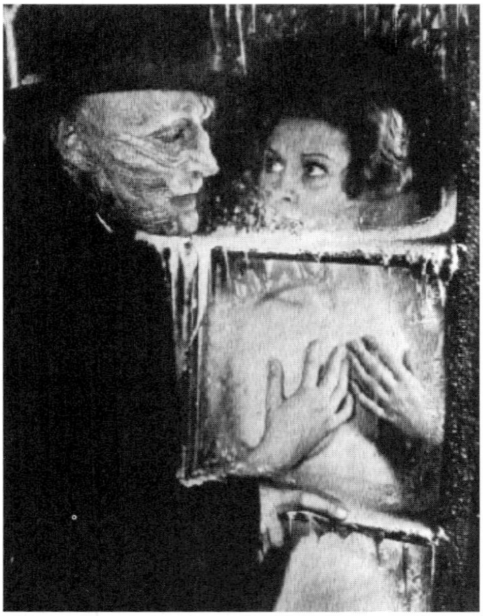

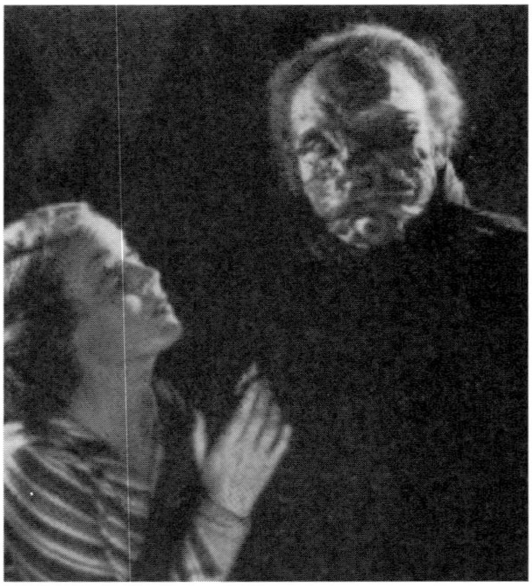

The Mystery Of The Wax Museum

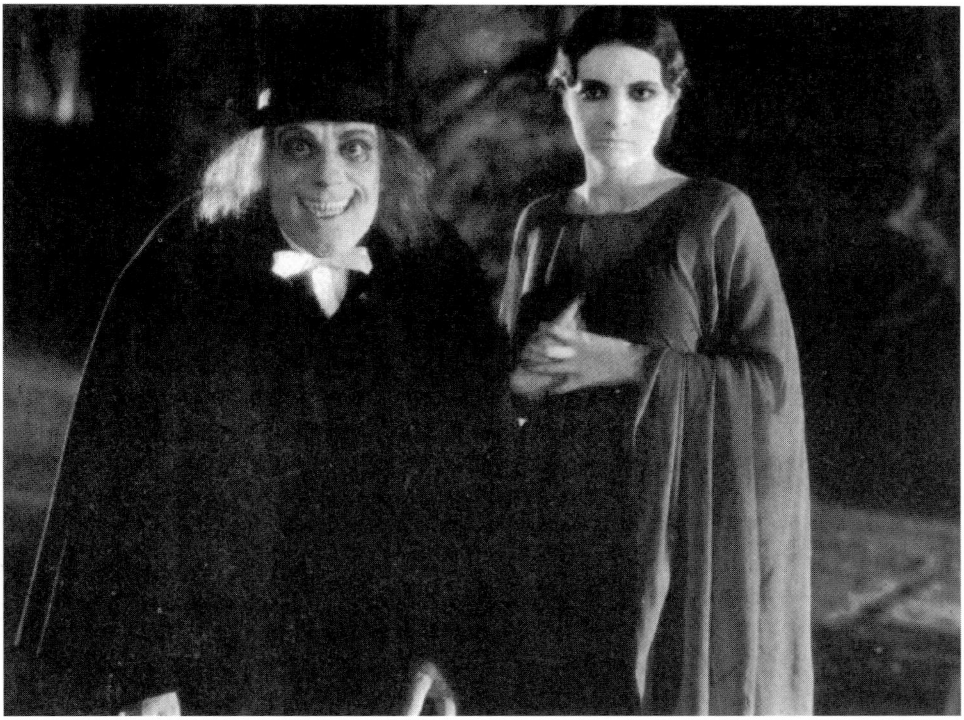

London After Midnight

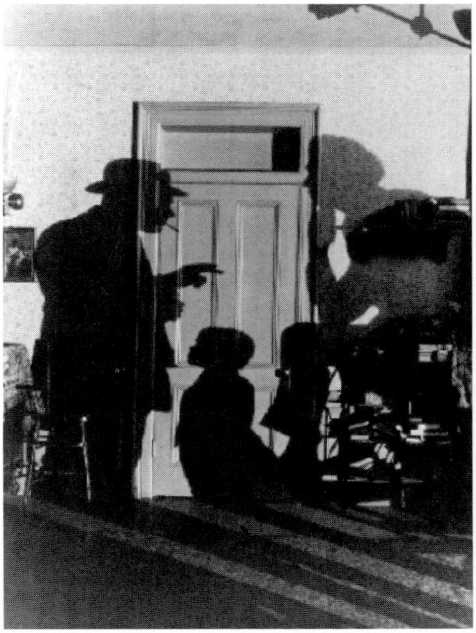

The Unholy Three

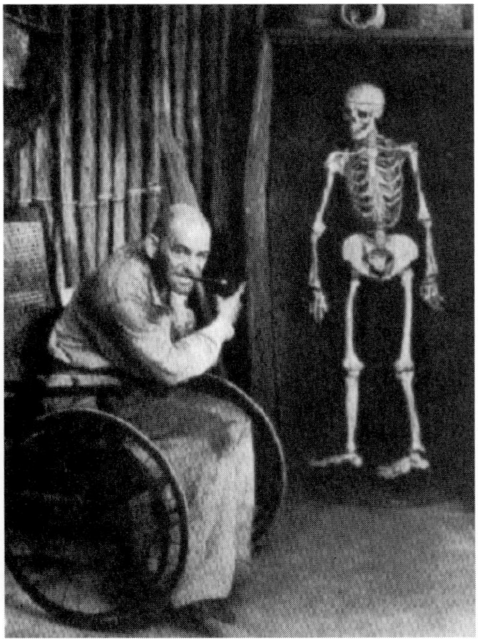

West Of Zanzibar

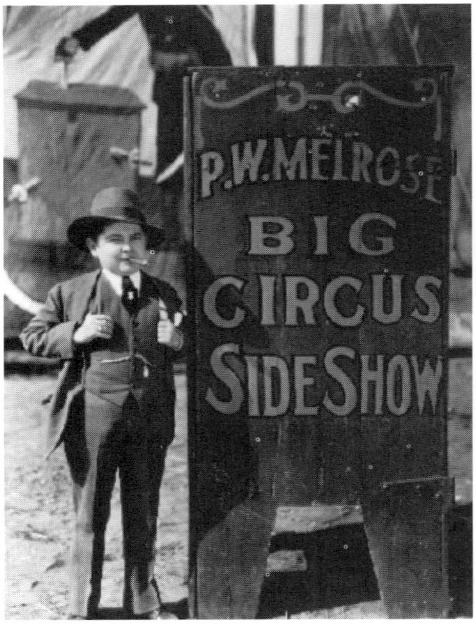

The Sideshow

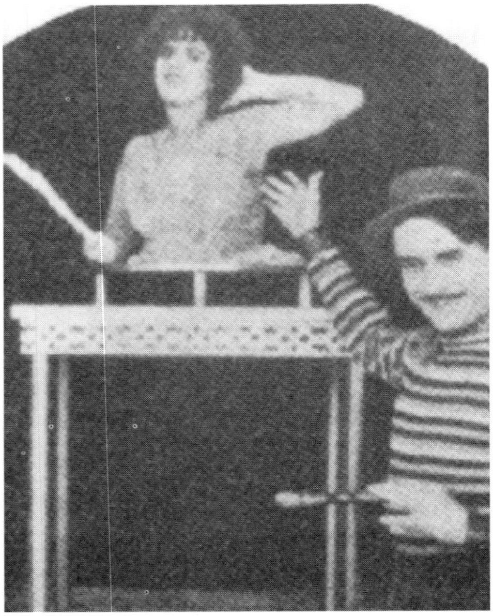

The Show

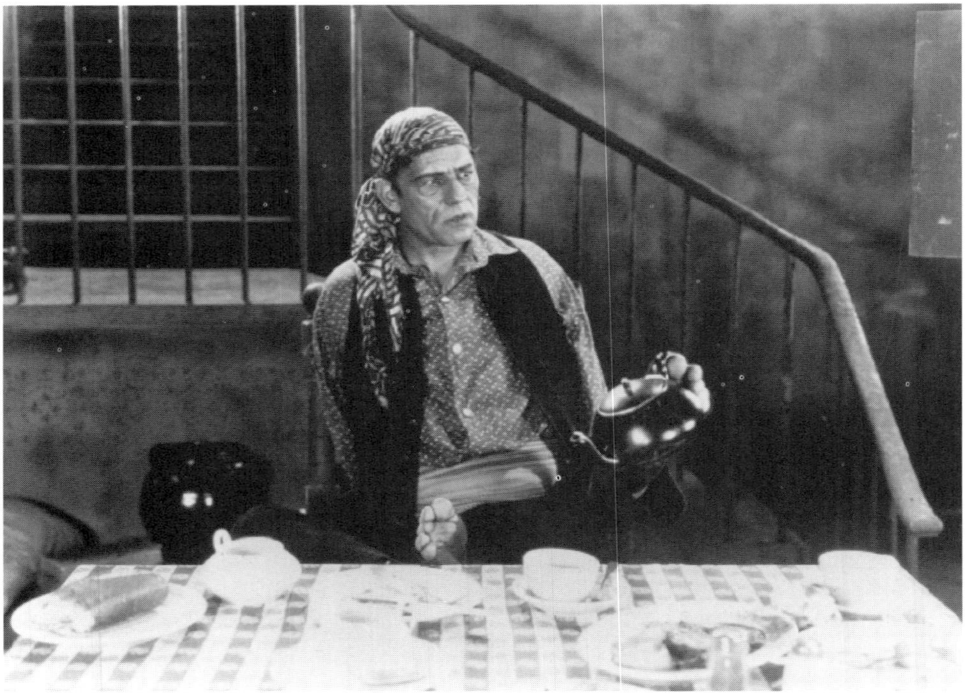

The Unknown

LOVE AMONG THE LIMBLESS

After Tod Browning's vast directorial success with Universal's *Dracula* (1931), MGM were desperate to capitalize on the moment and rushed through production on a film project of his which had been in development since 1929: *Freaks*.

The film was based on *Spurs*, a short story by Clarence A. "Tod" Robbins, whose story *Three Freaks* had earlier provided the inspiration for Browning's *The Unholy Three*. *Spurs* was an absurd, somewhat sadistic vignette concerning a circus midget who inherits great wealth and is accepted in marriage by the Junoesque bareback rider he is obsessed with. (The midget also rides in his act, but his mount is a wolfhound.) At their wedding feast she humiliates him in front of his peers, boasting she can carry him like a child from one end of France to the other. A year later she reappears, broken and aged. It seems that the midget has kept her to her word, renouncing his former steed in her favour and driving her with his spurs along country roads until she has indeed carried him the exact distance she boasted of.

Browning, in collaboration with main screenwriters Willis Goldbeck and Leon Gordon, kept the bones of this tale but went on to flesh them with an even more extreme tale of sexual humiliation and revenge, set in a harrowing milieu of circus freaks and their secret codes of honour. Once the script was completed, Browning set about holding auditions for 'actors' to populate this sideshow world. He ended up with the very cream of top-line show-freaks from carnivals around America; most 'self-mades' were rejected, and only the most outlandish of genuine human anomalies made the final cast.

From the outset it was clear that Browning's vision for *Freaks* was extreme; it seems that many exceptionally nasty or grotesque scenes and dialogue had to be excised during shooting. Even the finished version apparently included much more 'hardcore' footage of the freaks themselves, footage included for road show audiences but deemed too much to stomach for regular cinema viewers. Shooting took around 9 weeks, from October to December 1931, and was often fraught; regular film people objected to the presence of the freaks in the studio canteen, and there was also some hierarchical friction within the sideshow performers themselves. At one point, MGM executives even tried to shut the film down, while Browning kept the publicity machine rolling regardless, flooding an eager press with tales of hermetic freak colonies and bizarre rituals.

When the film was finally completed, early censor-board and press reactions were decidedly mixed. After various required cuts had been made (the New York State censor demanding some thirty minutes be removed), the film eventually opened across America from the early to middle part of 1932. A reviewer for one leading trade journal swiftly declared the film as *"so loathsome that I am nauseated thinking about it. The producers give an excuse that these creatures are all in the circus, implying that the characterizations are not that out of keeping with the conditions that may be imagined as existing in a circus. But this does not give them the right to do with them what the picture does. It is not fit to be shown anywhere"*. The *Herald Tribune* remarked that *"Mr Browning has always been an expert in pathological morbidity, but after seeing Freaks, his other films seem like whimsical fairytales"*, while the *New York Times* added: *"The difficulty is in telling whether the film should be shown at the Rialto Theater – where it opened yesterday – or in, say, the Medical Center."*

The *New Yorker* was kinder, calling the film *"a little gem"*, the *Motion Picture Herald* conceded *"...the production is bold and novel in conception and execution"*, and Louella Parsons was surprisingly supportive, saying *"For pure sensationalism, Freaks tops any picture yet produced... a weird nightmare... a picture so different the public will want to see it"*. For once, she was proved wrong. *Variety*, in its summary of the film's opening months, encapsulated the extremes of reaction it engendered: *"Planned by Metro to be one of the sensation pictures of the season, Freaks failed to qualify in the sure-fire category and has been shown in most parts of the country with astonishingly variable results. In spots it has been a clean-up. In others it was merely misery."*

"We didn't lie to you, folks," the fairground barker shouts inside the sideshow at the opening of *Freaks*. "We told you we had living, breathing monstrosities! But for an accident of birth, you might be as *they* are." The audience shifts uneasily. "They did not ask to be brought into the world." Now the hustler moves the people forward. "Their code is a law unto themselves. Offend one – and you offend them all." He takes the crowd to the edge of an open pit, where something squats at the bottom. There is a scream, but we cannot see what is at the bottom of the pit. "She was once a beautiful woman," proclaims the barker. "She was once known as the Peacock of the Air..."

With that, the film dissolves to a shot of an artist on the trapeze – the beautiful Cleopatra. She is played by Olga Baclanova with an air of studied sleaze, blonde and stealthy and predatory. Watching her from below is the midget Hans, played by Harry Earles (the thuggish 'baby' from Browning's earlier *The Unholy Three*). He is the epitome of the American hero, only he happens to be three feet tall. Yet his mannered playing and instinctive courtesy make him sure of winning the sympathy of the viewer during the events to come.

Cleopatra descends, and drops her cloak in front of him; he is too short to replace it on her shoulders. It is a moment of social embarrassment as great as the Stroheim sequence when the society lady drops her glove and a cloaked man fails to retrieve it, being later revealed as armless. Cleopatra laughs at Hans, then patronises him by kissing his cheek like a schoolboy, despite his assertion that "I'm a *man*." Having established the core of his drama, Hans' hopeless infatuation with an unfeeling 'big' woman, Browning then introduces us to his real world of freaks, when he shows us a flock of pinheads and midgets, some of the 'family' of sideshow artists, being taken for a walk along a sunny lakeside by their 'mother', Madame Tetrallini. This kind matriarch is touchingly played by Rose Dionne, an actress from the Sarah Bernhardt troupe. She soon has to defend her misshapen charges passionately against the verbal assaults of a passing game-keeper, who describes them as 'horrible, twisted things, crawling and gliding'. They are not monsters, but children, she counters, and they each have their place in God's world. After this speech, the viewer begins to feel more than mere pity for the freaks. They are so unselfconscious and innocent, that we begin to feel equally protective towards them.

Browning soon unveils the full repertoire of his sideshow cast, imported from all over the USA. Among those prodigies we meet are the Hilton sisters, the pretty Siamese twins Daisy and Violet, who bicker about the man one of them is to marry; five shy pinheads, the Snow Twins, Zip and Pip, and Schlitzie; a bearded lady (Olga Roderick), who is about to give birth to a (bearded?) baby; a skeleton man (Pete Robinson), who is the proud father; a merry, agile half-man called Johnny Eck, who moves about like a bird on his hands; a Living Torso, the 'Hindu' Prince Randian, who has only a trunk and head and wriggles along the ground like a caterpillar; a half-man half-woman named Josephine-Joseph, whose female side has fallen in love with the circus strongman, Hercules; two armless girls, Martha Morris and Frances O'Connor; Koo Koo, the bird-woman; the midget Frieda, played by Daisy Earles (Harry's sister); and several dwarfs, including Angelo Rossitto. We also meet Phroso the Clown (Wallace Ford), and his girl Venus (Leila Hyams), their only other 'normal' friends.

The freaks are worried by Hans becoming increasingly infatuated with Cleopatra. The midget is lending her money and even buying her expensive gifts. As one of the dwarfs remarks, "Cleopatra isn't one of us. We're just filthy things to her." Still, she continues to take presents from Hans, leading him on, whilst secretly carrying on with her regular lover, the strongman Hercules. Hercules is equally calculating, and shrewd enough to realise that Hans' gifts, a platinum necklace, is worth thousands of dollars. The midget must be rich; he is worth exploiting. A plan begins to hatch...

Frieda, the tiny bareback rider who is in love with Hans, tries to reason with Cleopatra, pleading with her to release the hapless midget from her web. Frieda is all too aware that Cleopatra is only after the fortune which Hans has inherited, and inadvertently reveals the extent of his wealth. Cleopatra is merciless; she mocks Frieda, and drives her away. Then she settles down with Hercules, and they begin to plot in earnest. The only way to get the midget's fortune is for Cleopatra to marry him, and then get rid of him so that she and Hercules can enjoy the spoils together. They decide that this is the best course; after all, midgets are not strong, and can easily grow sick.

And so the great wedding-day approaches, and the freaks, desperate for Hans to be happy, have planned a special wedding feast to welcome Cleopatra to their ranks. A table is prepared in the big top, and so the scene is staged for Browning to produce the first of two stunning set-pieces: one of the most potent, memorable and alarming sequences in cinema, a grotesque rivalled only by the beggars' orgy in Buñuel's *Viridiana*, or supper-time with Leatherface in Tobe Hooper's *Texas Chainsaw Massacre*. The festivities begin with sword-swallowers and fire-eaters, who perform as the freaks applaud. Cleopatra is seated at the head of the table, flanked by Hans and Hercules, quaffing liberal glasses of champagne. Soon she, and the freaks, are intoxicated. She grows more and more uninhibited, laughing at Hans' declarations of love and openly kissing her strongman lover, threatening to reveal her true colours; the freaks meanwhile work themselves into a tribalistic frenzy, beginning to thump on the table in accompaniment to the weird, strangulated wedding song they have devised for Cleopatra: "Gooba gabba, gooba gabba, gooba gabba, one of us; gooba gabba, gooba gabba, gooba gabba, one of us; gooba gabba, we accept her, we accept her, one of us; gooba gabba, gooba gabba, we accept her, *one of us!*" The limbless, the crawling, the crazed, all join in the refrain (sung in what director Browning would describe to the press as the "secret gibberish of the show-freaks") and sip in turn from the huge goblet of champagne carried by a dwarf who shuffles across the table (initial shots had him drooling into the cup). Finally, it is Cleopatra's turn to drink from the chalice, her time to be initiated into the ranks of the deformed. In a moment of drunken revelation she sees the full horror of her situation and, wracked with sudden revulsion, draws back and hurls the tainted champagne over her guests with a shriek of disgust: "Freaks! Freaks! Dirty, filthy, stinking *freaks!*" The assembly falls into stunned silence, then begins to scatter; Cleopatra picks up the comatose Hans, drapes him about her shoulders like a little boy, and exits followed by Hercules who blows a mocking farewell on his trumpet.

Weeks pass. Hans is growing inexplicably weaker and weaker, the doctor cannot find remedy; only Cleopatra can help him, nursing him and giving him his daily 'medicine'. But all the time, she is being watched. Dark shapes stir in caravan shadow as she visits Hercules, perch on steps and sills overhearing plot, peer from wagon windows as she administers the deadly medication. Hans, at first unbelieving, is finally alerted to the truth by his friends. Now it is their turn to conspire, to wreak revenge on the murderous lovers.

Hans surreptitiously stops taking the poison, while the others arm themselves with guns, knives and razors. Finally, the time for retribution is at hand. The carnival ups and moves on in the teeth of a midnight thunderstorm; we glimpse Johnny, running on his hands beneath Cleopatra's caravan. Just as she goes to give Hans more poison, his loyal friends appear from concealment. Just then the caravan hits a tree, splinters. Hercules comes to his shrieking lover's aid, freaks spilling out into the churning mud. As Cleopatra runs for safety, Hercules slips. He is surrounded by slithering, crawling, hopping shapes, their jagged weapons glinting in the lightning. Even Randian is there, a cut-throat razor clenched between his teeth. Darkness descends upon the strongman's final scream... Next, Cleopatra is shown stumbling through a nearby wood. Like night-demons, the freaks are on her trail; then she too topples, pinned by a falling branch; the blades begin to flash once more. Blackout.

The film resumes where Browning first left off to tell his tale, with the barker at the geek-pit. His pitch continues:

"...how she got that way will never be known. Some say a jealous lover. Others... *the code of the freaks!*"

At last, the freaks' handiwork is revealed. Cleopatra (barely recognizable) has been butchered and mutilated, truncated and disfigured; she is now nothing more than a squawking human chicken, shuffling and pecking at worms in the bone-pit. Not only has she become "one of us" to the freaks, she has become even less than they are, a true sub-human, the geek to end all geeks. The film fades on this startling image.

So ends *Freaks*, where Tod Browning's amputation/castration fixation had finally achieved delirium pitch. With Johnny Eck and Randian as his very own personal "evil mirror" eidolons, the director was able to give full rein to this bizarre fetish. Not content with the presence of these limbless protagonists, Browning makes it as implicit as possible that Hercules is ultimately emasculated in the mud; even the 'normal' Phroso implies his own impotence, quipping: "You should have caught me before my operation" to a female admirer. Sexual inadequacy and frustration (even perversion) drive the entire story. The Siamese twins gasp at the penetration of each other's lover; the hermaphrodite dreams of auto-copulation; Hans, with his infantile genitalia, can never consummate his Oedipal love for Cleopatra; jealousy and loss haunt the midway.

A creeping duality is omnipresent in *Freaks*. Although Browning wins our sympathy towards his twisted protagonists early on in the film, both the wedding-feast and the lightning-illuminated shots of them at the climax, slithering through the mud with vengeful intent, are truly shocking and re-establish an ambiguity toward their role; are they heroes or, ultimately, monsters? Is their dismemberment of Hercules and Cleopatra an act of righteous retribution, or in fact a resentful savagery perpetrated to bring these normal people down to their own level, to 'cut them down to size'? Audiences seemed to think the latter, and many left the cinema screaming. This, coupled with poor reviews, proved disastrous. MGM panicked and withdrew the film, reputedly cutting a great deal of the more explicit footage before re-releasing it variously (and under the aegis of exploitation mogul Dwain Esper) as *Nature's Mistakes*, *Forbidden Love*, and *The Monster Show*. Lurid posters begged such dilemmas as: "Do Siamese Twins Make Love?", "Can A Full Grown Woman Truly Love A Midget?", "Do The Pin-Heads Think?", and "What Sex Is The Half Man Half Woman?", while an apology was tacked on at the start of the film, assuring the viewer that *"...the majority of freaks are endowed with normal thoughts and emotions... never again will such a story be filmed, as modern science and teratology is rapidly eliminating such blunders of nature from the world."* [They spoke too soon.] But even cuts, re-titling, *and* the addition of a moralistic prologue could not salvage Browning's maligned masterpiece. Seldom shown again in America and completely banned in England, *Freaks* was to prove the undoing of its maker. The outrage surrounding the film effectively finished Tod Browning's career; he made a few more films, including *Mark Of The Vampire*, *The Devil Doll* (1936), and a last foray into the world of performers, *Miracles For Sale* (1932), but then faded into obscurity.

Freaks finally enjoyed a retrospective success, and new cult status, when fresh prints were circulated in the early '60s, the film being 're-discovered' by a successful showing at the Venice Film Festival of 1962 and gaining an eager new audience. It found instant acceptance amongst the New York underground film set, and played the midnight movie circuit there for years to come. *Freaks* was even allowed to be shown in England, after 30 years, where – thanks to the efforts of young film-maker Antony Balch – it ran at the Paris-Pullman in London, duly receiving such compliments as *"Touching, funny and delicate"* from the *Evening Standard*, and *"Extraordinary! A plea for understanding"* from the *Times*. Mindful perhaps of the thalidomide scandal, Nina Hibbin countered in the *Daily Worker*: *"To release Freaks in the '60s, when misuse of science has produced its own appalling tragedies of deformation, I find hard to take"*; but the film's new credibility was finally summed up by Penelope Gilliat in the *Observer*: *"The film is moving, harsh, poetic, and genuinely tender. It triumphs at once over your nausea... What Browning has made is really a fable, concerned like most fables with pure ideas of trust and betrayal and revenge."*

There is a final bitter irony to the story: Tod Browning, long-believed dead after his Hollywood career was cut short, was eventually found to be still living in 1962; yet he died from throat cancer, aged 80, on the 6th October that year, just months too soon to appreciate the rehabilitation of the film which had caused his earlier decline.

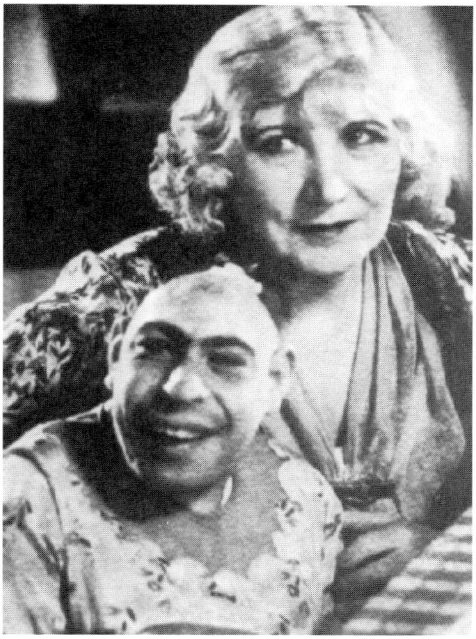

Rose Dionne with Schlitzie

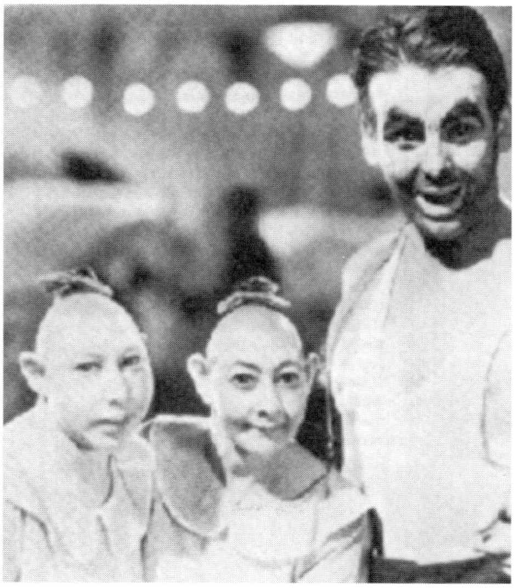

The Snow Twins and Phroso

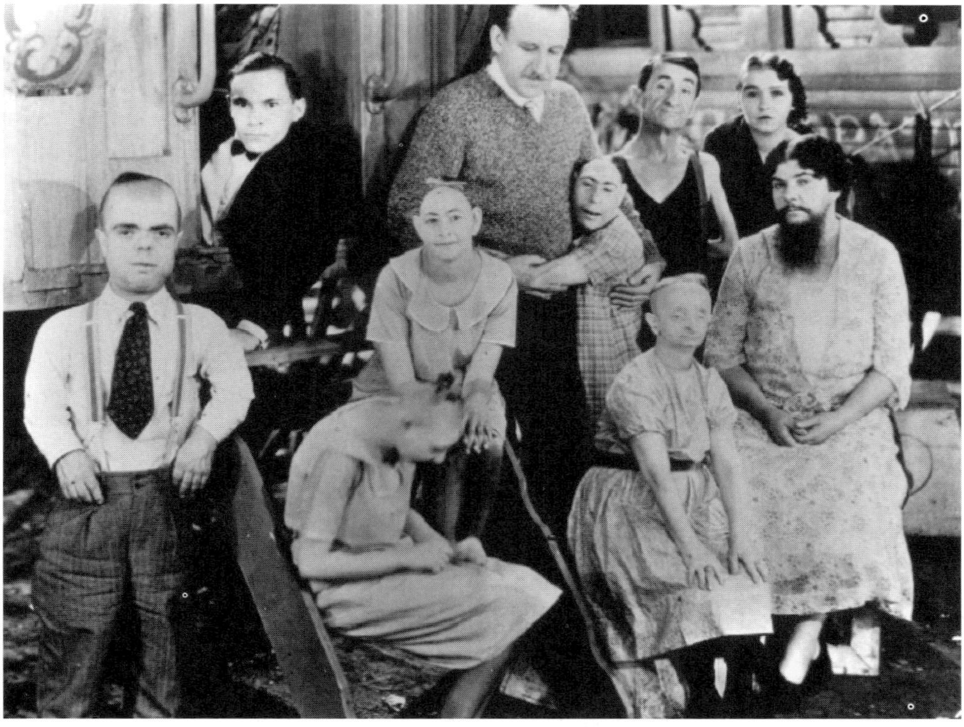

Tod Browning with the cast of *Freaks*

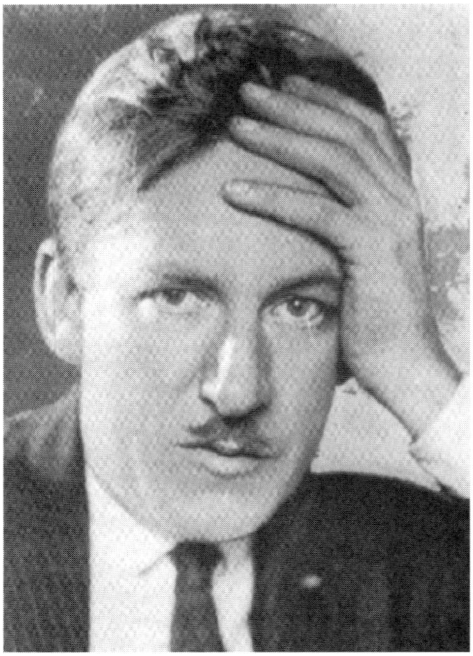

Tod Browning

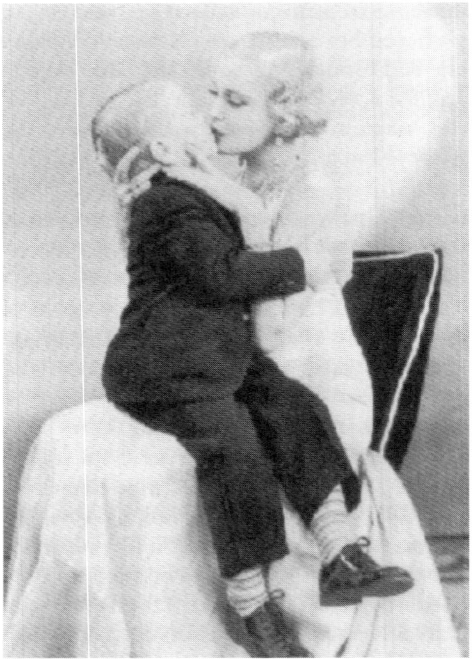

Harry Earles, Olga Baclanova

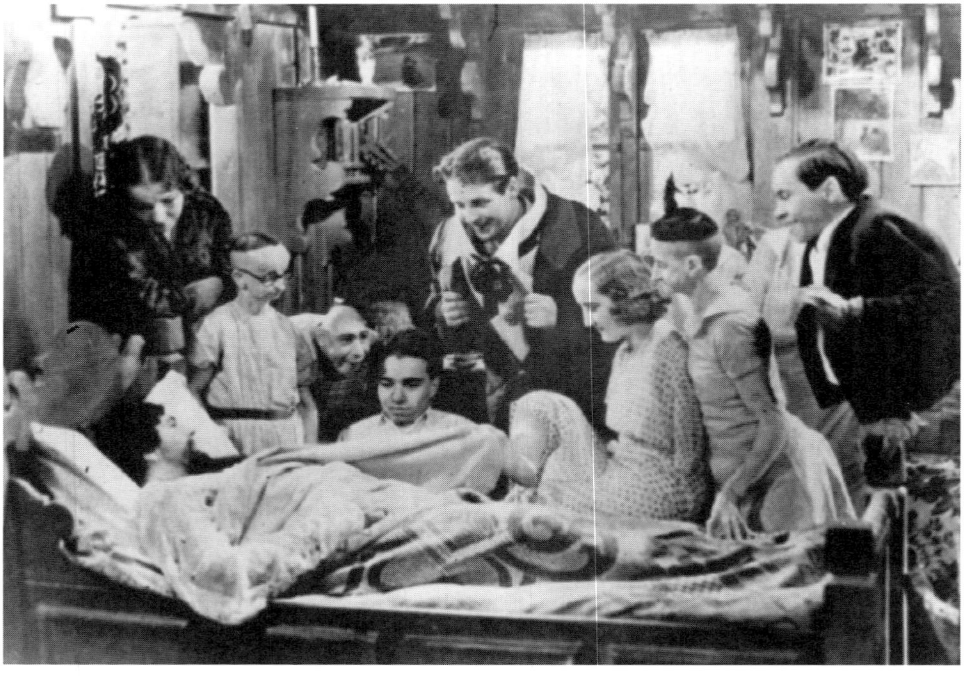

The Bearded Lady gives birth

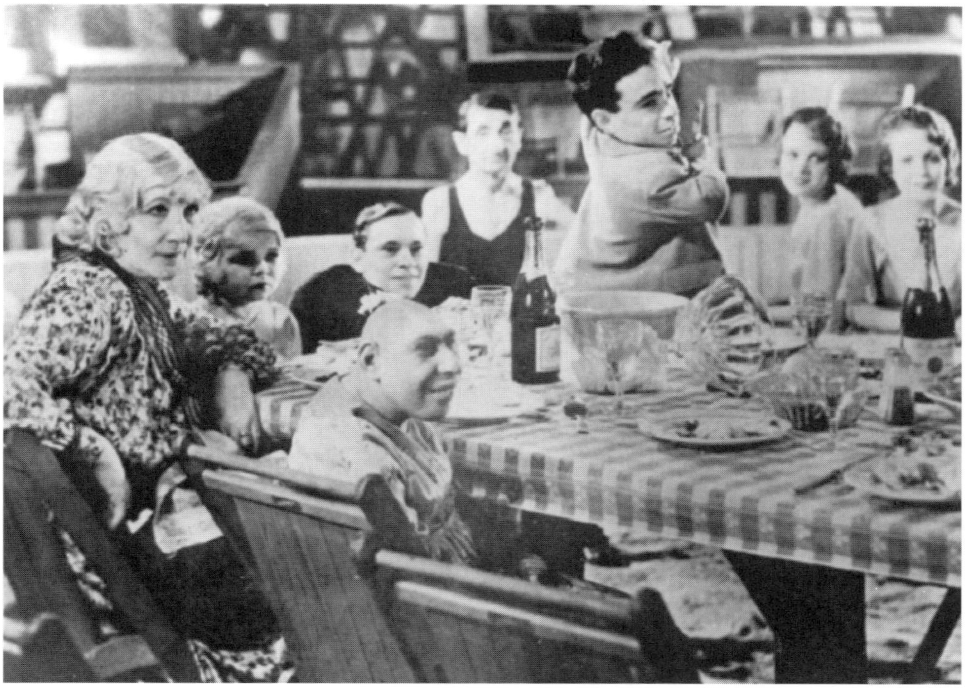

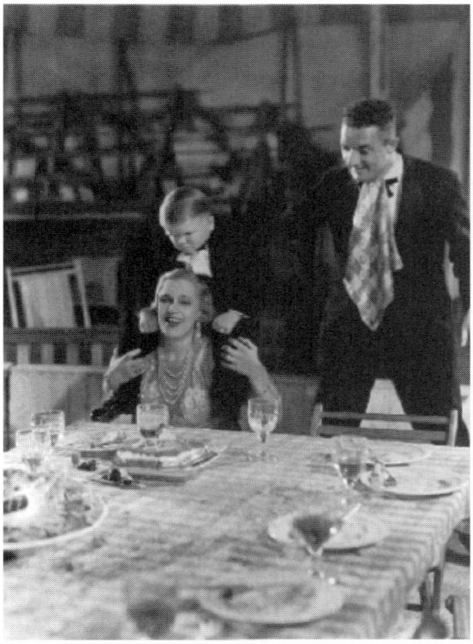

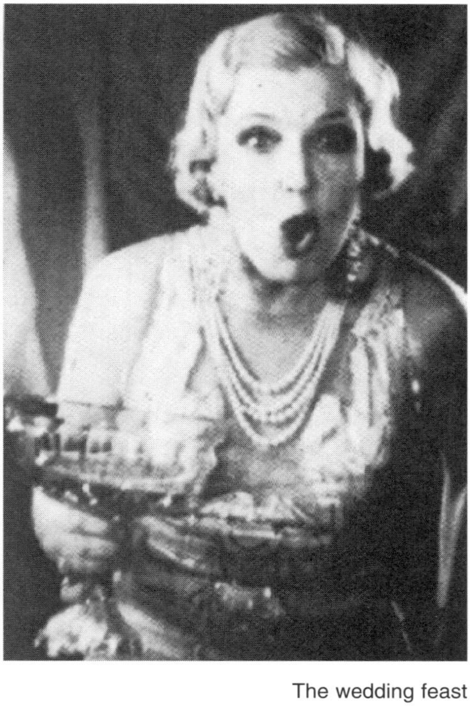

The wedding feast

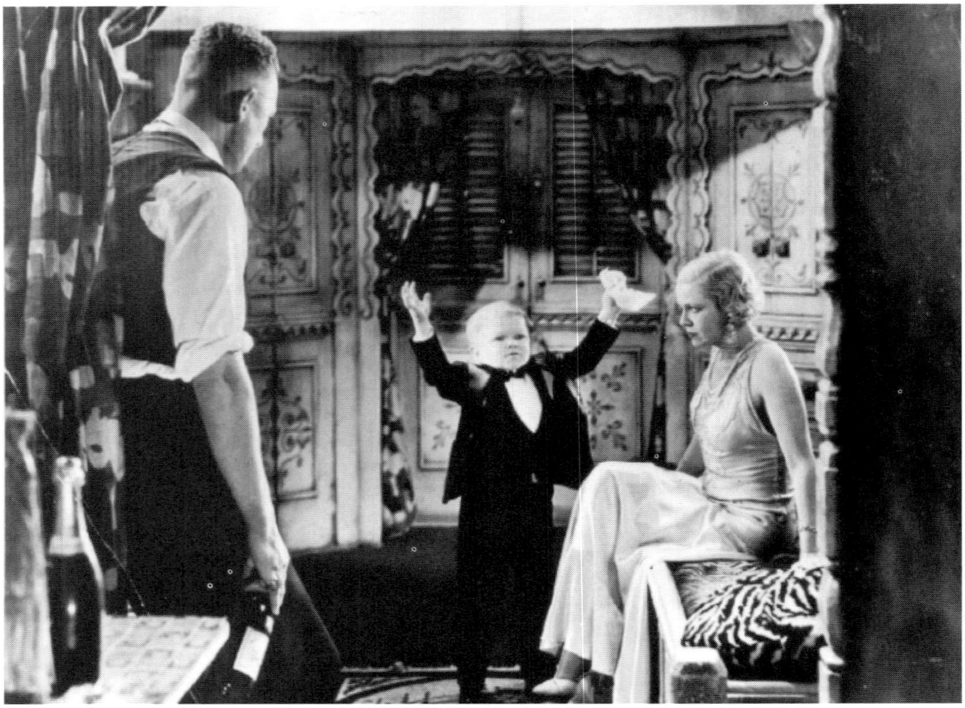

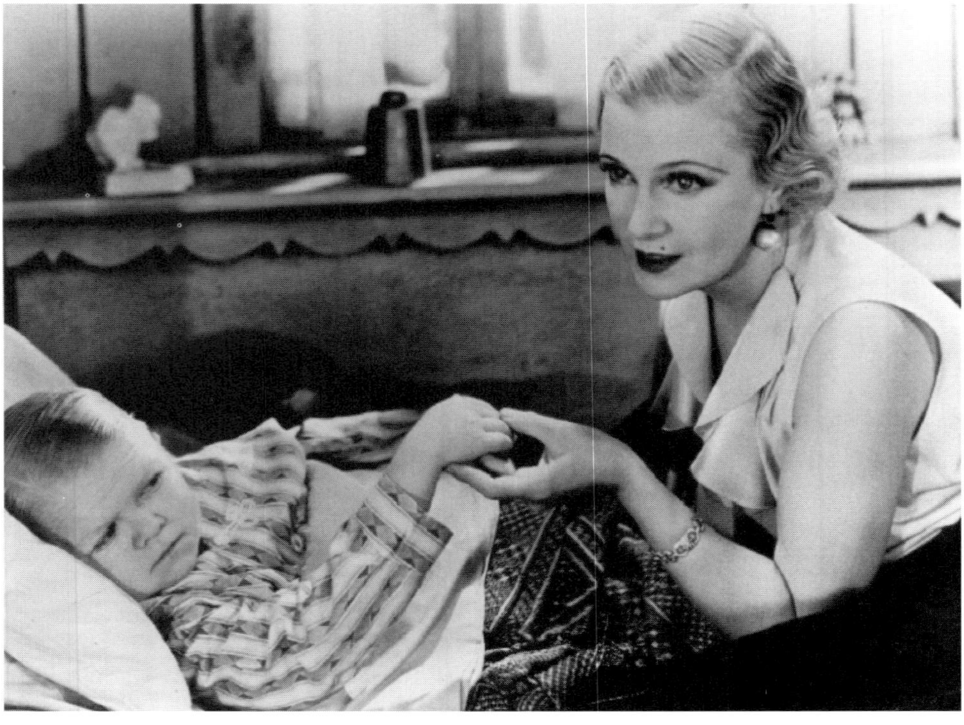

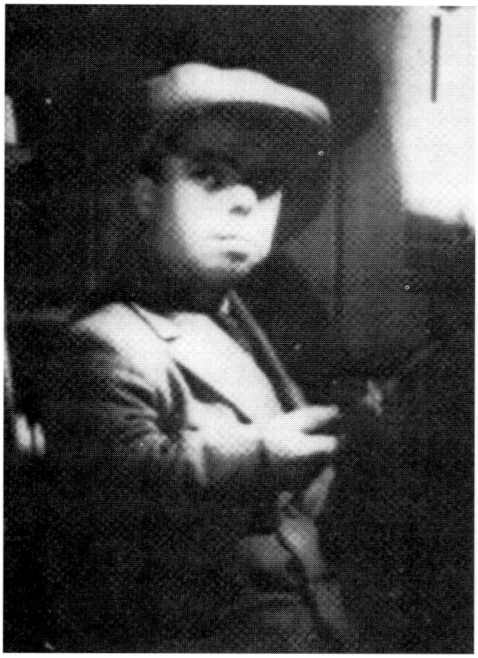

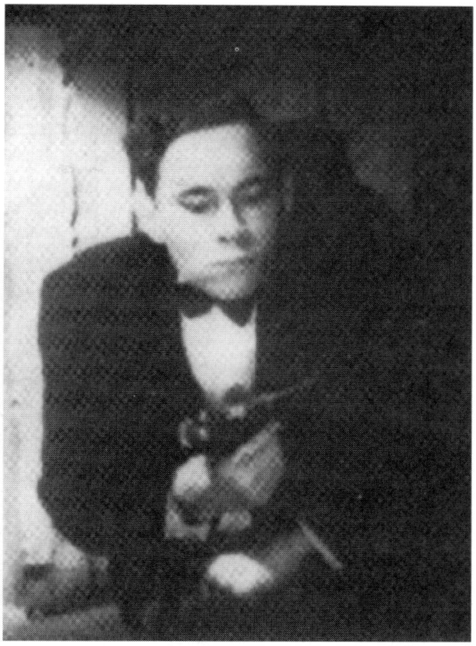

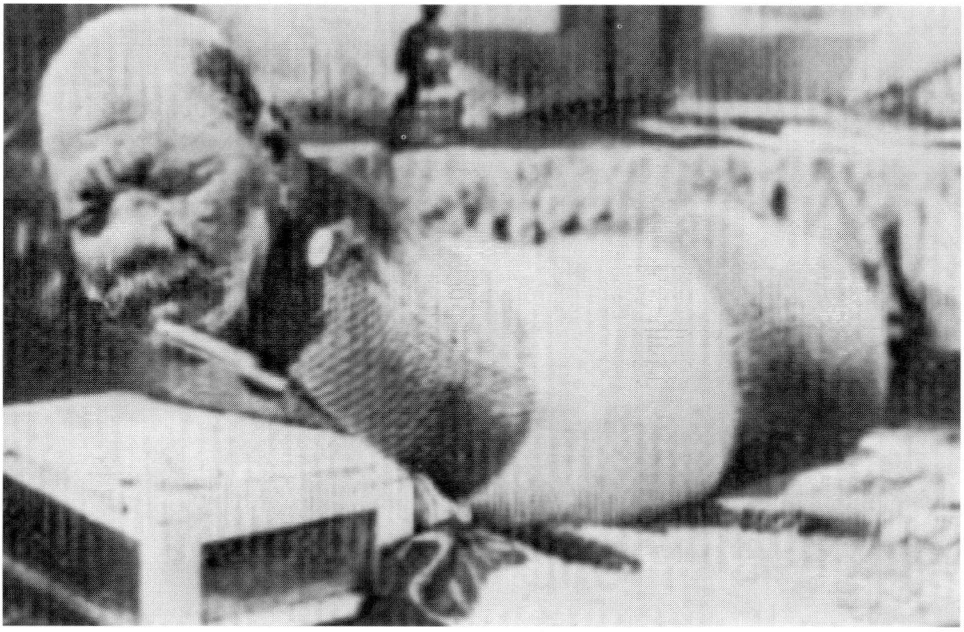

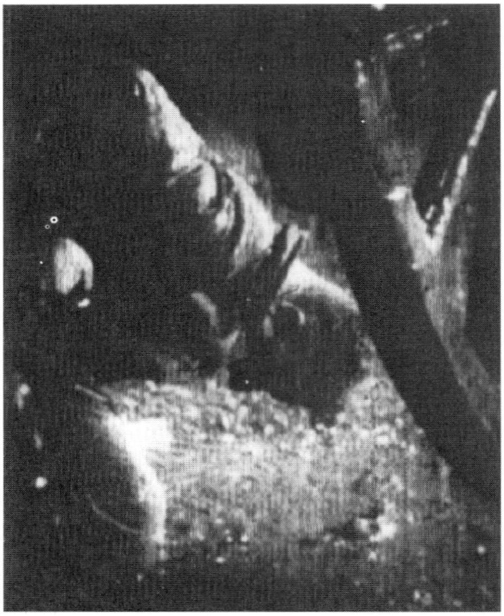

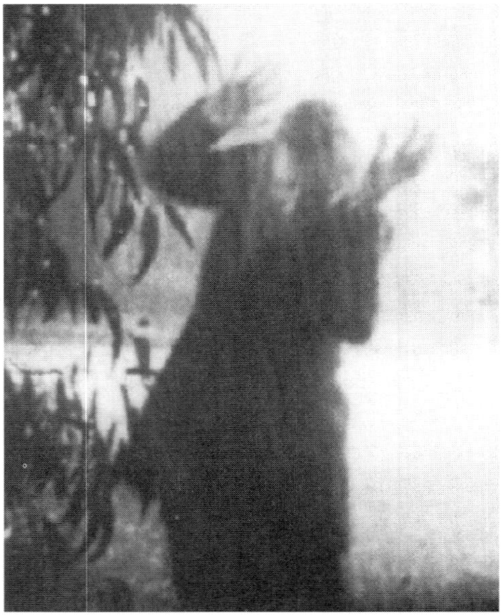

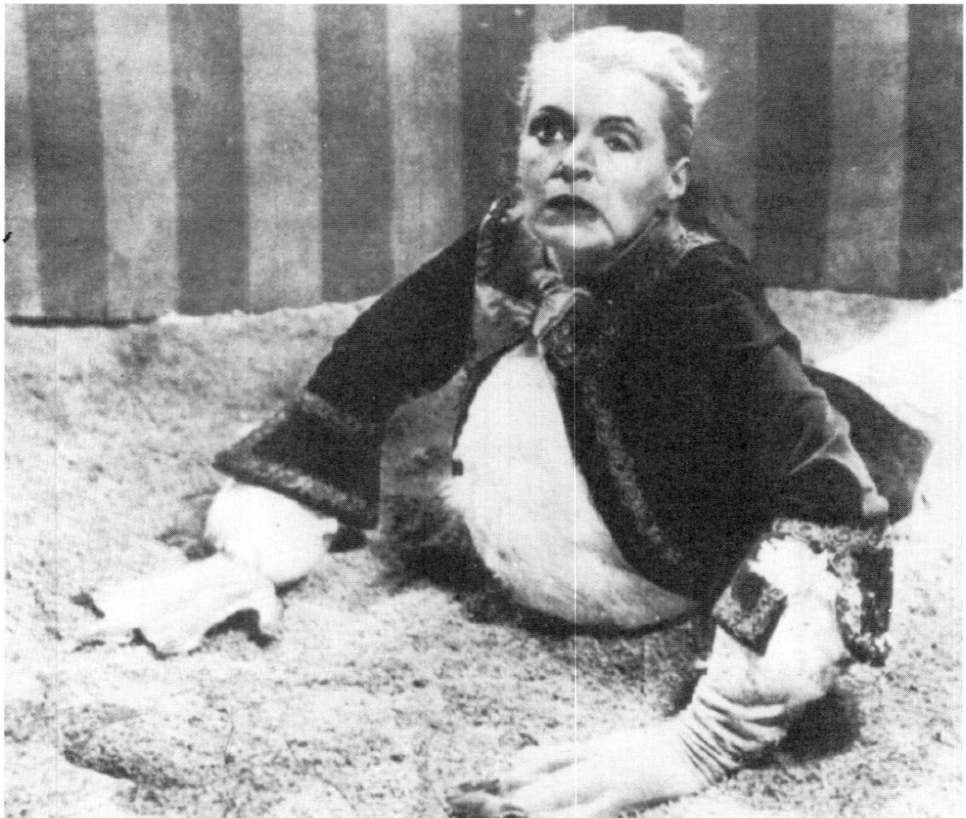

The revenge of the Freaks

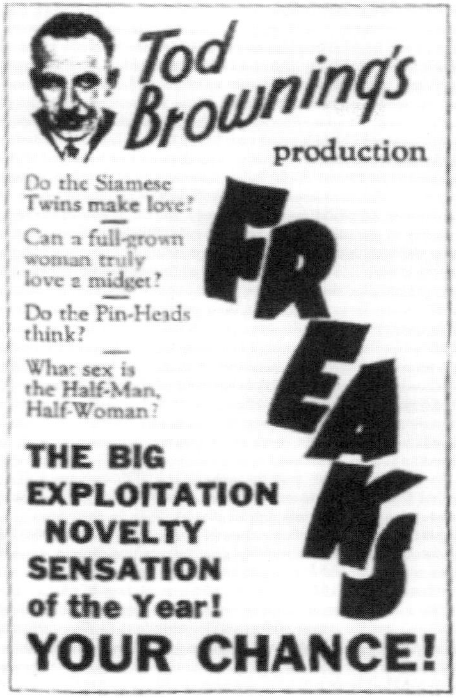
Tod Browning's
production
Do the Siamese Twins make love?
Can a full-grown woman truly love a midget?
Do the Pin-Heads think?
What sex is the Half-Man, Half-Woman?
FREAKS
THE BIG EXPLOITATION NOVELTY SENSATION of the Year!
YOUR CHANCE!

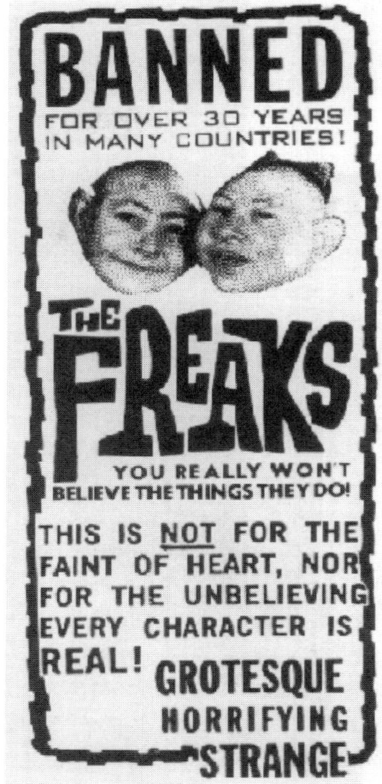
BANNED
FOR OVER 30 YEARS IN MANY COUNTRIES!
THE FREAKS
YOU REALLY WON'T BELIEVE THE THINGS THEY DO!
THIS IS NOT FOR THE FAINT OF HEART, NOR FOR THE UNBELIEVING EVERY CHARACTER IS REAL!
GROTESQUE
HORRIFYING
STRANGE

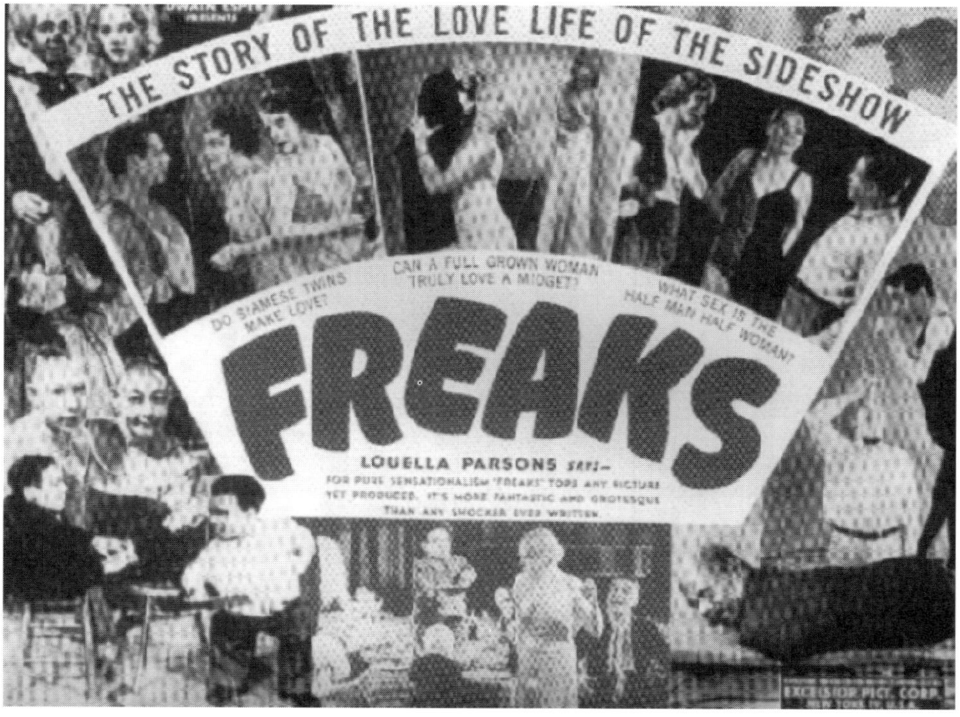
THE STORY OF THE LOVE LIFE OF THE SIDESHOW
DO SIAMESE TWINS MAKE LOVE?
CAN A FULL GROWN WOMAN TRULY LOVE A MIDGET?
WHAT SEX IS THE HALF MAN HALF WOMAN?
FREAKS
LOUELLA PARSONS SAYS—
FOR PURE SENSATIONALISM "FREAKS" TOPS ANY PICTURE YET PRODUCED. IT'S MORE FANTASTIC AND GROTESQUE THAN ANY SHOCKER EVER WRITTEN.

HELTER SKELTER

The sinister aspect of the fairground, travelling carnival, circus and *théâtre macabre* has remained a perennial theme in bizarre cinema. Evil doings under the Big Top have featured in such films as *Circus Of Horrors* (1960), with Anton Diffring as a circus owner/plastic surgeon who arranges fatal accidents for his reconstructed patients, *Circus Of Fear* (aka *Psycho Circus*, 1967) with Christopher Lee and dwarf Skip Martin as 'Mr Big', *Beserk* (also 1967), with Joan Crawford, and even Hammer's *Vampire Circus* (1972), in which a travelling show is the cover for a coven of shape-shifting sex-vampires. The nadir of this particular sub-genre would appear to be *Terror Circus* (aka *Barn Of The Naked Dead*) (1973), a Z-movie concerning a madman in the US desert who captures women for his own private circus; some are devoured by animals, while the man's father, a homicidal monster deformed by radiation, is kept locked in a shed between slaughter sprees.

Shady showmen have featured in the likes of Robert Florey's *Murders In The Rue Morgue* (1932), with Bela Lugosi as Dr. Mirakle, whose prize exhibit is a freak, homicidal ape; *House Of Frankenstein* (1945), with 'Professor Lampini's Chamber Of Horrors'; *Torture Garden* (1967), an Amicus anthology linked by one Dr. Diablo (Burgess Meredith); and, more benevolently, *The Seven Faces Of Dr. Lao* (1964), in which Tony Randall appears as a snake-haired Medea, the Great God Pan, the Abominable Snowman and other man-beasts.

Grand Guignol, the theatre of violent illusion, features in Karl Freund's classic *Mad Love* (1935), and in such intriguing later films as *The Hypnotic Eye* (1959), *Theatre Of Death* (1966), with Christopher Lee, and Gordon Hessler's *Murders In The Rue Morgue* (1971); but it has perhaps most noticeably formed the backbone of two very bizarre and extreme 'Z-movies': Herschell Gordon Lewis' *The Wizard Of Gore* (1970) and Joel M. Reed's *Blood-Sucking Freaks* (1978). It might be said that all Lewis' films are an attempt to translate the effects of Grand Guignol (in particular bloody dismemberment, as in *Blood Feast* [1963]) to the screen. *Wizard Of Gore*, which recalls the premise of *The Hypnotic Eye*, is especially pertinent. The story concerns Montag the Magician (played by Ray Sager), whose violent show includes the vicious murder of women by cutting in half with a chainsaw, staking through the head with a steel spike, eviscerating with a punch-press, and impaling with swords down the throat. Although the women leave the stage intact, they later succumb to the injuries inflicted on them – presumably when the hypnosis wears off. Lewis illustrates this with typically vile gore effects, such as the chainsawed victim collapsing in a restaurant in a pile of her own entrails.

TV hostess Sherry Carson, impressed by Montag's illusions, invites him onto her show. He proceeds to hypnotise not only the studio audience, but all the home viewers (with the exception of Sherry's boyfriend Jack, who has recognized the corpse in the restaurant). Montag's next 'trick' is to lead the occupants of the TV studio towards certain death in a flaming inferno. Jack arrives just in time, and pushes the magician into the flames. This appears to be the end of the story, but then Lewis and his scriptwriter Alison Louise Downe pull off their surprise punch: as Jack and Sherry later ponder events, Jack peels off his face to reveal that he is, apparently, in fact Montag, and then rips out Sherry's guts with his bare hands; Sherry however does not die, she merely laughs, brushes her intestines aside and informs Montag that *he* has been *her* illusion all along. They are then transported back to the start of the film for the cycle to begin again.

Wizard Of Gore is remarkable for its wantonly unexplained symbols and events (such as bloody stigmata which appear spontaneously on hands), its extreme violence and sadism and, above all, its blatant flaunting of notions of 'illusion' and 'reality', all presented with Lewis' customary disregard for cinematic niceties. Yet somehow it works, sucking the viewer into its madness, and asserting itself on its own claustrophobic, nightmare level.

Blood-Sucking Freaks (aka *The Incredible Torture Show*), remains one of the sickest, most absurd sex and gore films ever made. The mad magician here is the Great Sardu (convincingly played by Seamus O'Brien), who swears revenge on the critic who condemns his hideously gruesome torture show as fake (it isn't); abetted by Ralphus, his sadistic dwarf assistant, he proceeds to kidnap a famous ballerina and keep her locked up to be brainwashed in his den of vice. This establishment is the setting for some outrageously unnerving scenes; Ralphus, who keeps a harem of cannibal girls in cages, indulges in practices which seem to have come straight from the pages of de Sade's *120 Days Of Sodom*. People are violently tortured and decapitated (enabling the dwarf, at one point, to fuck a severed head), brains are sucked out through drinking straws, limbs amputated, eyes gouged out, women used as human dart-boards or ashtrays, *ad infinitum*. In the grand finale, the caged women are released and fall upon their captors in a feeding frenzy, tearing them to shreds and devouring them (one loving close-up shows teeth sinking into Sardu's ripped-out genitals). This film goes beyond anything dreamed up by H G Lewis, beyond Jose Larraz' *Vampyres*, beyond mere pornography; in Sardu's dungeons an atmosphere of complete, wanton amorality is established and, despite the trash aesthetic at work, this may well be, in its very darkest moments, the nearest thing since Pasolini's *Salo* (1975) to a cinematic recreation of the terrifyingly nihilistic microverse of de Sade's Château de Selliny.

A sadistic stage act is also at the centre of one of the very strangest of bizarre films: Jess Franco's *Necronomicon (aka Succubus)* (1969). Nothing to do with H. P. Lovecraft, this confusing work is something of a meditation on subjective reality, and seems to operate mostly in an arcane zone where dreams and waking have irrevocably blurred. Nightclub performer Lorna (Janine Reynaud) plays out various bloody acts of torture and fake (?) murder on her manacled victims. These become inseparable from her fantasies and dreams, in which she also participates in sex and slaughter orgies. Fearing herself in the sway of a demon, she consults a psychiatrist – to little avail. Eventually the viewer loses track altogether of the 'reality' of events on screen, and is left to ponder on the obscure dialogue, incisive jazz score, and sado-erotic imagery.

The darker side of another freakish sideshow and stage institution, ventriloquism – only touched upon in Browning's *The Unholy Three* – was fully explored in the final, and by far the best, segment of the 1945 British ghost/horror compendium film, *Dead Of Night*. This film's dark endpiece – and the only story conceivably set within the bounds of psychological possibility – is a terrifying, genuinely disturbing tale directed by Cavalcanti and starring Michael Redgrave as the ventriloquist convinced that his dummy, Hugo Ffitch, is alive. We see the dummy's personality begin to dominate more and more in this bizarre symbiosis, until finally the man succumbs to complete mental breakdown and ends up in prison, arrested for a murder which he believes Hugo has committed. Though he destroys the dummy, Ffitch's personality is seen to have taken him over completely in the devastating climax, a scene which in its intimations of insanity and mental possession both harks back to *Caligari* and clearly anticipates Alfred Hitchcock's *Psycho* (1960). The basic premise was reprised to unnerving effect in *The Devil Doll* (1963), and rather less successfully in *Magic* (1978), with Anthony Hopkins as the deranged ventriloquist.

Numerous films, including Hitchcock's *Strangers On A Train* (1951) and Byron Haskin's *The Power* (1967), have utilised the superficial gaity of the carnival to counterpoint scenes of despair, violence or murder; drawing on that pool of dark energy which bubbles invisibly beneath the surface. Some of the most effective, poetic films to have tapped this source more directly are *Nightmare Alley* (1947), Curtis Harrington's *Night Tide* (1961), and Jack Clayton's *Something Wicked This Way Comes* (1983). In the first, based on William Lindsay Gresham's bleak *roman noir* of the same name, Tyrone Power plays a sideshow grifter who bluffs and deceives his way to a position of wealth and social status as spiritual adviser to a millionaire. Finally exposed as a fraud, he returns broken and alcohol-addicted to the carnival, where in return for his daily bottle he takes the most degrading position in the show – the geek, whose 'act' is to bite the heads off live chickens. *Nightmare Alley* is a particularly dark film, unusually faithful to its source material, a frightening glimpse at the ulcered underbelly of carnival life and mores.

Night Tide is less nihilistic, a strange fantasy starring Dennis Hopper as the sailor on leave in a Californian coastal resort who comes to frequent a sideshow, where he becomes obsessed with the young girl who plays a mermaid. It turns out that the girl (Luana Anders) truly believes herself to be descended from a race of sea-people, and that she must kill during the full moon as the result of an ancient pelagic curse. The sailor finally finds her dead, drowned in her tank. Recalling Val Lewton's *Cat People* in mood and tone, *Night Tide* is an enigmatic piece which effectively utilises its carnival and littoral setting to establish an other-worldly, fatalistic tension.

Something Wicked This Way Comes is an adaptation of the classic novel of the same name, a meditation on childhood in which Ray Bradbury distils the dark essence to its most perfect crystallisation. Bradbury himself wrote the film-script, and though it suffers a little by comparison to his original, it still manages to capture much of the original's fantastic mood. When the mysterious Pandemonium Carnival rolls into a sleepy mid-western town, miraculous events begin to occur; the town's occupants are getting younger. Inevitably, the carnival's ringmaster Mr. Dark (Jonathan Pryce) has his own sinister price to exact in return, as Jason Robards discovers. Dark is finally defeated by means of his own magic, time-defying calliope.

Another Bradbury adaptation with 'magical' carnival connections, *The Illustrated Man* (1969), starred Rod Steiger and Claire Bloom in a film of three self-contained story segments, linked by Steiger as man tattooed from head to foot, in the manner of P. T. Barnum's Frank Hayes. The difference here is that his tattoos tend to come alive, depicting strange stories to the beholder. The stories, unfortunately, are fairly average. The more sinister, obsessional aspect of tattooing was explored in some detail by Bob Brooks' *Tattoo* (1983), featuring Bruce Dern in psycho mode as a tattoo artist with a fetish for decorating female flesh. He finally abducts a beautiful model (Maud Adams), and they enter a twilight, claustrophobic sexual relationship centred around the tattoo machine with which she ultimately stabs him. An apparent attempt to recreate the monomania of Oshima's *Ai No Corrida*, the film fails to convince on a more than superficial level.

Tobe Hooper's *Funhouse* (1981) is more upfront, transposing the basic post-*Halloween* slasher formula to a funfair setting and thereby benefitting from that milieu's unwritten lore of dread. The simple plot involves a group of youngsters trapped in the deserted funfair (whose displays include an impressive family of embalmed freaks) after dark, where they are stalked by a homicidal maniac who turns out to be a deformed, cleft-headed albino retard (apparently part-modelled on the legendary Bill Durks). There are several effective moments, although one would have expected the director of *The Texas Chainsaw Massacre* to have wrung more fear from such a potentially nightmarish story.

On a lighter note, Ray Dennis Steckler's notorious Z-movie, *The Incredibly Strange Creatures Who Stopped Living And Became Mixed-Up Zombies* (aka *Teenage Psycho Meets Bloody Mary*) (1963), used a carnival setting to tell its legendarily confused story about a gypsy fortune-teller with her own retinue of acid-scarred zombies, who hypnotizes a man (Cash Flagg, *aka* Steckler) into committing a string of murders. The zombies finally break loose and kill everyone in sight. Billed as 'the first monster musical', this unclassifiable absurdity is redeemed only by exquisite, saturated colour photography from Vilmos Zsigmond and Laszlo Kovacs.

More recently, the ludicrous *Howling VI: The Freaks* (1991) has an English vampire and werewolf frolicking in a travelling sideshow in Texas, while *Freaked* (Tom Stern and Alex Winter, 1993) is a sick comedy concerning a truly bizarre freak show in the South American jungle, whose inmates include Keanu Reeves as a Dog Boy and Mr T as the Bearded Lady(!).

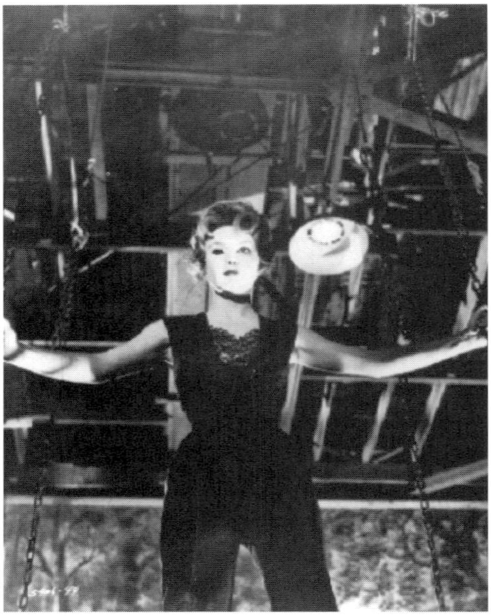

The Hypnotic Eye

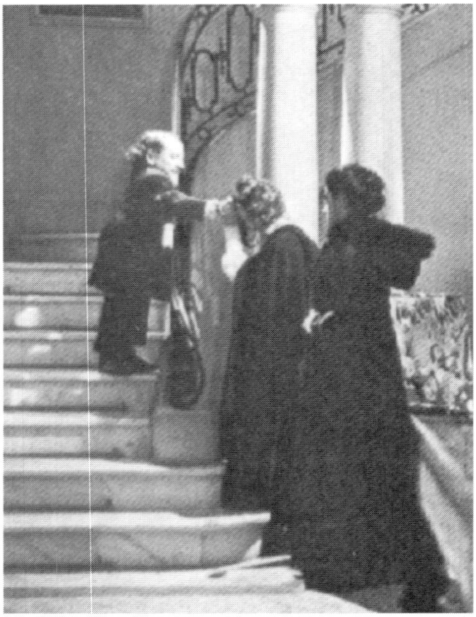

Murders In The Rue Morgue

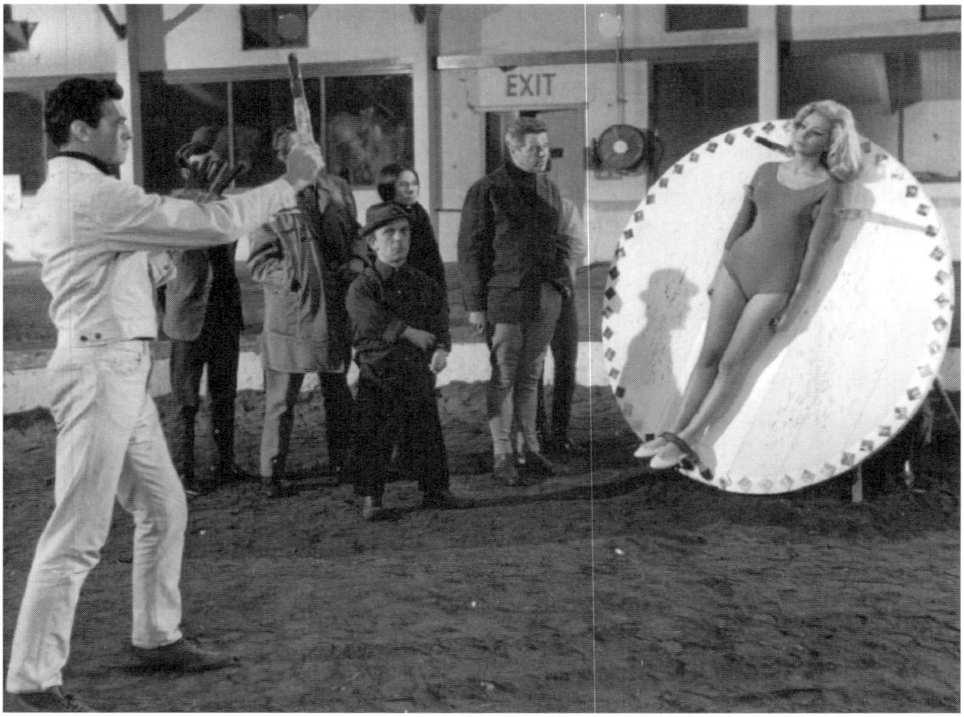

Circus Of Fear

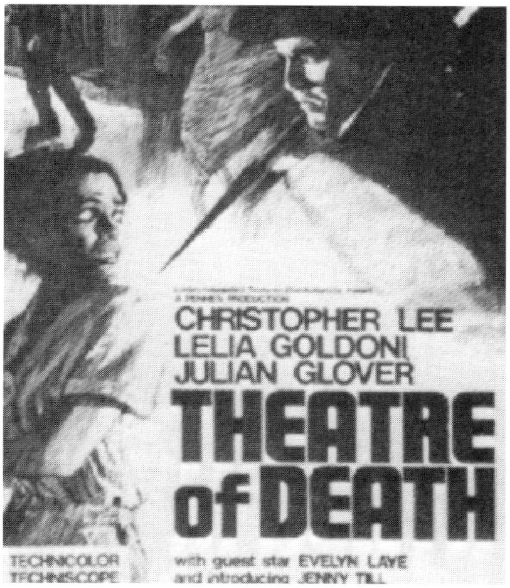

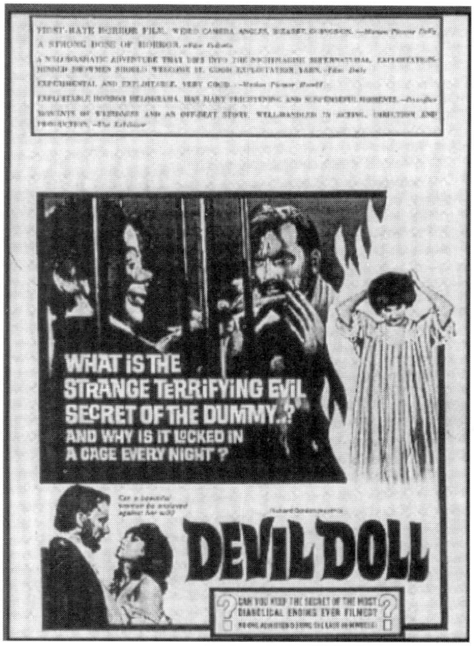

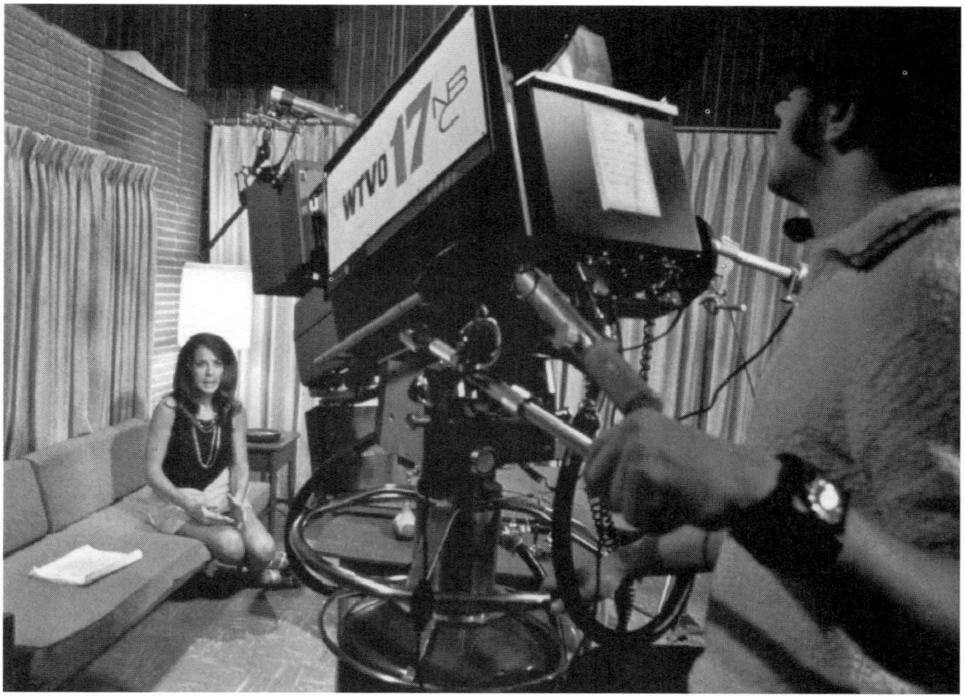

Wizard Of Gore

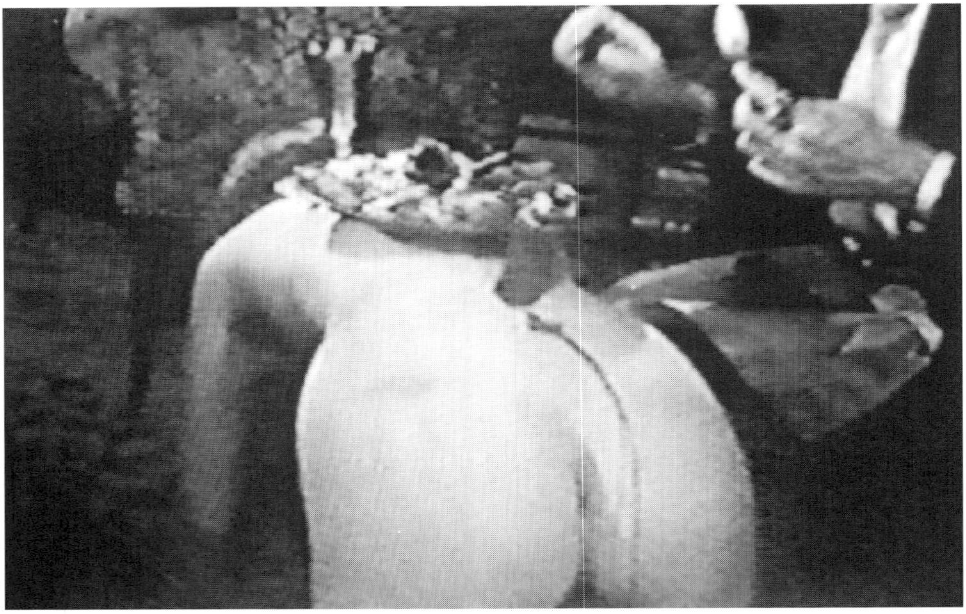

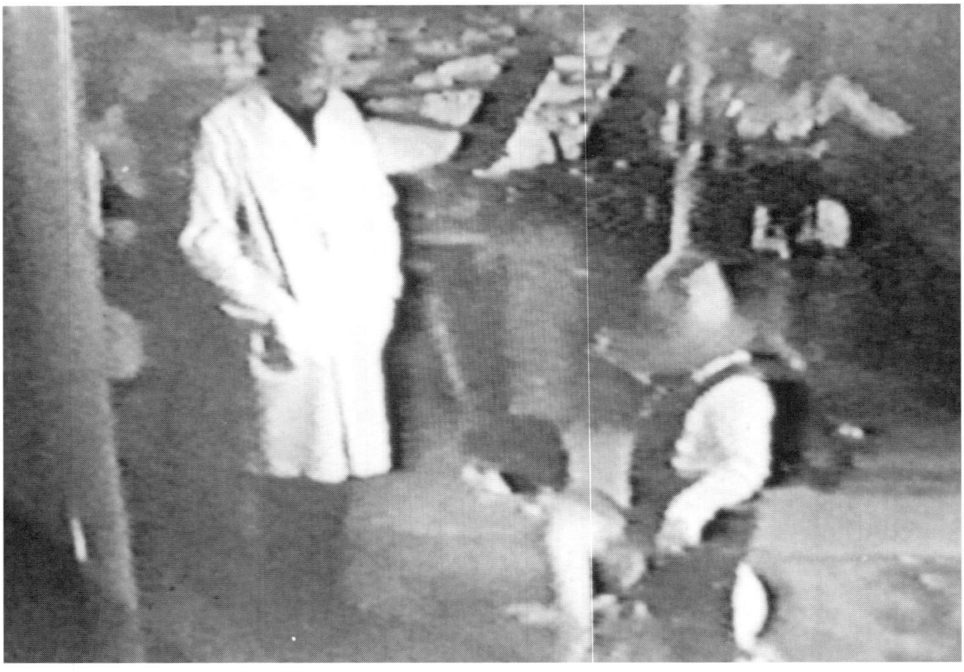

Blood Sucking Freaks

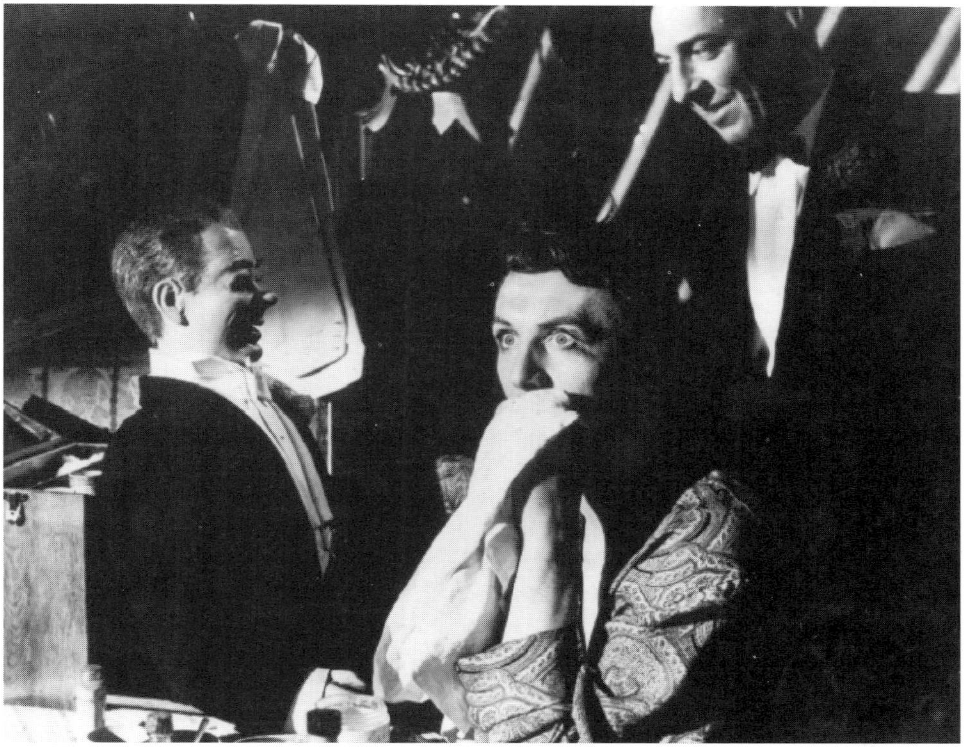

Dead Of Night

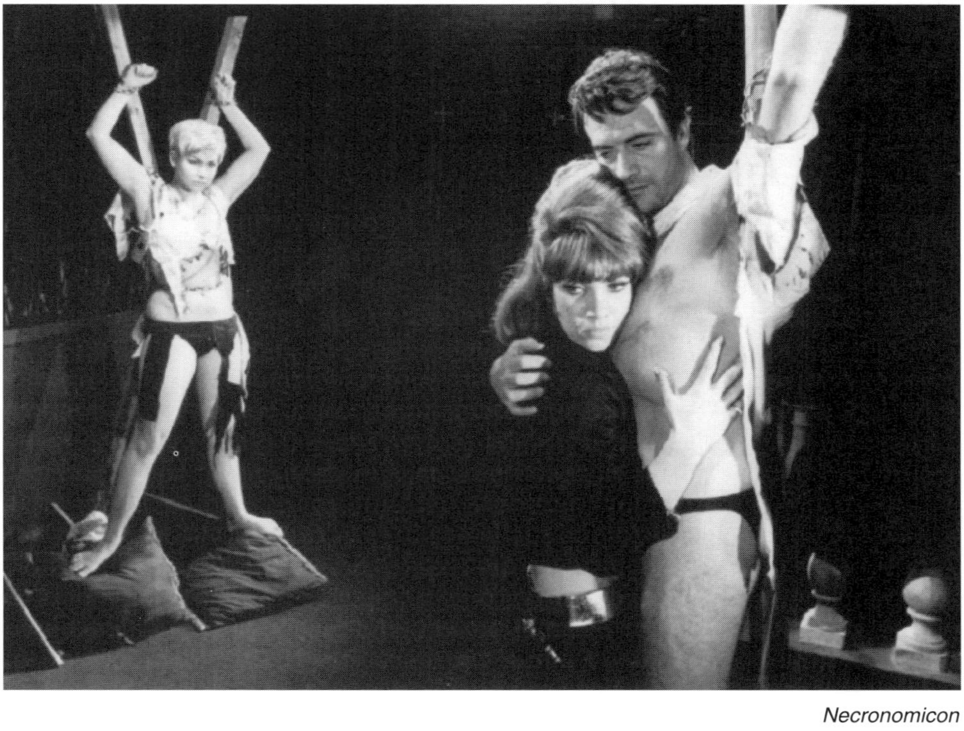

Necronomicon

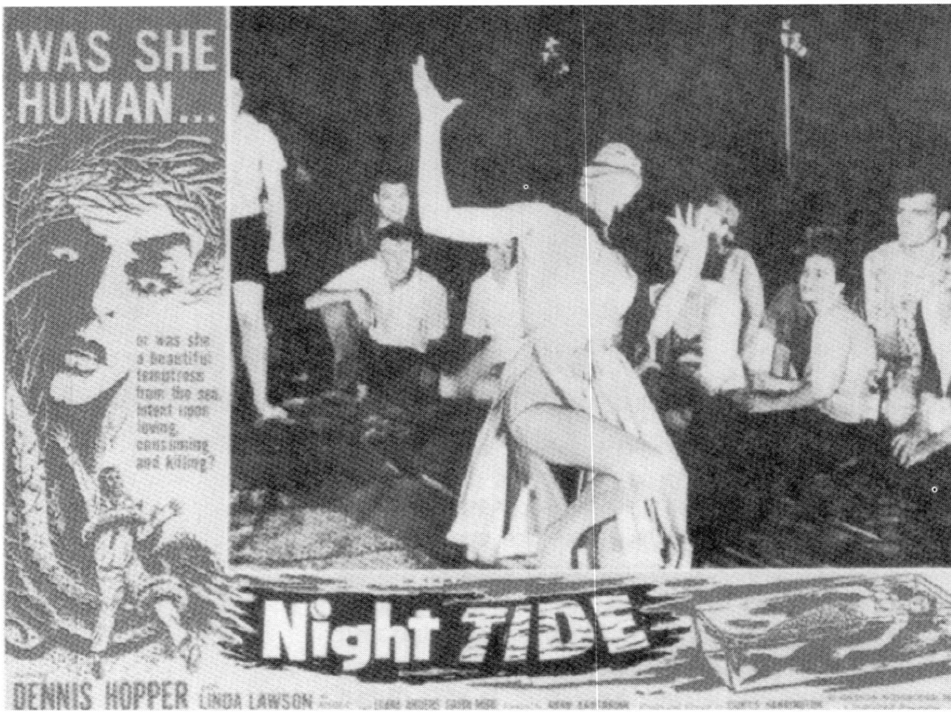

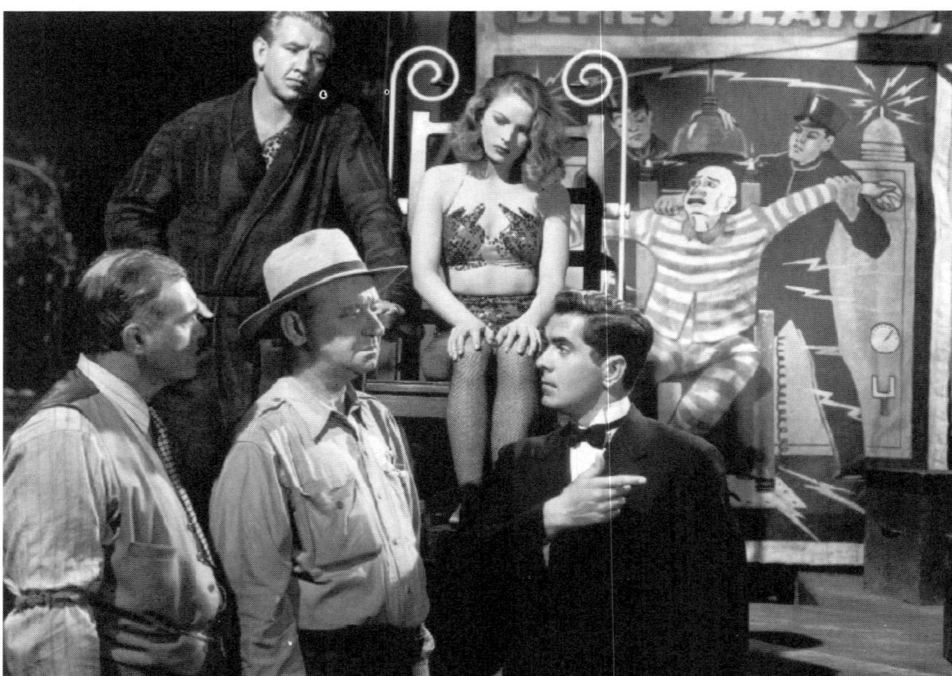

Nightmare Alley

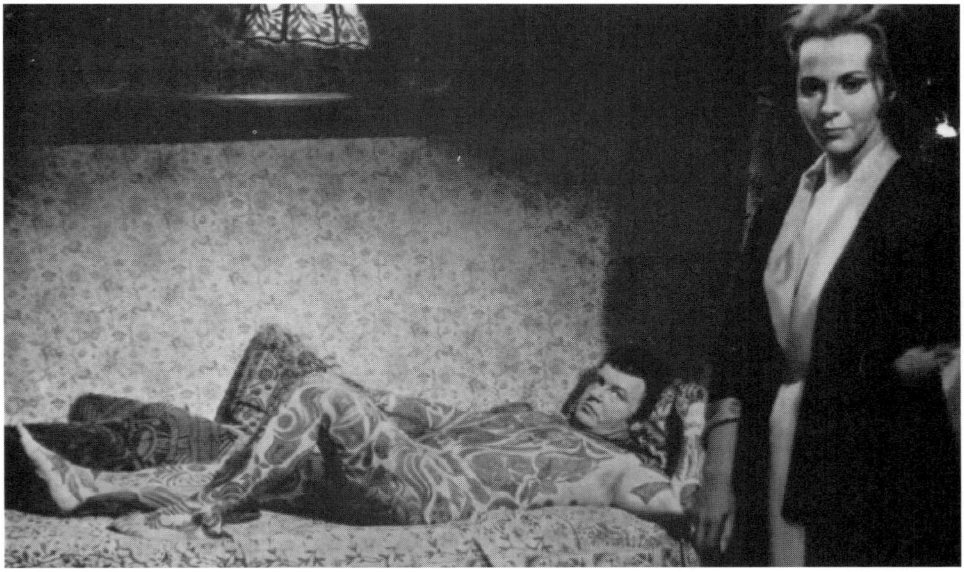

The Illustrated Man

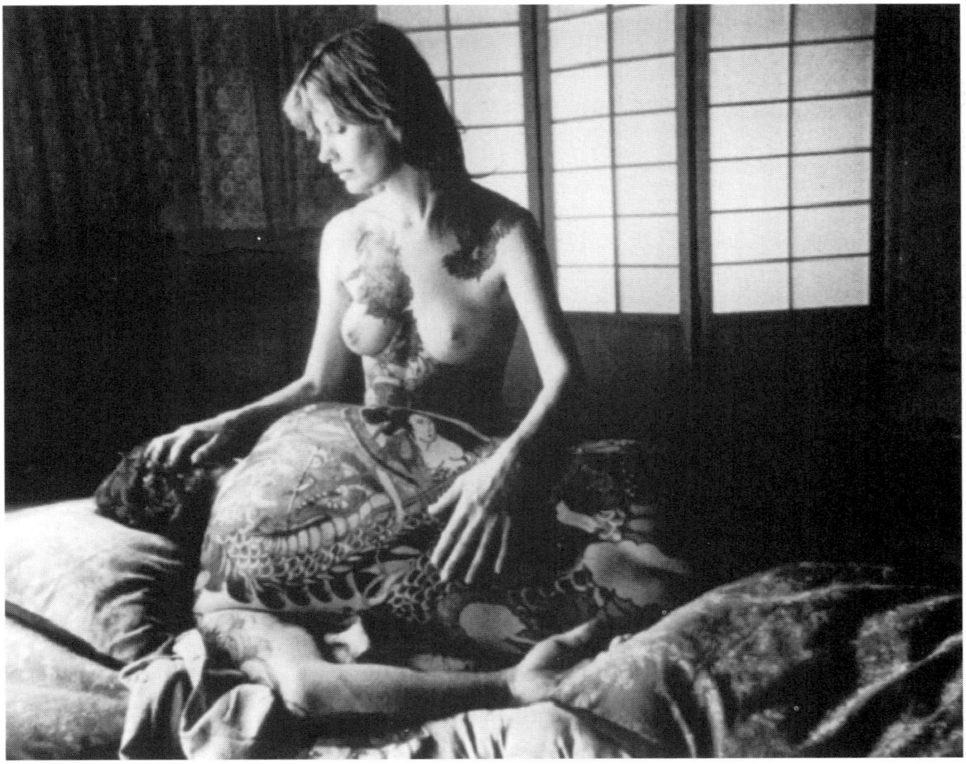

Tattoo

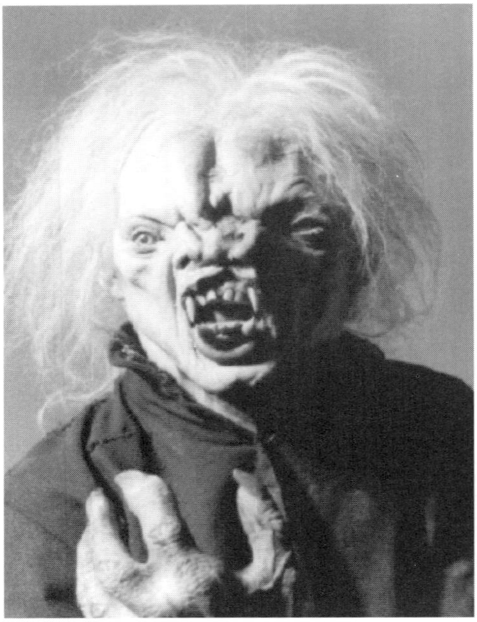

Funhouse

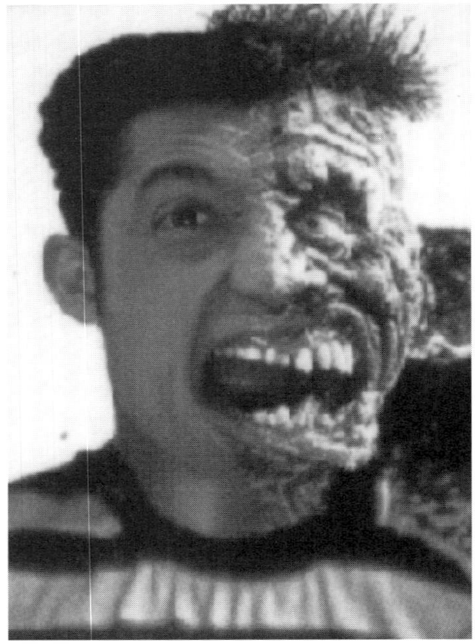

Freaked

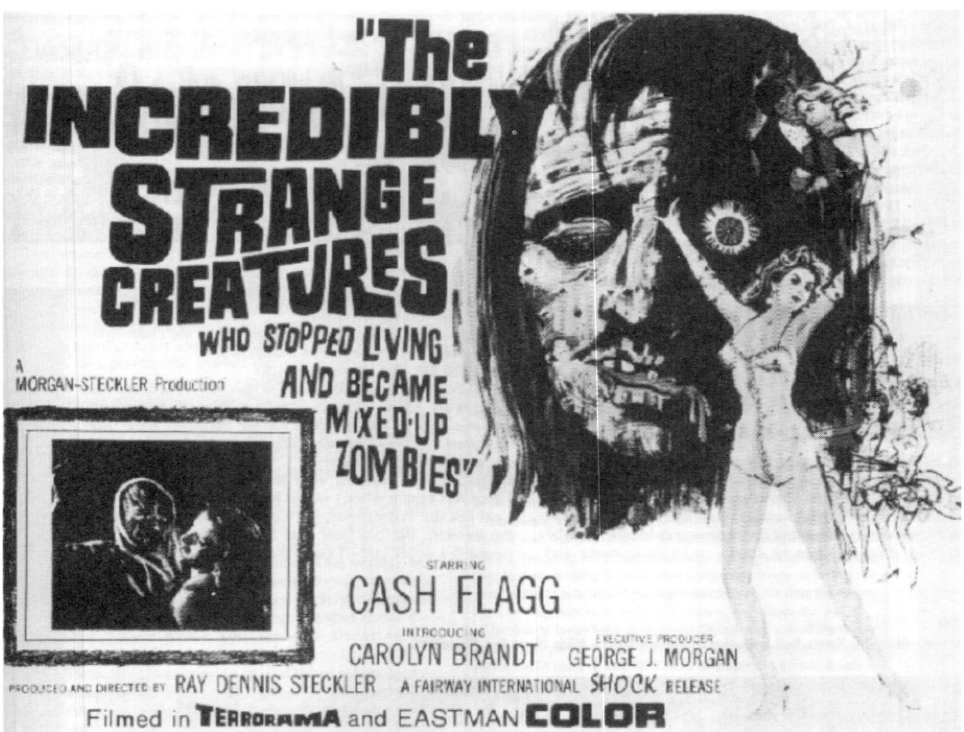

IN THE SHADOW OF THE SUN

None of the circus- or carnival-orientated films discussed above, as bizarre as they may be, dared to transgress as far as *Freaks*; the themes examined in Tod Browning's twilight masterwork would not be so explicitly addressed again until some 30 years after that film's release. A few notable works – of variable merit – have emerged from that particularly murky area.

In *House Of The Damned* (1963), a couple visiting an old mansion formerly owned by a sideshow boss become seeming victims of homicidal ghosts. The 'ghosts' turn out to be a retinue of freaks, hiding out in the house since the showman's death. Real 'freaks', including legless people, are featured, as well as an early appearance by giant Richard Kiel, who went on to play Jaws in the Bond films.

La Donna Scimmia/The Ape Woman (1963) is a fairly straight retelling of the real-life story of Julia Pastrana: a sleazy showman (Ugo Tognazzi) discovers the hair-covered woman (played by Annie Giradot) at a poorhouse, exploits her as an 'ape-woman'/stripper and finally resorts to marrying her when she threatens to quit. Finally agreeing to have sex with her, he impregnates her and she and her deformed baby die during childbirth; he happily embalms and exhibits the freak corpses, milking them for dollars even after death. This Italian entry is a downbeat, sensationalistic film which also includes gratuitous slideshows of naked African women. Upon its first release in America, a ridiculous 'happy ending' was substituted; the spectre of moral outrage over *Freaks* evidently still held sway – though not for much longer.

She Freak (1966), produced by exploitation doyen David F. Friedman (also responsible for such delights as Herschell G. Lewis' *Blood Feast* and *Two Thousand Maniacs*), is a low-budget, low-life partial re-make of *Freaks*. A waitress (Claire Brennan) marries the owner of a down-at-heel freakshow, whose exhibits include a two-headed foetus. She then has an affair with a ferris-wheel operator, whom the husband murders in jealous rage. When he goes to jail, she takes over the show, soon making the mistake of firing one of the dwarfs. As in the original film, the freaks take their terrible revenge and turn her into one of them, a hideous half-beast doomed to see out her miserable existence at the bottom of the snake-pit. As the fairground barker proclaims: "There are only two sorts of monster, Ladies and Gentlemen; those who God made and those who were put together by me. I think there are both sorts in what you are looking at in there..."

Jack Cardiff's *The Mutations* (1972) goes even further in its depiction of sideshow horrors, although here a scientist (Donald Pleasance) is using a freakshow as a cover for his experiments on living people. Attempting to create hybrids of humans and plants, he consigns his many failures (known as "The Royal Family of Strange People") to perform in the show, which is operated by a sadistic dwarf (Michael Dunn). Tom Baker plays his disfigured assistant. Real-life 'freaks' and sideshow performers were used in the film, including a monkey woman, frog boy, human skeleton, alligator lady (Esther Blackman) and human pin-cushion. The doctor's one success, a venus flytrap-man, was (hopefully) achieved by make-up. *The Mutations* has it all: the mad scientist, disfigurement and sadism, mutilation and murder, human oddities; the apparent dead-end for the fairground/freak sub-genre of bizarre cinema.

Two outstanding, transcendent films have, however, since appeared which deal explicitly with abnormal people, and the bizarre world of the travelling sideshow with its tormented denizens, yet which have both in their own ways managed to slip the boundaries of that world. Both come from 'cult' directors who first made their names with relentlessly grotesque early features of extraordinary imagination: David Lynch and Alejandro Jodorowsky. Lynch, who attained renown through his nightmare classic *Eraserhead* (1977), went on to direct *The Elephant Man* (1980), the story of England's most famous human anomaly John (born Joseph Carey) Merrick, also known as the Elephant Man due to his advanced condition of congenital neurofibromatosis. The film is based on the true account published in 1923 by surgeon Sir Frederick Treves, in which he described the unfortunate young man, who was born in 1862, as follows:

"He had a fleshy appendage hanging down from his forehead like an elephant's trunk. A spongy growth covered his neck. He was completely hairless. His forehead covered one eye. A mass of bone from the roof of his mouth projected out from his upper jaw. He had no nose. His body was hung with sacks of wrinkled skin. His right hand resembled a fin. His feet were too swollen to allow him to walk except by a shuffling gait. In addition, he had been dropped when a baby and his backbone was twisted out of shape."[3]

Lynch introduces us to Merrick as an exhibition in a seedy Victorian sideshow. The show is presided over by the sadistic Bytes (played by Freddie Jones), and The Elephant Man – a wretched, hooded figure – is his prized 'performer'. When Treves (played by Anthony Hopkins) visits the show and sees Merrick's unprecedented condition, he persuades Bytes to allow him to borrow the 'freak' to be examined by his students at the Royal Hospital. Treves soon becomes sympathetically involved with Merrick (brilliantly portrayed by John Hurt), recognizing that beneath his monstrous exterior lies a sensitive and intelligent man, and manages – despite initial opposition from the hospital governor F. C. Carr Gomm (Sir John Gielgud) – to procure him a permanent residency at the hospital.

Merrick makes swift progress, and even achieves a certain celebrity; but his new happiness is destroyed by two horrific events. An unscrupulous hospital porter (Michael Elphick) obtains the key to Merrick's room, and starts to make an illicit living by charging the drunken clientele of local pubs to come in and look at the famous patient. The scene where this practice finally gets out of hand, resulting in a drunken, vicious, jeering gang entering Merrick's room, dousing him with whisky, assaulting him and smashing his belongings, is one of the most harrowing ever filmed; like Michael Powell's *Peeping Tom*, it underlines the voyeuristic nature of the cinematic experience, forcing us to confront the cynicism inherent in our own interest in the film – like these scum, we too have paid to witness the moment of the Elephant Man's unmasking, to ogle at his deformity, and our shame is even more heightened by the sympathy we have now developed for the victim.

The porter is discovered by Treves and sacked, but has his revenge by betraying Merrick to Bytes, who steals his former charge from his haven and takes him off to a squalid carnival in Belgium, where once again he is subjected to ridicule, beatings and starvation. Finally, while Bytes languishes in a drunken stupor, the other circus freaks mutiny, freeing Merrick and helping him to a passage on a ship back to London. After narrowly escaping death at the hands of a brutal mob, the Elephant Man is finally reunited with Treves. He resumes his happy life in the hospital until, after a visit from a famous actress who reminds him of his mother, he decides to sleep on his back, as she would have, and dies during the night, asphyxiated by the weight of his distorted cranium.

Photographed in austere monochrome by Freddie Francis, *The Elephant Man* achieves a similar atmosphere of bleak, filthy industrial ruin to that in *Eraserhead*; the oneiric ambience of the latter work is also recalled in Merrick's several dream sequences, chiefly involving his mother, stampeding elephants, and nebulous celestial panoramas. Largely avoiding gratuitous sentimentality, Lynch is able to transmute the twilight melancholy of his earlier film into a poignant affirmation of the ability of one man's inner feelings and visions to survive the inhumanities inflicted upon him by his fellows.

Alejandro Jodorowsky achieved an overnight, if underground, notoriety with the release of his second feature, the strange and violent 'metaphysical Western' *El Topo/The Mole*, in 1971. He later made a few less widely-seen pictures, before creating what many consider to be his masterpiece: *Santa Sangre* (1989). This extraordinary film tells the story of Fenix, a child of the circus, from traumatic boyhood to psychotic manhood. We first see Fenix (played by Jodorowsky's son, Axel) as a troubled patient in an asylum; perched at the top of a tree in his bare cell, eating only raw meat. Then back some ten years or more, and we find him as a boy, rolling into town with the travelling carnival owned by his knife-thrower father, the Great Orgo. His companions are Aladin, the dwarf elephant-trainer, and Alma, the young mute girl, her face a white mask, with whom he is in love. She is the ward of the voluptuous tattooed lady, who ceaselessly teases and arouses Orgo as they rehearse his deadly act.

Meanwhile, Fenix's mother, Concha – a repressed religious fanatic – holds court in the shanty church of Santa Sangre, a bizarre Frieda Kahloesque shrine to an armless martyr, erected around a font of 'holy blood'. Soldiers and bulldozers wait without; when the church is duly condemned as heretical by a visiting priest – the holy blood turns out to be red paint – they advance upon the sisters of Santa Sangre and the sheet-metal temple is demolished. Concha returns distraught to the circus, where Fenix is horrified to see her being brutally fucked by Orgo, screaming as if in pain. The blood motif reoccurs as a circus elephant dies in a pool of its own haemorrhages; the funeral of this wretched pachyderm, pushed into a ravine to be quickly dismembered and eaten by hordes of ravenous peons, provides another typically Buñuelesque glimpse of Mexico.

Orgo decides the come has come for Fenix to become a man; he must undergo a ritual tattooing, performed by Orgo himself, and be marked with the same great bird which adorns his father's chest (the first in a series of avian motifs which run through the film). Soon afterwards, Orgo finally succumbs to the charms of the tattooed lady. Concha stumbles across them and, seeing her worst fears realised, lashes out in blind revenge, dousing her husband's genitals in hydrochloric acid. Destroyed, Orgo takes his own vengeance – dragging her into the deserted ring and shearing off both her arms at the shoulders with his heavy throwing knives. At the moment of dismemberment, Concha's face is imbued with religious ecstasy – she has become the living embodiment of Santa Sangre. Orgo, no longer a man, staggers outside the tent and kills himself, slicing through his own throat as Fenix watches helplessly from the confines of his trailer. The tattooed lady flees the scene, taking her young ward with her, and Fenix catches his last glimpse of Alma's white face in the rear of their speeding car. Darkness.

Forward to the asylum, where the grown-up, taciturn Fenix has become a messiah to mongoloids. Taking them on a trip to the cinema at night, he is exposed to the urban Mexico of criminals, cripples, transvestite hookers and human oddities. This whole nocturnal episode, culminating in a set-piece knife homicide, seems like some grotesque, evil hybrid of Buñuel, David Lynch and Dario Argento. The tattooed lady has become a crazed prostitute servicing deformed clientele; her ward Alma, now a young woman, suffers at the hands of these drunken wretches. Repulsed by the attentions of a misshapen giant, she flees into the night, narrowly escaping the clutches of an earless man. Meanwhile, the tattooed lady has a visitor; we see her viciously, bloodily hacked to death by the feminine hands of an unknown assailant.

Soon afterwards, a rope appears at the window of Fenix's cell; he escapes to the street below, where he is met by the armless figure of his mother. Fenix is soon re-united with the dwarf Aladin, then he and Concha take to the stage as a double act, with Fenix providing arms for his mother. This relationship also extends into their bizarre private life, and it is obvious that Fenix, totally dominated by Concha, sees this as his only role in life. Later, he even takes to totally bandaging the rest of his body, imitating the Invisible Man in an apparent attempt to negate his body, his identity, everything but his arms.

Inevitably, Fenix finds a female admirer – a voluptuous stripper – through his stage-act. Dressing in the costume of the Great Orgo, he holds an afterhours audition for a knife-throwing act, hypnotising the girl. Concha appears and, finding Fenix about to engage in a sexual act with the stripper, wills him to impale her with his knife. In a scene reminiscent of *The Wizard Of Gore*, she falls dead and bleeding only when the hypnotic spell is broken.

Thereafter, mother, son and dwarf once more abandon the world of performance and retreat to Concha's home, a new shrine to Santa Sangre, where Fenix is tortured by visions of severed limbs, crashing temples, birds, dead brides, and tattooed horses.

It is not long before Fenix, wandering the town, comes across another woman who attracts him; this time she is a huge, female wrestler, whom he invites to his home that evening. Again, Concha appears at the first onset of lust and wills him to kill. He butchers the wrestler with a samurai sword, but the murder is witnessed by another house-guest who flees to alert the police.

Meanwhile, Fenix is finally discovered by Alma, who has been searching for him all these years. In the final battle of wills, Fenix cannot carry out his mother's order to kill Alma, and he instead plunges a knife into her chest with her own (his) hand. At once, she fades away into nothing. Likewise Aladin, and the other friends from his childhood who have come with Alma; they were all hallucinations, and Fenix has been manipulating a ventriloquist's dummy which he believed to be his Concha. At last liberated from his trauma and the repressive spectre of his dead mother, Fenix regains his hands and his will, and he and Alma give themselves up to the police.

Despite its flash-frozen visual mnemonics for a whole pantheon of grotesque cinema from *Caligari* and *Mad Love* through *Psycho* to *Blue Velvet*, *Santa Sangre* remains very much a pure Jodorowsky vision, a typically phoenixological celebration of one man's *rite-de-passage* through mayhem and psychosis to re-birth. Its infernal synthesis remains, as yet, unchallenged; we await the first true freak-film of the '90s.

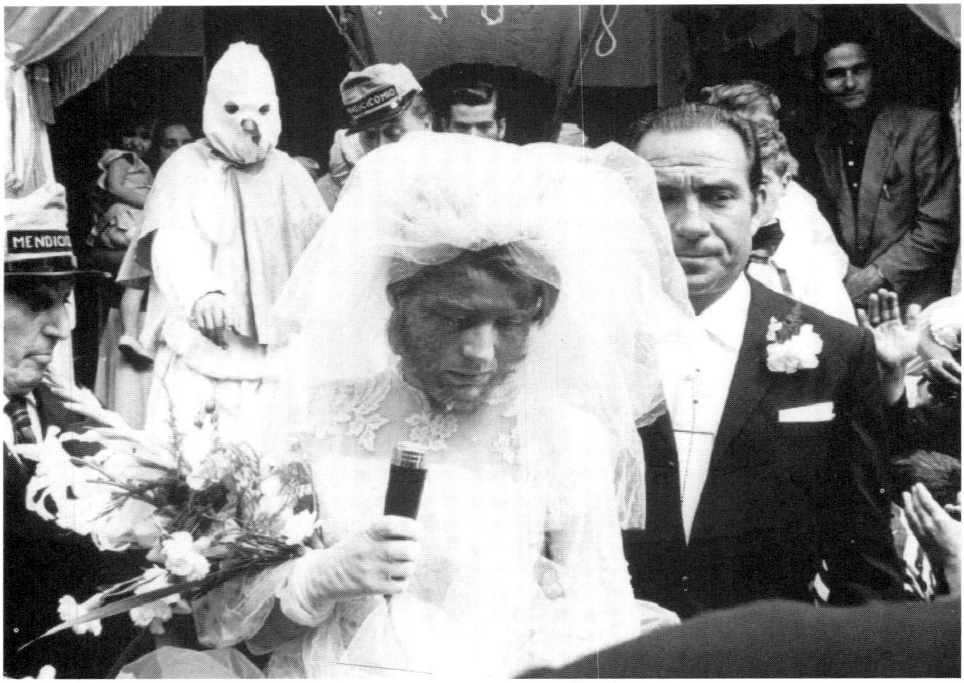

La Donna Scimmia

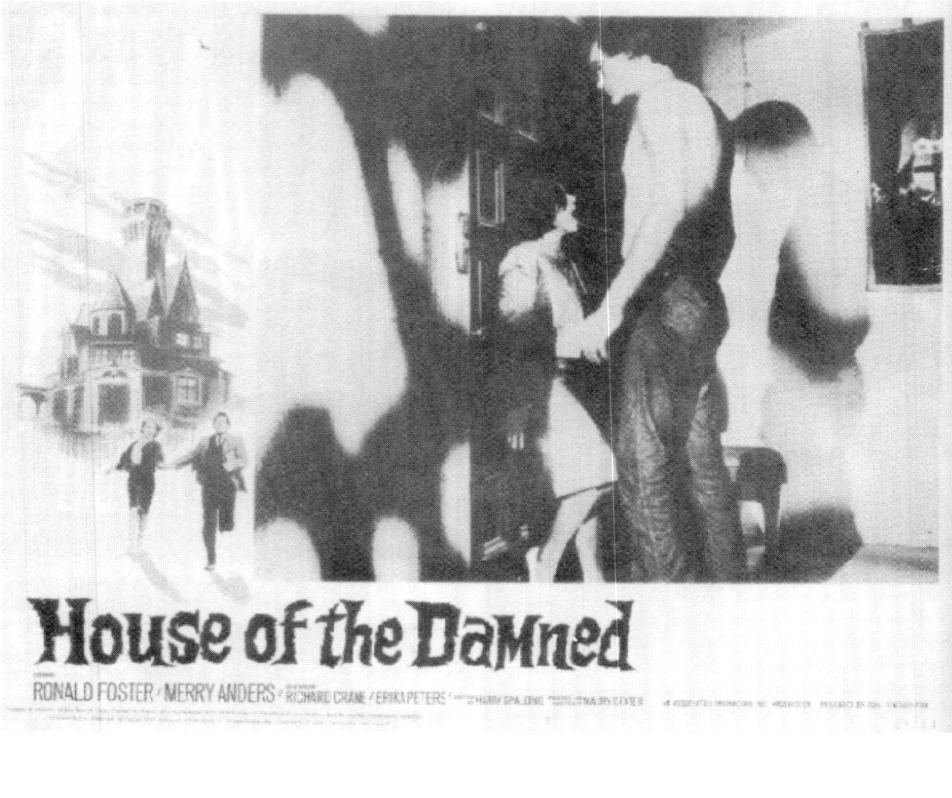

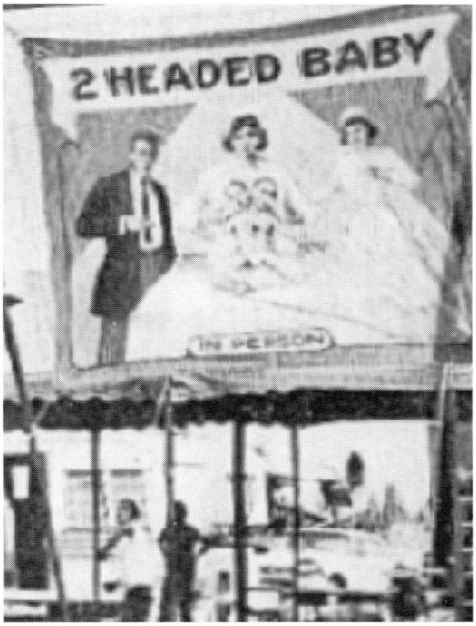
2 HEADED BABY
IN PERSON

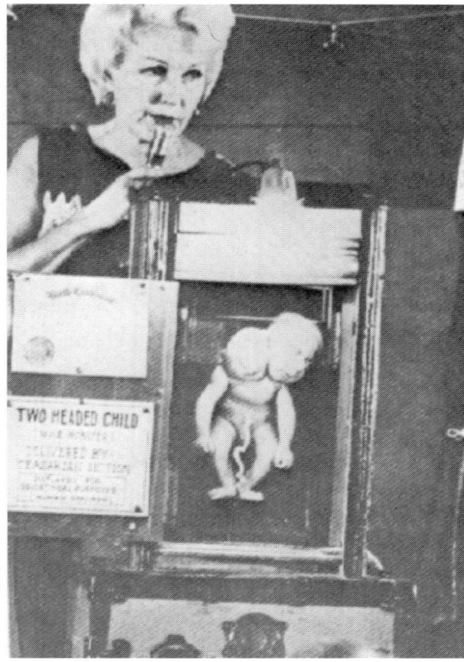
TWO HEADED CHILD

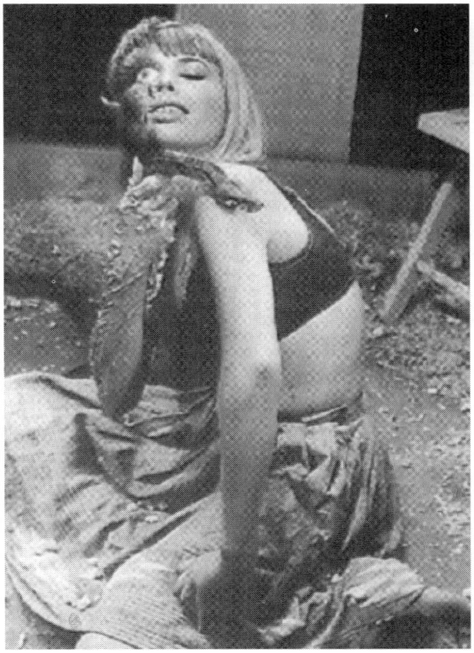

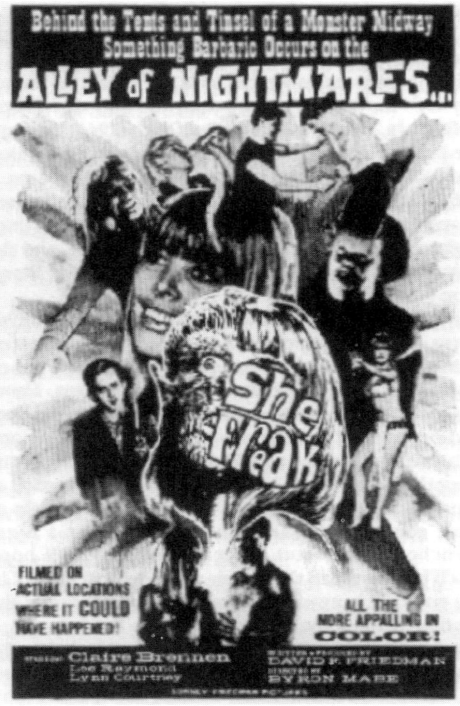
Behind the Tents and Tinsel of a Monster Midway
Something Barbaric Occurs on the
ALLEY of NIGHTMARES...
She Freak
FILMED ON
ACTUAL LOCATIONS
WHERE IT COULD
HAVE HAPPENED!
ALL THE
MORE APPALLING IN
COLOR!
Claire Brennen
Lee Raymond
Lynn Courtney
DAVID F. FRIEDMAN
BYRON MABE

She Freak

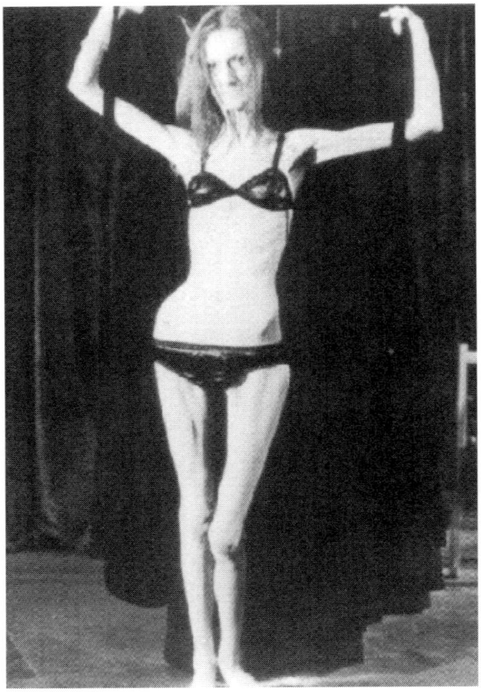

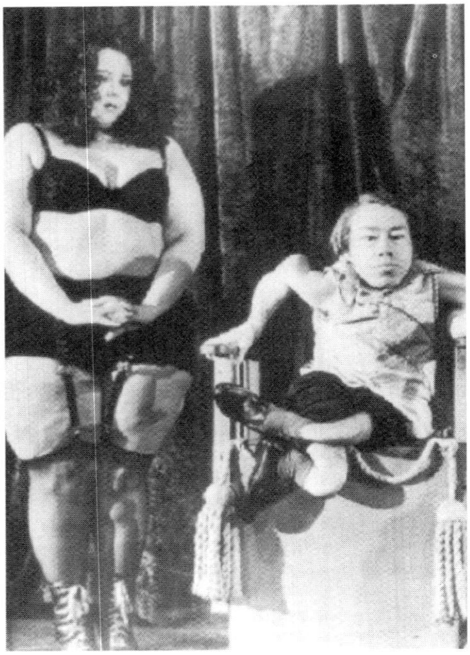

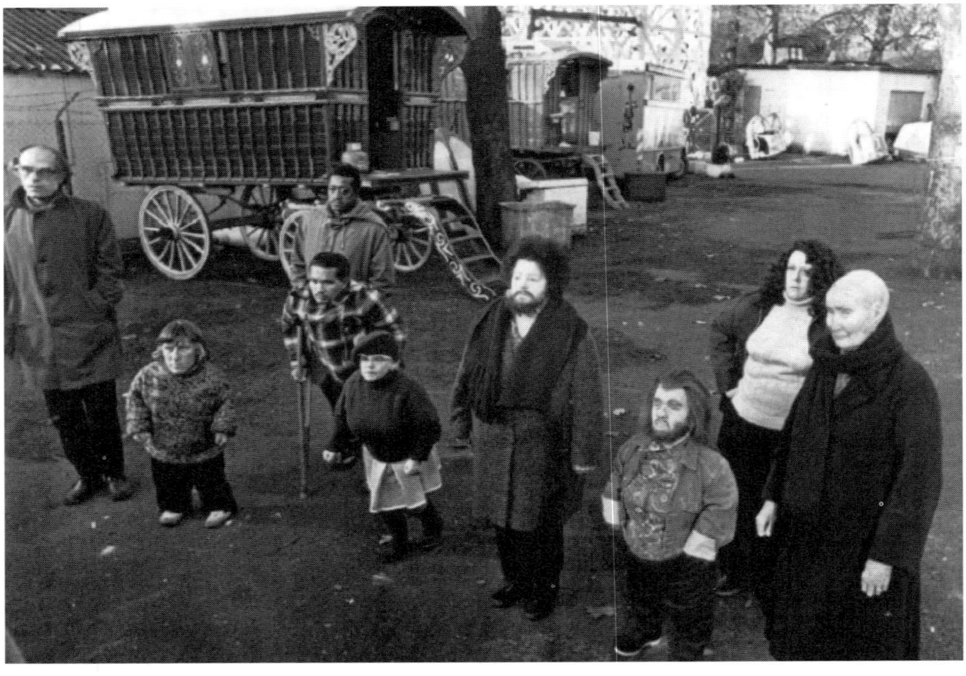

The Mutations

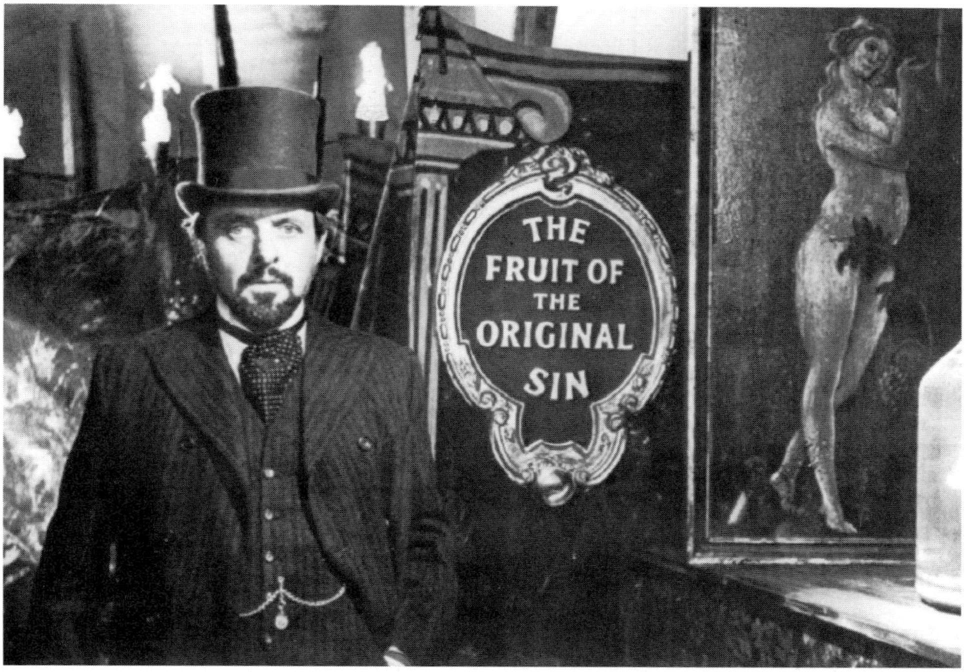

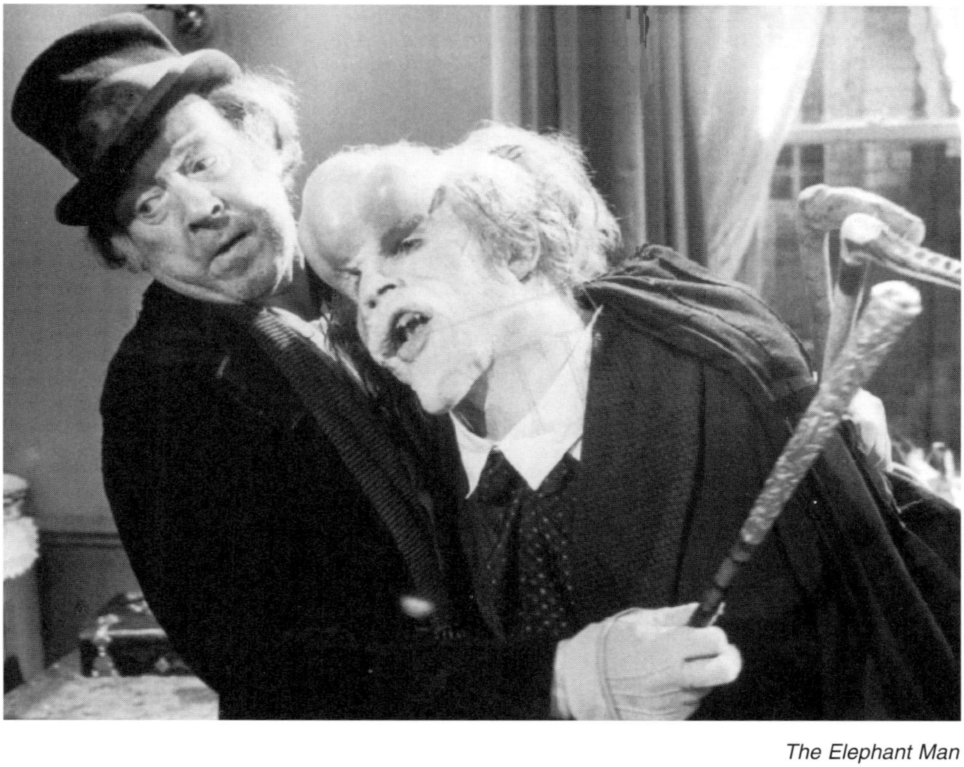

The Elephant Man

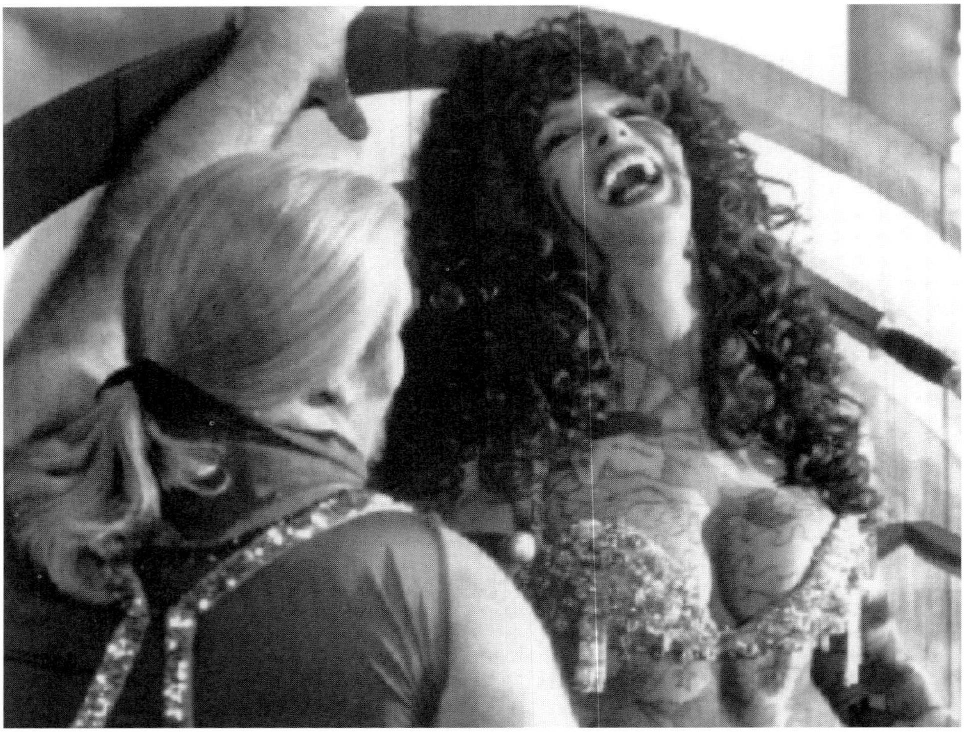

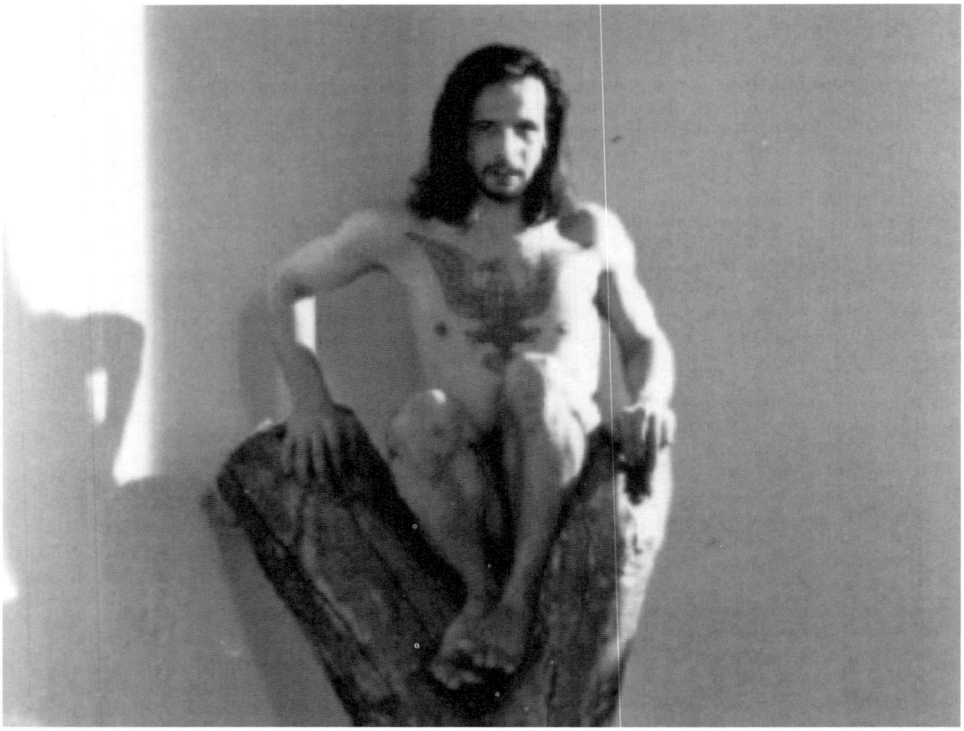

Santa Sangre

NOTES

1 Browning even reverberated subtle echoes of his stock iconography throughout *Dracula*: the vampire, who penetrates his 'lovers' by fang alone, can easily be perceived as being dead below the waist; while the exceptionally grotesque, fly-eating and incarcerated Renfield is an archetypal pit-bound geek.

2 The basic formula of these films, the demented homicidal sculptor working with human materials, has been diluted even further over the years in such works as Roger Corman's *A Bucket Of Blood* (1959), Herschell G. Lewis' *Color Me Blood Red* (1965), the Canadian oddity *Playgirl Killer* (1965), *Cauldron Of Blood* (1967) with Boris Karloff, Stephanie Rothman's *Blood Bath* (1966), Joseph Adler's *Scream Baby Scream* (1969), and the British Mike Raven vehicle *Crucible Of Terror* (1971).

3 Treves first wrote about Merrick, in strictly medical terminology, in "A Case Of Congenital Deformity" (*Transactions Of The Pathological Society*, 1885).

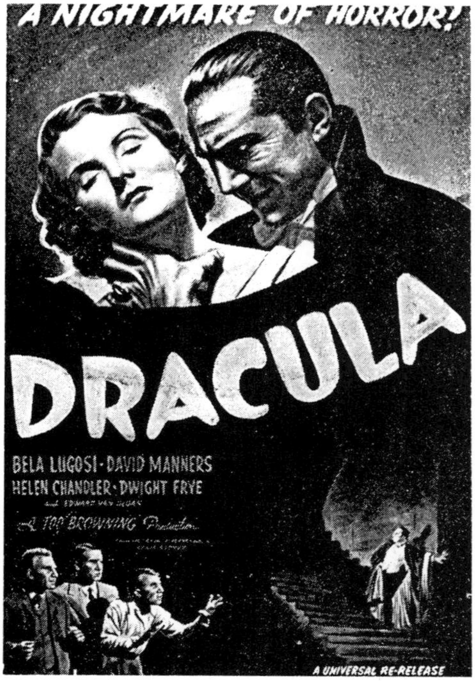

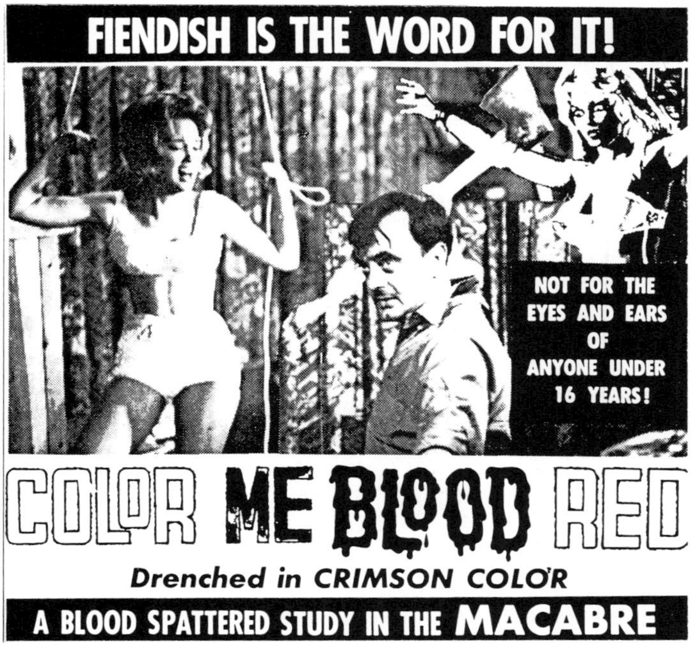

Chapter Two:

FLESH INFERNO

(Geeks, Freaks, And Fetishes)

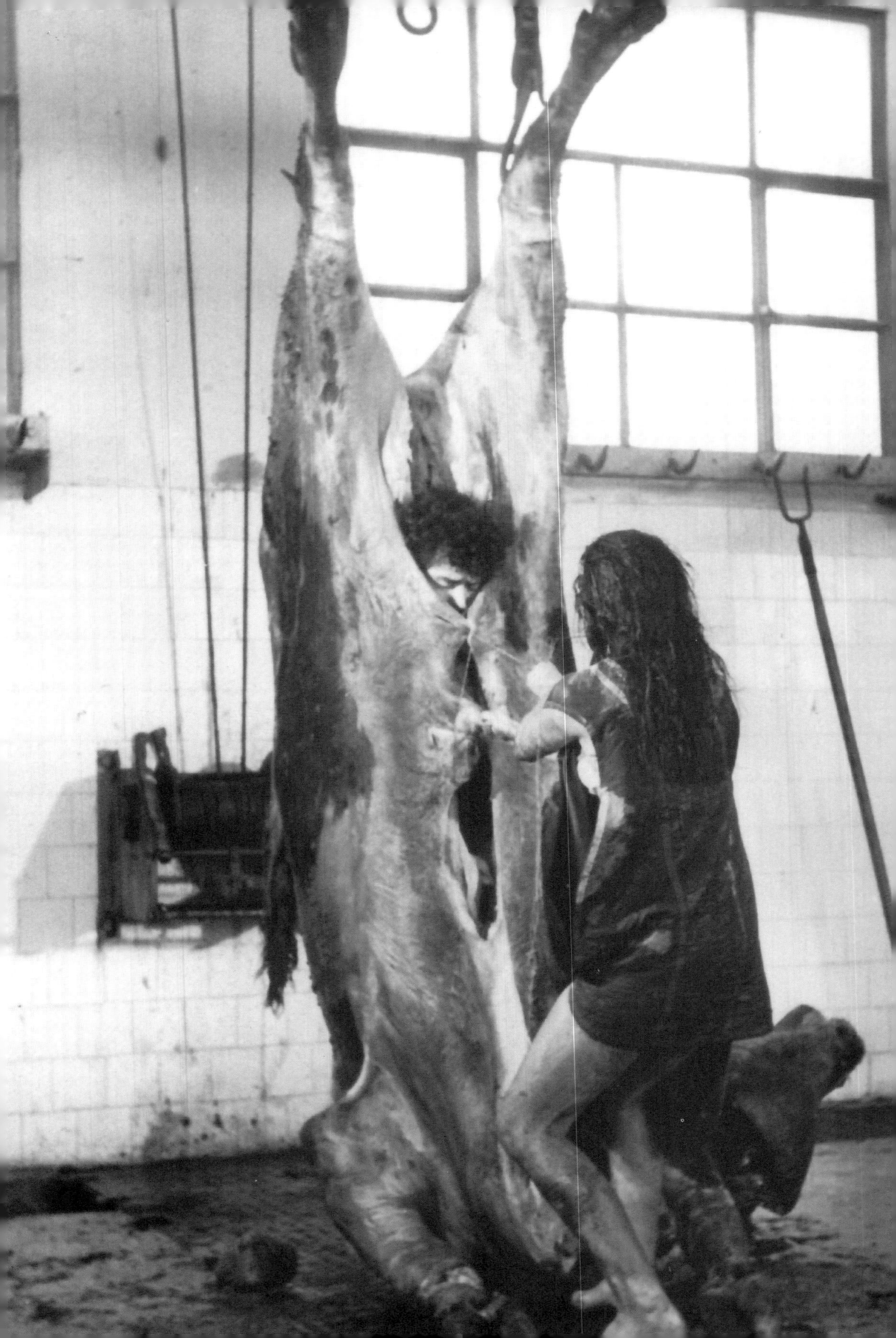

HIDDEN FACES

After the furore surrounding *Freaks*, film-makers became, for a while at least, more sensitive to the issue of employing real human anomalies in their productions. This is reputedly why Cecil B. de Mille withdrew from his *Sign Of The Cross* (1932) the undoubtedly outlandish sequence depicting vicious Amazon women fighting achondroplasic dwarfs in the Roman arena. Yet human prodigies never completely disappeared from the screens; giants, such as Jack Earl or the 7′ 8" Max Palmer (star of *The Killer Ape* [1953]) and, in particular, dwarfs, have continued to appear, largely in films of a bizarre or fantastic nature.

Dwarfs first appeared in films as far back as *The Haunted Curiosity Shop* (1901) and *The Dwarf's Cakewalk* (1905). They were later used to portray creatures such as the Munchkins in *Wizard Of Oz* (1939) and goblins in *A Midsummer Night's Dream* (1935). Rumour also has it that midgets were responsible for the moving props in certain Busby Berkeley extravaganzas. In 1938, they were finally accorded their own bizarre tribute: *The Terror Of Tiny Town*, directed by one Sam Newfield, was the first (and last) all-midget Western. Billy Curtis, John Bambury and Little Billy are amongst those involved in this stilted tale of a minuscule range war (Curtis would return more respectably to this milieu as Mordechai in Clint Eastwood's *High Plains Drifter* [1973]). After that, it was mostly back to being used as Hollywood extras in jungle adventures such as *Jungle Moon Men* (1953, dressed up as animals or painted black as pygmies), or in commonplace circus dramas.

Dwarfs have, however, played more important roles in a number of films. In 1933, French director Jean Vigo employed the celebrated dwarf actor Delphin to play Headmaster to brilliant effect in his anarchistic classic *Zéro De Conduite*; another French dwarf, Piéral, featured in films such as *Eternal Retour* and *Princesse De Clèves*. Dwarfs figure as courtiers in period dramas such as Walerian Borowzcyck's *Blanche* (1970) and Franklin Schaffner's *The Warlord* (1965); circus dwarfs appear in several of Ingmar Bergman's films, including *The Seventh Seal* (1957) and *The Silence* (1963); Donald Sutherland is butchered by a sinister, red-cowled (female) dwarf in Nicholas Roeg's *Don't Look Now* (1974); Anna Karina is threatened by a midget thug with an out-sized revolver in Godard's *Pierrot Le Fou* (1965); Volker Schlöndorff's *Die Blechtrommel/The Tin-Drum* (1979) uses David Bennent, a child actor with arrested growth, to portray the dwarf Oskar, and also features Roswitha, a midget somnambulist; and in Terry Gilliam's *Time Bandits* (1981), a boy is whisked from his suburban home into a series of outrageous adventures through time and space by a whole crew of dwarf thieves, including actors Malcolm Dixon, Mike Edmonds, Jack Purvis, Tiny Ross, and David Rappaport (who took his own life in 1992). *The Great Rock'n'Roll Swindle* (1978, resurrected from the ashes of Russ Meyer's *Who Killed Bambi?*) featured dwarf actress Helen of Troy.

Other notable examples of dwarf actors have included Marcel Guegan, Franco Drago (the 'heart-breaker of Italian cinema', who claimed few women of any size could resist his charms), Jerry Austin, Skip Martin ('Hop-Frog' in Roger Corman's excellent *Masque Of The Red Death* [1964]), Billy Barty (as seen in Roger Corman's *The Undead* [1956]), Michael Dunn, Hervé Villechaize (Nick-Nack to Christopher Lee's three-nippled Scaramanga in *The Man With The Golden Gun* [1974], and an evil dream-figure in Oliver Stone's *Seizure* [also 1974]), and Kenny Baker (R2D2 in *Star Wars* [1980]). Exploitation mogul William Castle investigated the love-life of midget Paul Dale in *It's A Small World* (1950). Angelo Rossitto, one of the cast of *Freaks*, went on to appear in a succession of B-movies such as *Scared To Death* (1947), a strange Bela Lugosi vehicle, and *Sherlock Holmes And The Spider Woman* (1944), in which he played an African pygmy carried around by the arachnoid villainess in her vanity case. In 1980 he cropped up in *Galaxina*, alongside the late Dorothy Stratten, as a tiny alien, and shortly before his death featured as half of MasterBlaster, a giant/dwarf team, in George Miller's *Mad Max 3: Beyond Thunderdome* (1985). One of the most disturbing recent uses of a dwarf occurs in Giuliano Carnimeo's *Rat Man* (1987), in which the tiny, deformed Nelson De La Rosa plays the monstrous title role.

Yet the ultimate film to utilise dwarf actors remains Werner Herzog's *Auch Zwerge Haben Klein Angefangen/Even Dwarfs Started Small* (1970). This merciless work is undoubtedly Herzog's bleakest, most paralyzing vision of humanity; even *Freaks* pales beside its horrifying intensity. The locale for the events we witness is an institutional home for dwarfs, controlled by (unseen) normal-sized people. It soon becomes apparent that the dwarfs, once docile, are in revolt. The 'normal' people have fled, leaving in charge a senior dwarf who has in turn been imprisoned in his office, shunned for his complicity. The lunatics have taken over the asylum. But from this point on, events become decidedly grimmer.

The dwarf society starts to break down; chaos and bitterness erupt as the dwarfs realise that despite their 'freedom' they are powerless, directionless – Herzog's metaphor for godless, existentially impotent mankind. The newly-elected leaders are ridiculed and humiliated, a pair of blind dwarfs are persecuted; a sow nursing her litter is butchered, chickens are killed and a savage cock fight instigated; finally, a monkey is crucified. The oppressed have become the oppressors; there is no hope. Herzog dwells again and again on scenes of grotesque, relentless cruelty, lingering over the carnage and madness. Most terrifying of all are the shots of mocking, malicious, pinched little faces, the terrible engulfing laughter of the dwarfs, the repeated image of the dwarf who stands back and cackles with nihilistic abandon as this holocaust continues to consume Herzog's shattering microcosm of humanity.

Human anomalies have cropped up in many other films; most – though by no means all – have been contributions to exploitational cinema. The Hilton Sisters Daisy and Violet, the Siamese twins from *Freaks*, were given their very own 'starring vehicle' in 1950. *Chained For Life* (aka *Love Among The Monsters*) basically retold the real-life case of (male) Siamese twins Lucio-Simplicio; one twin was tried and found guilty of murder, yet the innocent twin could scarcely be sent to jail alongside the other. The judge imposed a hefty fine instead, but from then on their 'act' was dogged by misfortune and squabbles. This scenario was scarcely more horrifying than the Hiltons' real story. They were born in England in 1908, and sold by their mother (a barmaid) to an American promoter who treated them like animals, growing rich by exhibiting them at freakshows until they were finally able to gain their liberty. Little-seen, *Chained For Life* is a classic example of the exploitation film masquerading as social document.

Meanwhile, a formerly handsome actor now struck down with acromegaly (a hideously disfiguring disease) was making a short but renowned career for himself as a movie 'heavy': Rondo Hatton, who appeared in numerous B-movies which openly exploited his facial deformity, such as *Pearl Of Death* (1944), *Jungle Captive* (1944), *House Of Horrors* (1946) and *The Brute Man* (1946). The last-named was to be Hatton's final role – the acromegaly killed him shortly after its completion. Although a number of actors have traditionally played on their 'ugly' looks to sustain careers as horror actors – more recent examples include Reggie Nalder (*Mark Of The Devil*, *Salem's Lot*) and Michael Berryman (*The Hills Have Eyes*, *Deadly Blessing*) – none has been as extreme a case as Rondo Hatton. This equation of physical ugliness with evil persists, sadly, to this day.

Occurrences of human anomalies in mainstream or big-budget films (except for dwarfs, and 'giants' such as Ted "Lurch" Cassidy or Richard Kiel) became increasingly rare after the '40s; only more marginal entries dared to enter this area without 'legitimate' cause. Federico Fellini's *Satyricon* (1969), his version of Petronius' ancient Rome, is one such case. Fellini wilfully fills the screen with a succession of grotesqueries, images both beautiful and bestial, ghastly and gorgeous; amidst the flagellation, pederasty, sodomy and bestiality we find dwarfs, hunchbacks, obese prostitutes and even a (fake) hermaphrodite (Pasquale Baldassare). Obese women also feature in Fellini's *8½* (1963) and *Amarcord* (1973, also notable for its dwarf nun). Italy was also responsible for such lesser items as *House Of Freaks* (1973, originally released as *El Castello Dell'Orrore*), a low-budget sex horror in which dwarf actor Michael Dunn (in one of his last appearances – he killed himself in 1974) may be found next to a giant, a 'missing link', and a bevy of naked girls.

Two or three other instances cropped up in the '70s, including Tinto Brass' *Salon Kitty* (1976) and Michael Winner's *The Sentinel* (1977). Brass' film, a sensationalistic treatment of the S.S.'s notorious Joy Division obviously designed to cash in on the publicity generated by Liliana Cavani's *The Night Porter* (1974), features an extraordinary early sequence where would-be whores for Nazi brothels are put through their paces. In order to possess the right stuff for the job, the women are expected to visit and service a succession of frighteningly deformed monsters in cages. Real 'freaks' are used in this harrowing section of the film. Brass went on to produce the infamous *Caligula* (1980), his apparent attempt to out-Fellini Fellini in depicting a savagely decadent Rome and its attendant retinues of the malformed.

The Sentinel, typically for Michael Winner, strays even further into the realms of bad taste. This over-the-top horror film concerns a very unusual house in New York; in its basement sits a mute priest (John Carradine), whose job is to guard the very gate of Hell. Bizarre residents include a pair of naked lesbian cannibals (Sylvia Miles and Beverly D'Angelo), and a woman (Christina Raines) who slices off her dead father's nose with a breadknife. The climax comes when another crazy tenant (Burgess Meredith) opens up the gate, and Hell's freakishly malformed occupants spill forth. Although Dick Smith's make-up accounted for some of these 'monstrosities', Winner also used a troupe of real human anomalies to portray the supposed embodiments of evil. Quite a stir resulted; whether genuine, or merely hype instigated by the director, remains open to conjecture.

As well as 'freaks of nature', those unfortunate enough to have been crippled through misfortune have appeared in many films. Anti-war films in particular have employed amputees to underline their message; the French director Abel Gance took this one step further. Re-making his classic anti-war film *J'Accuse* in 1938, Gance went to an exceptional extreme. For the climactic scene, which involves the vengeful war dead rising from their graves to prevent the living from precipitating fresh carnage, Gance employed as actors actual facially disfigured war veterans from World War I. Recruited from the *Union des Gueules Cassées* ('The Union of Ruined Faces'), these terribly maimed soldiers – to all intents and purposes playing zombies, but in a 'non-horror' scenario – provide a terrible real-life correlative to the visages of Chaney in *Phantom Of The Opera* and Atwill in *Mystery Of The Wax Museum*. The result was a blurring of reality and fiction, a nightmare vision of decades past – and to come.

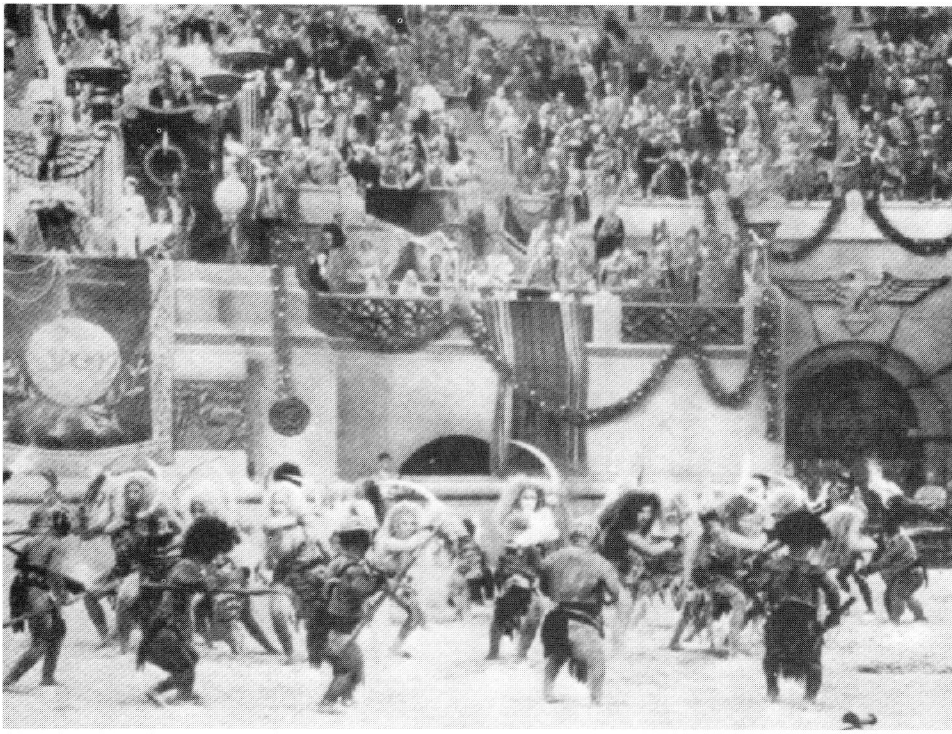

Sign Of The Cross

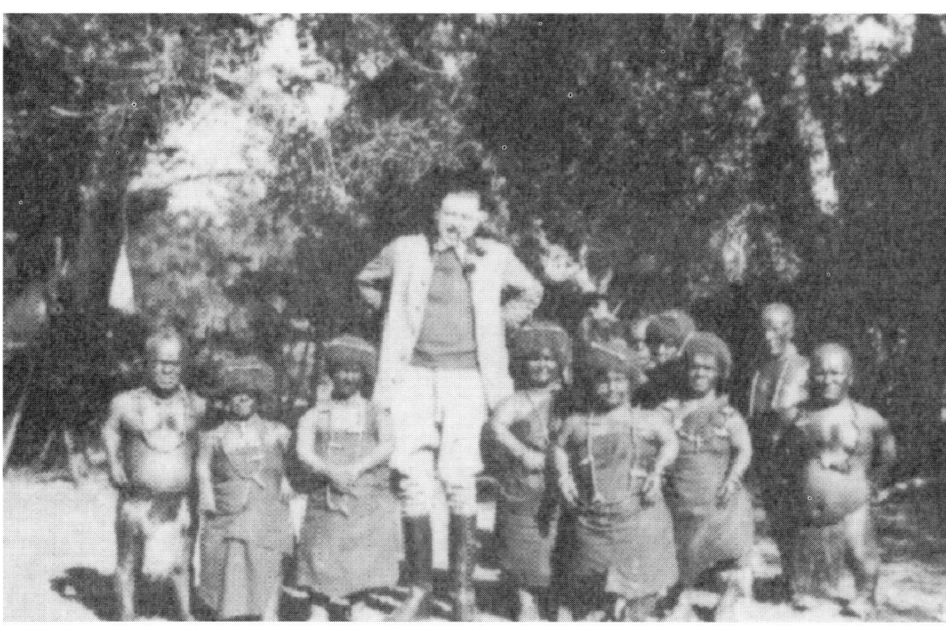

Hollywood Extras c.1935

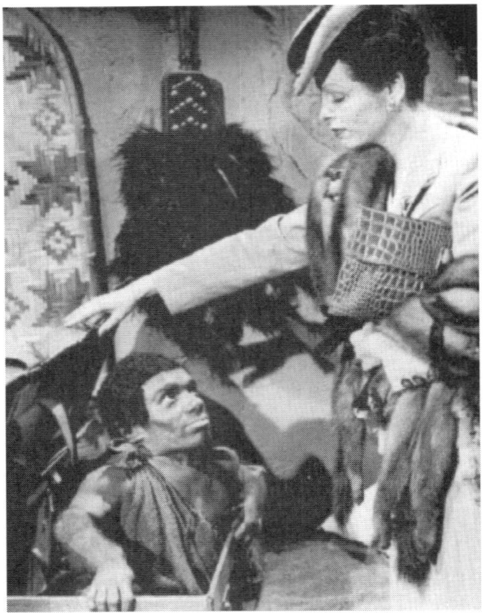

Sherlock Holmes And The Spider Woman

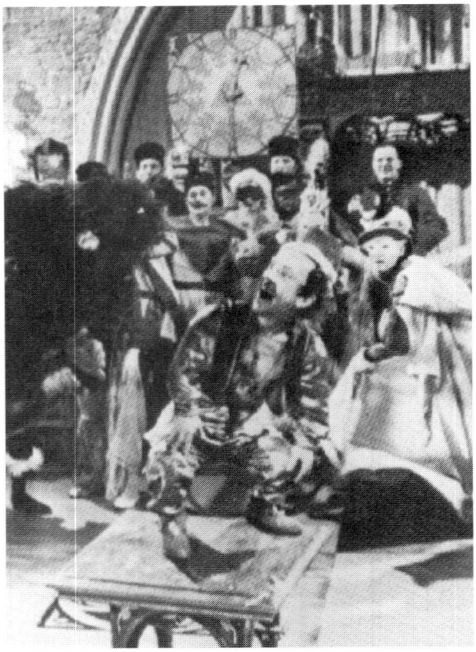

Masque Of The Red Death

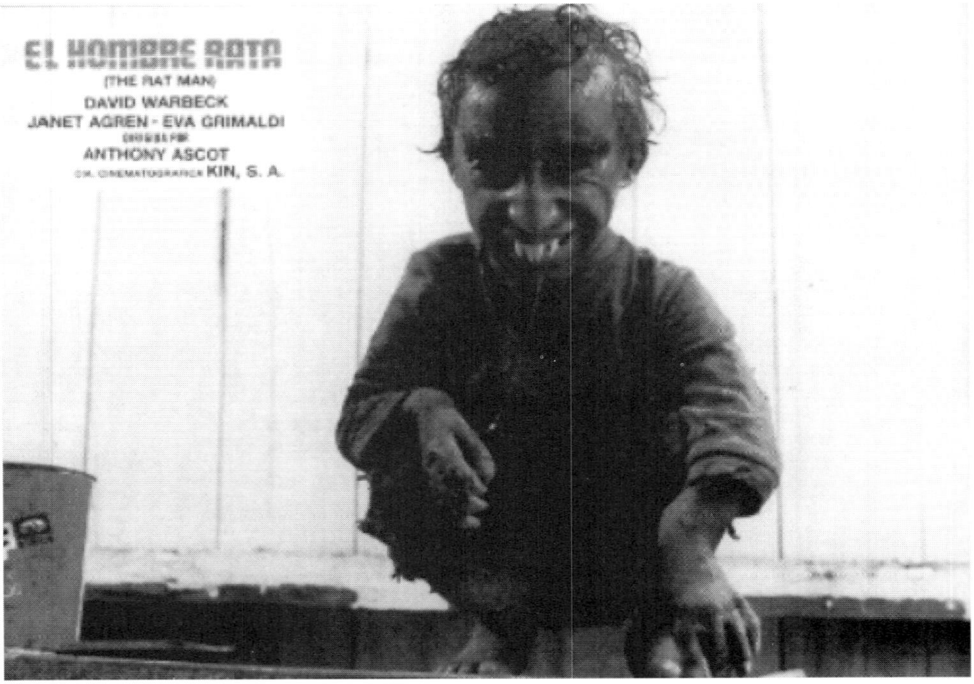

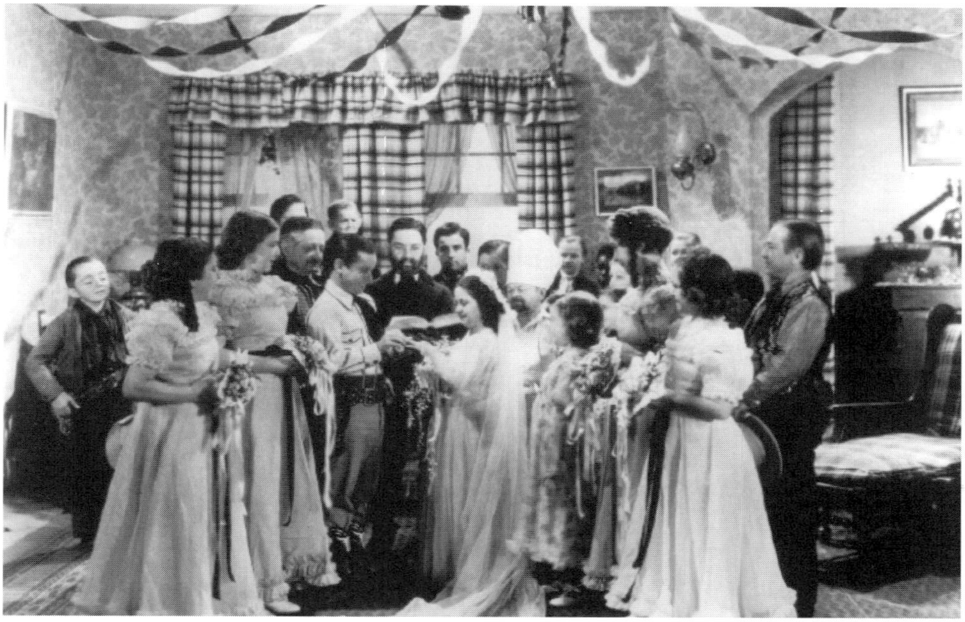

The Terror Of Tiny Town

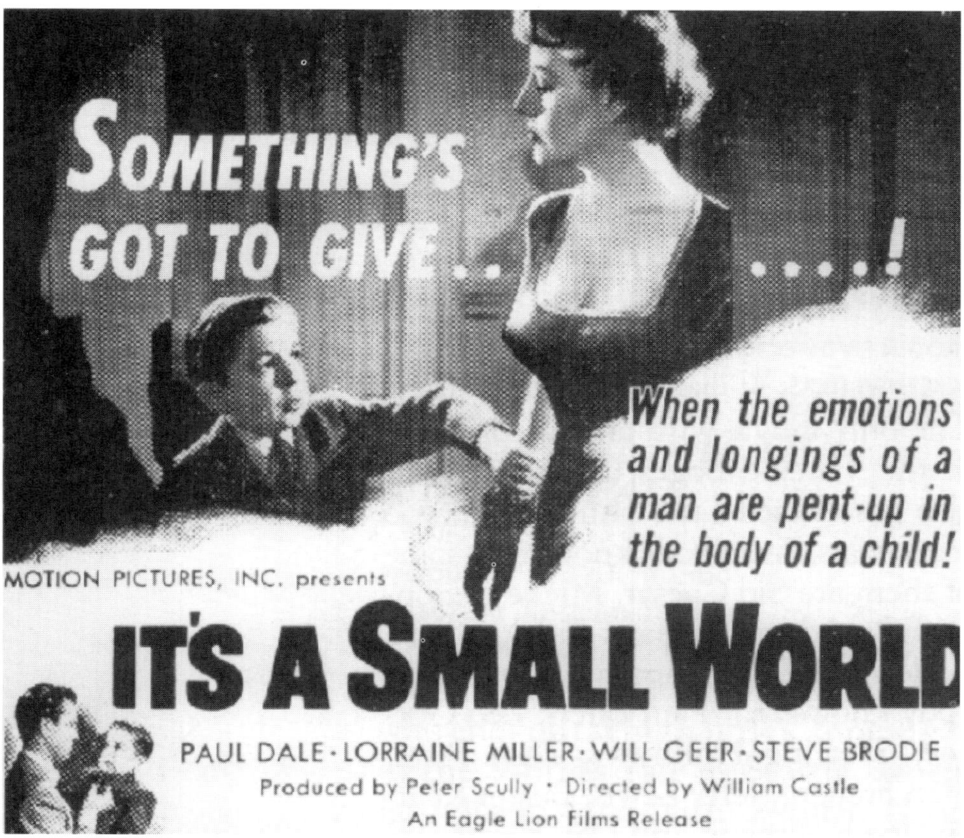
SOMETHING'S
GOT TO GIVE.. ....!
When the emotions
and longings of a
man are pent-up in
the body of a child!
MOTION PICTURES, INC. presents
IT'S A SMALL WORLD
PAUL DALE · LORRAINE MILLER · WILL GEER · STEVE BRODIE
Produced by Peter Scully · Directed by William Castle
An Eagle Lion Films Release

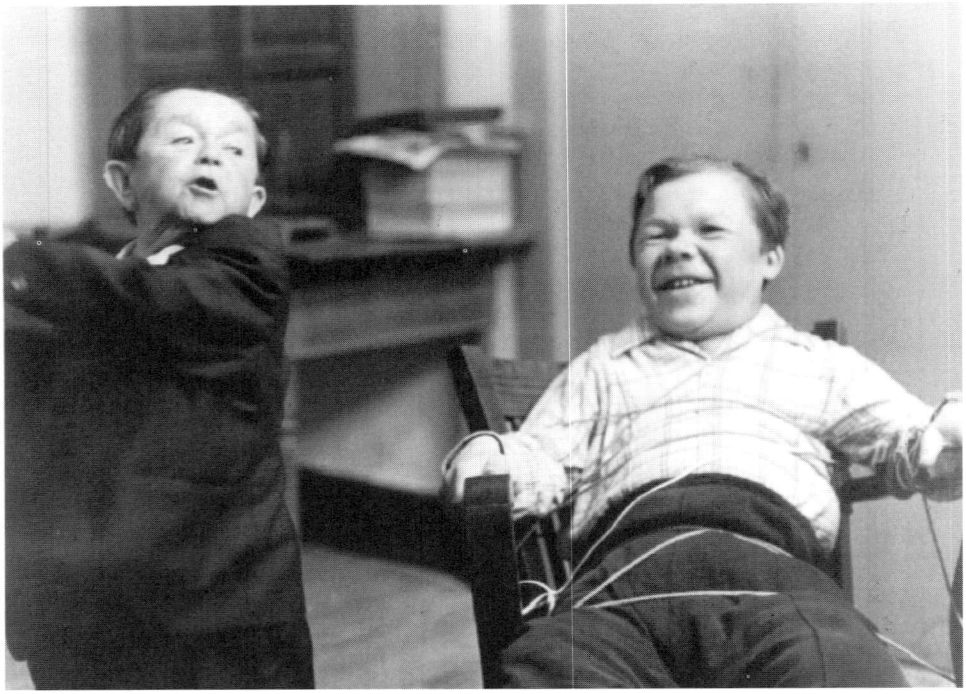

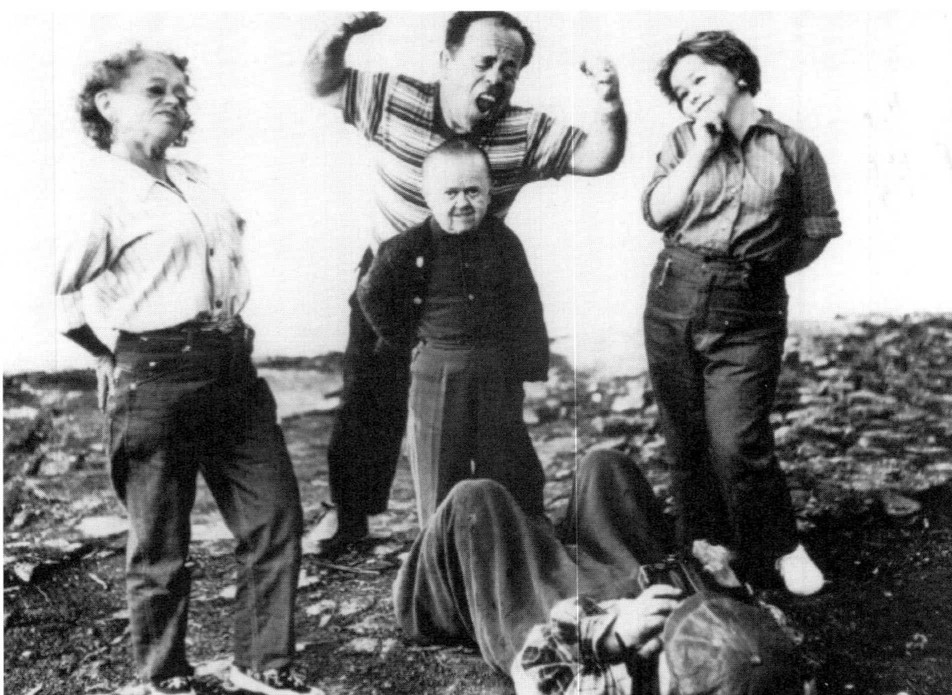

Even Dwarfs Started Small

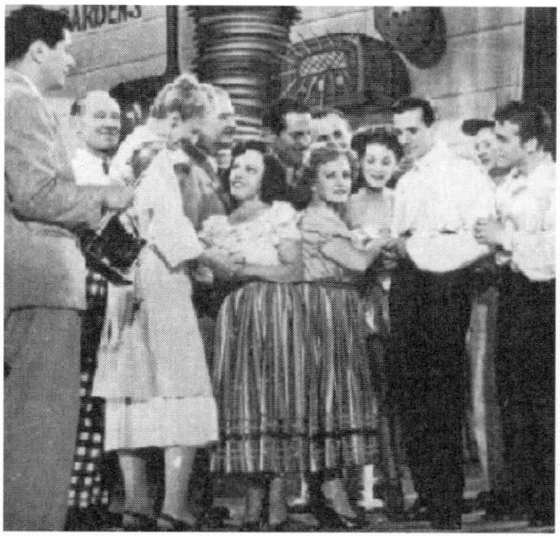

Chained For Life

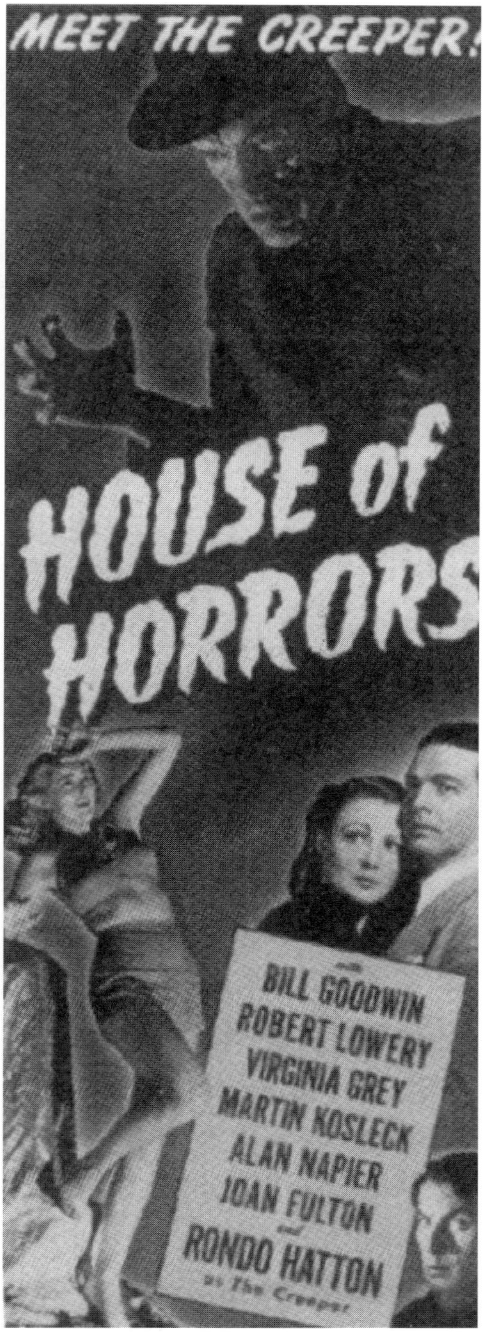

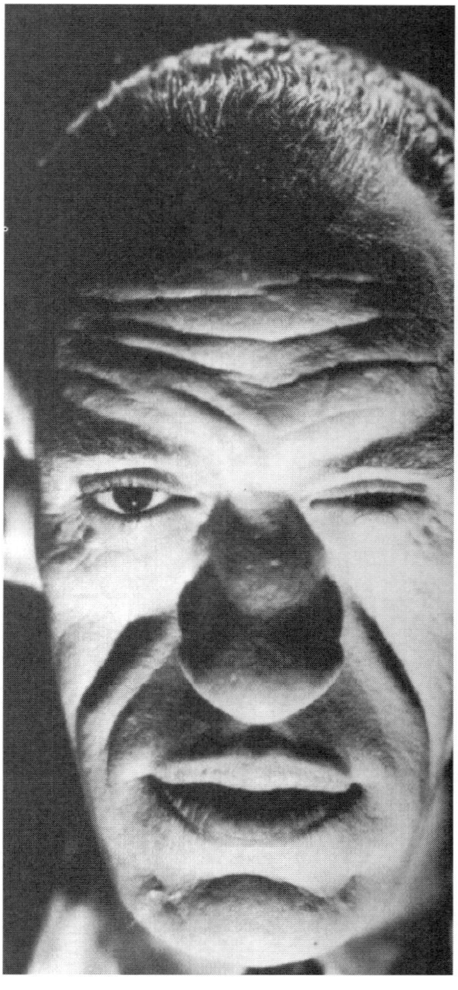

Rondo Hatton

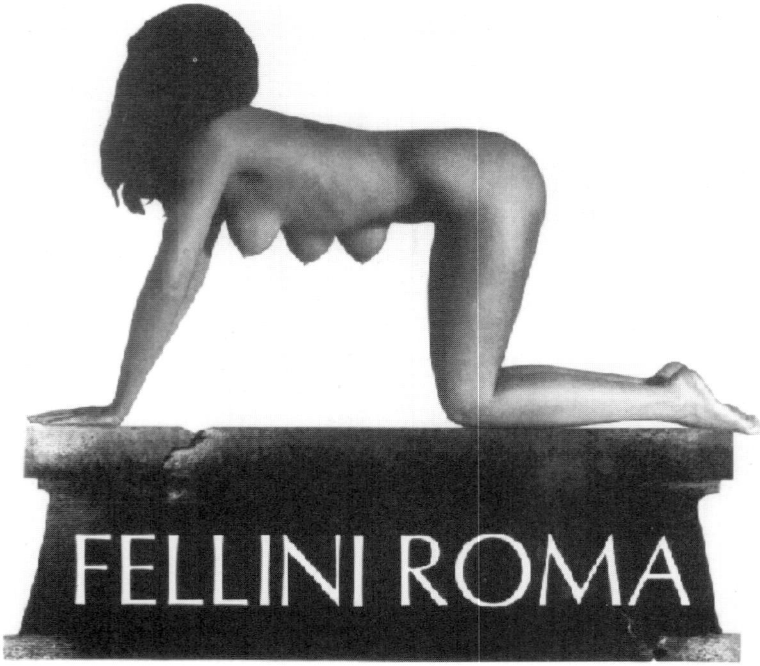

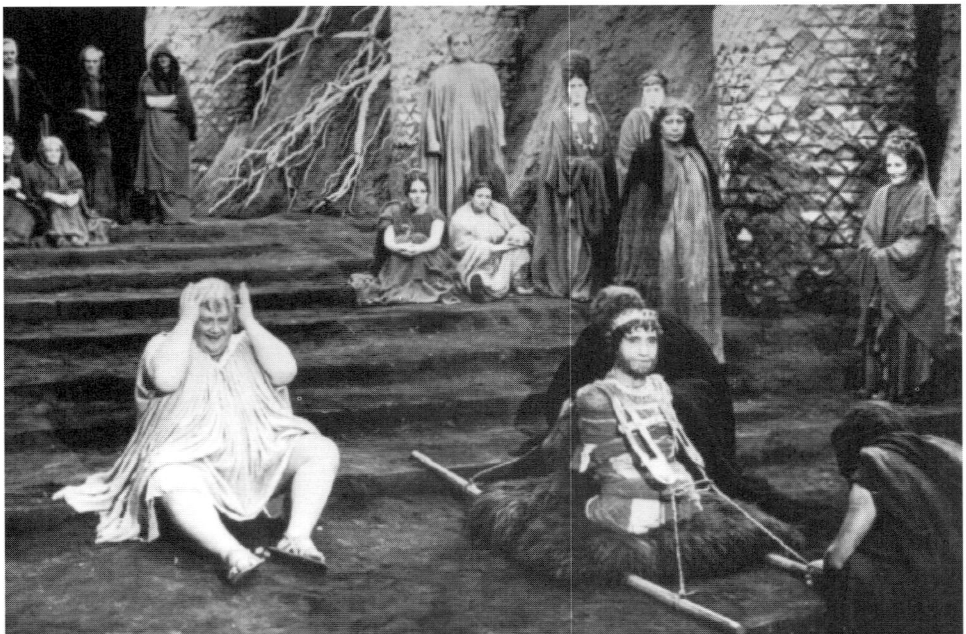

Satyricon

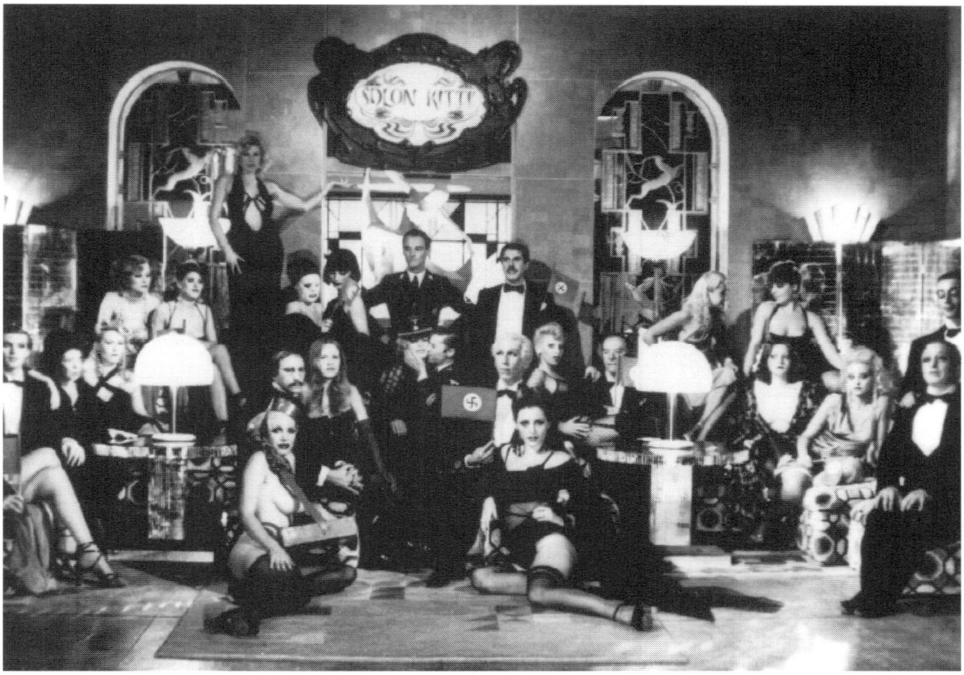

Salon Kitty

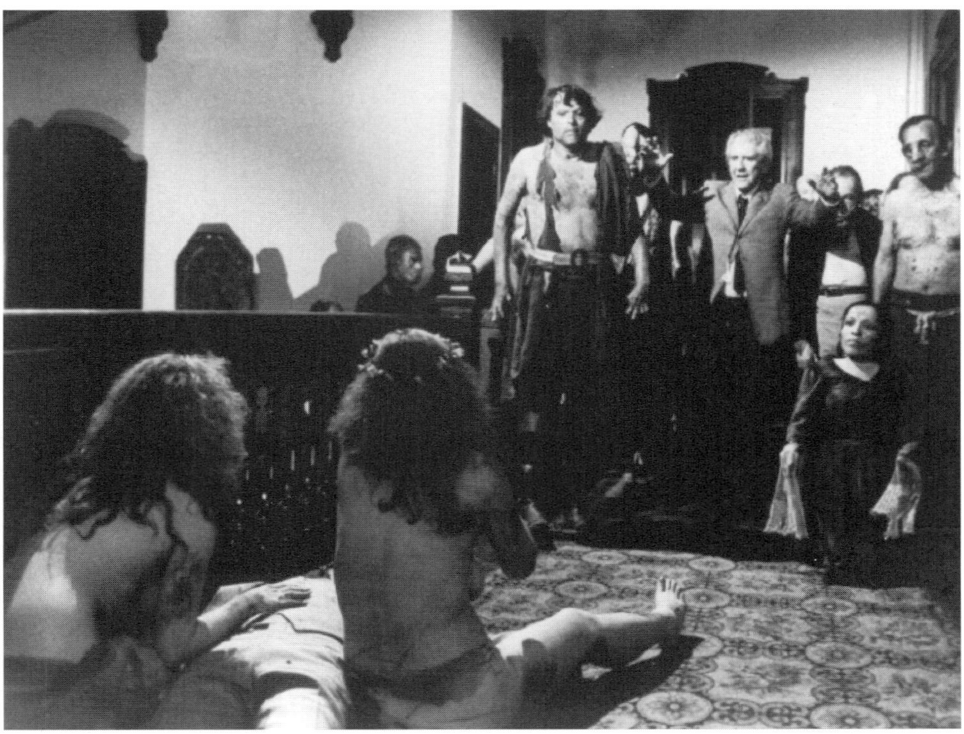

The Sentinel

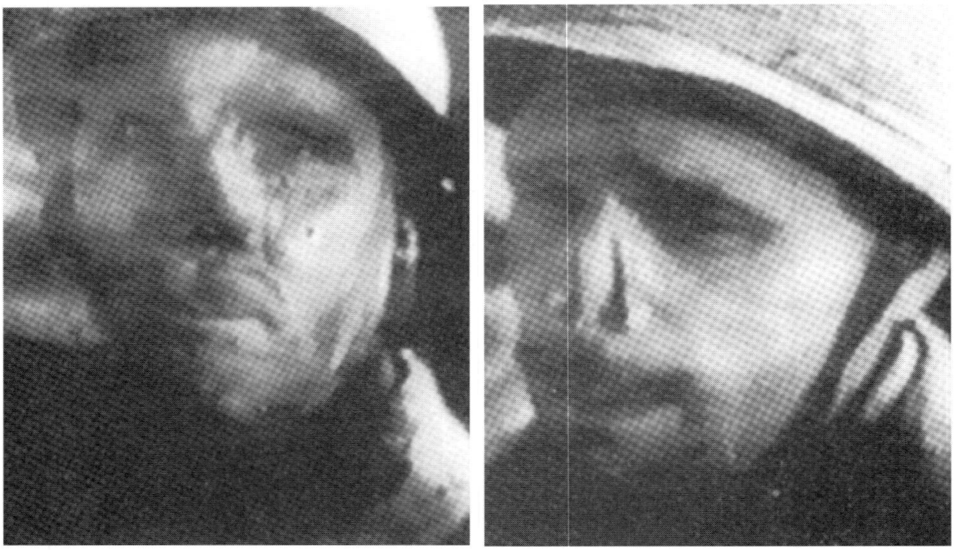

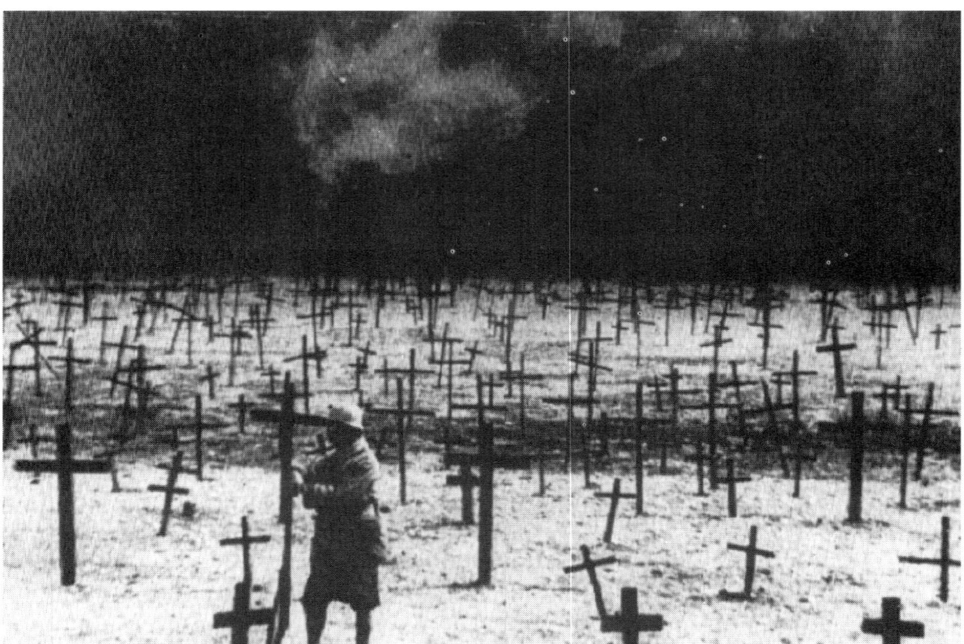

J'Accuse

SKIN SICKNESS

It could be argued that all Freak Film is, by its very nature, pornographic (certainly according to the term's literal meaning). It is undeniably voyeuristic, vicarious, and at times lascivious. Even David Lynch's unimpeachable *The Elephant Man*, as it leads us tantalisingly towards the final unveiling of John Merrick's twisted flesh, exercises the precise effect of a slow striptease. One serious film-maker, in particular, has continually and heavily featured, even eulogised, physical deformity and mutilation to the very point of sexual fetishization. Luis Buñuel, the Spanish master, made his first film, *Un Chien Andalou*, in 1929 with the assistance of the great surrealist Salvador Dalí. From the very start, this classic film assaults the viewer with violent and erotic images. A woman's eyeball is deliberately sliced through with a razorblade, a severed hand is found in the street, priests are chained to rotting donkeys; in one particularly disquieting scene, a man's hand turns into a stump as it caresses a woman's face. His next work, *L'Age D'Or* (1930) – involving Dalí to a lesser extent – was equally controversial; here we see carnal lust expressed as rampant foot fetishism, visions of churning excrement, an explicit reference to the Marquis de Sade (when Christ is depicted in the role of the Duc de Blangis, leaving the Château de Selliny after an abominable season of murderous orgies), and a typical example of Buñuel black humour when the film's hero brutally and gleefully kicks a blind man to the ground. Buñuel next made *Tierra Sin Pan*, another unflinching gaze at human cruelty, while Dalí confined his visions of mutant flesh to canvas;[1] having declared that "Hitler has four balls and six foreskins", he went on to depict a freak Lenin with grotesquely elongated buttocks (*The Enigma Of William Tell*), following works like this with the even more horrific autophagous apocalypses of *Soft Construction With Boiled Beans: Premonition Of Civil War* and *Autumn Cannibalism*.[2]

Buñuel, after a period of inactivity, repeated the sadism of his early films in *Los Olvidados* (1950), where a blind beggar is surrounded by jeering youths, knocked over and robbed (typically, Buñuel confuses our sympathies by making the blind man a paedophile). In the same film, a legless man is lifted bodily from his cart, stumps waggling in the air, and hurled into the gutter. The Sadeian theme is repeated in *El* (1953), as we see the protagonist, armed with rope, needles and thread, set off to sew up his wife's sexual organs;

Viridiana (1961) features a blasphemous parody of the Last Supper as a horde of filthy, lecherous beggars and cripples hold a drunken revel; dwarfs feature with religious significance in *Nazarin* (1958) and *La Voie Lactée* (1969); the severed hand crops up again in *El Angel Exterminador* (1962). Buñuel's apparent obsession with female feet and legs, demonstrated throughout these films by images of thighs bathed in milk, coated in crushed eggs, glimpsed teasingly between stocking and suspender and even splattered in blood, is emphasised by the shoe fetishes in *The Young Girl* (1960) and *Diary Of A Chambermaid* (1964), and reaches its culmination in *Tristana* (1970). Here, an old man's object of desire (Catherine Deneuve) has her leg amputated below the knee; the man drools over her stump, while she dreams of his severed head impaled on a bell clapper.

In his universe of perverse desires and suffering, peopled by cripples, amputees, dwarfs, priests and beggars, Buñuel has gone as far, if not further, than Tod Browning in attempting to express the outer limits of human obsession in transmutations of the flesh; the physical evidence of man's religious compulsions toward murder and mutilation, the poetry of the sado-masochistic impulse, are expressed with near-pornographic revulsion.

It is not surprising that a director of Luis Buñuel's stature should inspire imitators; that one of his apparent 'disciples' should turn out to become a powerful and original film-maker in his own right is perhaps more unusual. The Chilean director Alejandro Jodorowsky demanded immediate attention with his first professional feature, the fascinating *El Topo* (1971); like King Hu's *A Touch Of Zen* transposed to a Fellini-spaghetti Western, this audacious film is an incandescent attempt to define a new cinema of the psyche. Jodorowsky (who also plays the lead role) fills the screen with obscene beauties, dazzling grotesqueries and bloody, Biblical mayhem in depicting one man's odyssey in search of revelation. The story follows El Topo (The Mole) as he rides with his son through nameless desert landscapes pocked by disembowelled mules, raped and butchered brides, rivers of blood, and graves brimming with rabbits or bees, encountering transvestite bandits, ancient prostitutes, four Zen Masters and a labyrinth haunted by thousands of cripples, dwarfs, idiot children and other deformed beings. Jodorowsky's most alarming creation is the Double Man, composed of a legless man who rides strapped on the shoulders of an armless man to form a single entity. After a succession of violent events, including castration, rape, flagellation, and multiple assassinations, El Topo sires a new child by a dwarf and then sets fire to himself in a final act of self-immolation.

In defence of this unparalleled catalogue of atrocities, Jodorowsky has said: "With every new picture, I must change myself, I must kill myself, and I must be born. I must kill the actors and they must be born. And the audiences, the audiences who go to the movies, must be assassinated, killed, destroyed, and they must leave the theatre as new people. This is a good picture." For once, a director has achieved his aim. *El Topo* has been reviled by many as self-indulgent, blasphemous, and unintelligible; yet it remains a unique experience, and Jodorowsky's faithful were finally rewarded when he delivered his masterpiece to date, the previously-discussed *Santa Sangre*.

Traces of Buñuel may also be found in the universe of Jodorowsky's collaborator Fernando Arrabal (whose *Fando And Lys*, a tale of tar babies, was filmed by the Chilean prior to *El Topo*), both in his films as director (such as *J'Irai Comme Un Cheval Fou* [1973], in which he presents us with the uncomfortable juxtaposition of a razor blade and an erect penis, *Viva La Muerte* [1970]) with its cast of degenerates, and *L'Arbre De Guernica* [1975]) and as actor (he appears in Jacques Baratier's sado-masochistic trip *Piège* [1968] as a seller of man-traps).

One of the many scenes of blood and blasphemy in Peter Fleischmann's *Dorothea* (1973), showing a one-legged man crucified in a torture dungeon, also carries a distinct echo of the Spanish master, an explicit expression of the S/M fantasies hinted at in the latter's *Belle De Jour* (1967); this predilection also found full flower in the likes of Barbet Schroeder's *Maîtresse* (1976).

Physical fetishization was also present to a large extent in the films of '60s American exploitation directors such as Russ Meyer and Doris Wishman. Meyer's mammary obsession pervades every one of his monomaniacal films, from his early 'nudie' *The Immoral Mr. Teas* (1960), to 'roughies' like *Lorna* (1964) and *Faster, Pussycat! Kill! Kill!* (1965). In the latter, Tura Satana leads a trio of super-fit, dominating women in an assault against a crippled old man in a wheelchair and his musclebound, moronic son, known as Vegetable. Most men might hesitate to describe Lorna Maitland, Tura Satana or Kitten Natividad (hyper-pneumatic star of *Beneath The Valley Of The Ultra-Vixens* [1979]) as 'freaks', but in Meyer's oeuvre they have become precisely that; women deliberately chosen, displayed and exploited for their physical abnormality. This mammary madness was taken to its probable ultimate by Doris Wishman in her films *Double Agent 73* (1972) and *Deadly Weapons* (1973), starring the uniquely endowed Chesty Morgan, whose bust measured in at an astonishing 73". In these paeans to male infantilism Chesty, playing a secret agent, gets to smother men to death with her giant breasts, and even has a hidden camera installed in one of them.

Moving into the area of hardcore pornography, we find Chesty Morgan's male counterpart: the late, legendary Johnny 'The Wad' Holmes. Probably the first genuine hardcore superstar, Holmes' unique attribute was his 14" penis, which certainly qualifies him as a genuine human anomaly; meanwhile, the initial publicity for the notorious *Deep Throat* (1972) was based around the claim that its star, Linda Lovelace, had her genitals in her throat – a freak condition which has yet to actually make the medical textbooks. Just as live sex peepshows have replaced the traditional sideshows, so the basic achievement of hardcore porn – the reduction of the human form to meat – is arguably on a par with the dehumanizing tendencies of the old-style, more easily identified freak movie. When hardcore strays into areas such as coprophilia and bestiality (*The Pig-Fucking Movie*, *Dog Fucker* [Lovelace again]), or mutant S/M as in *Sex O'Clock USA*, *New York City Inferno*, *Slave Sex* or *Born To Raise Hell*, the 'geek' connection is made even more apparent.[3]

The final word in excess meat goes to Walerian Borowczyk, whose *The Beast* (1975) sees a maiden literally fuck to death a creature with a horse-sized member, and in whose surreal, caged apocalypse of a film *Blood For Dr Jekyll* (1981), a psychotic stalker (Udo Kier) literally impales and gores the women of a sunken house with his rampant and murderous foot-long penis.

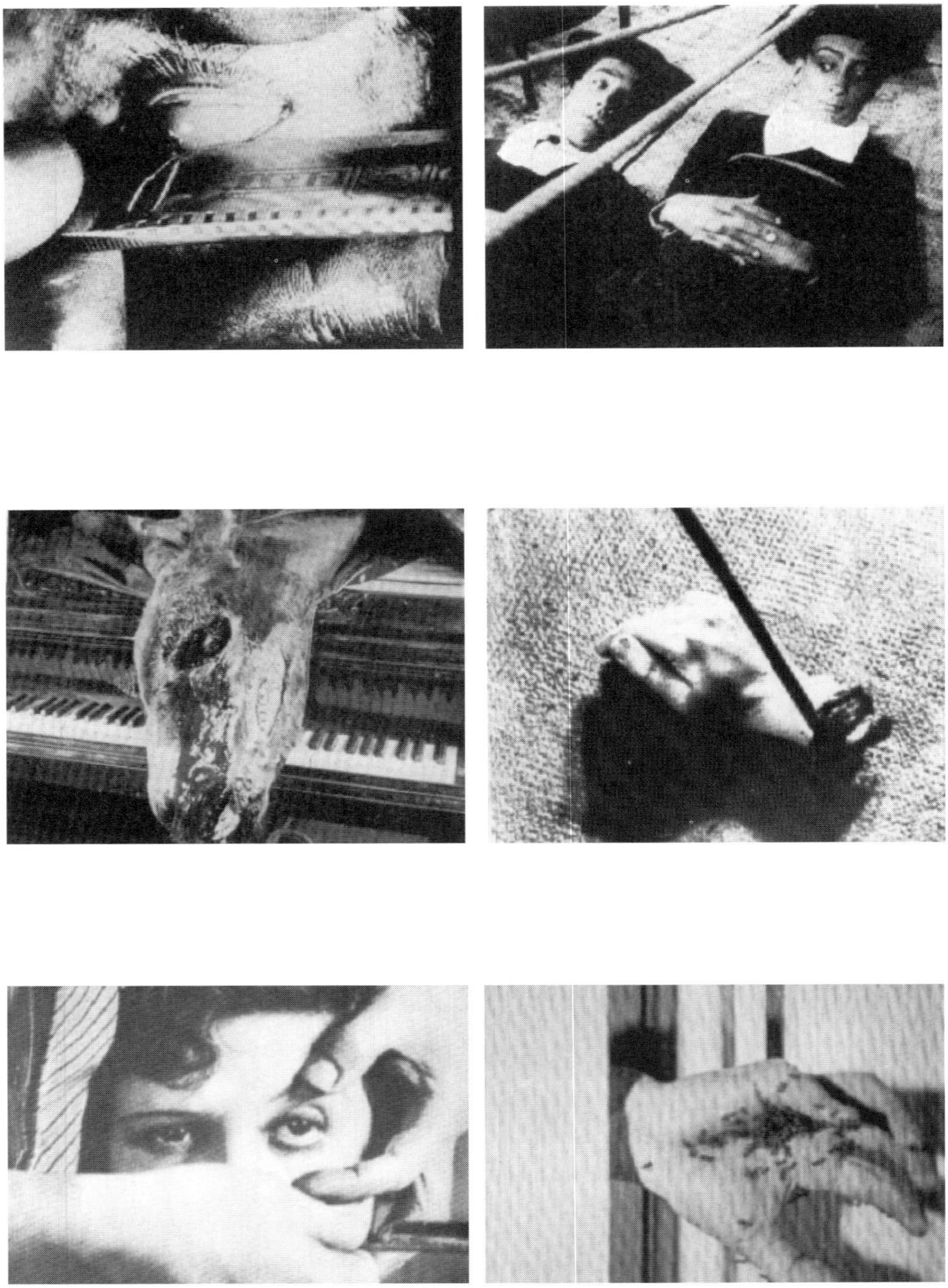

Un Chien Andalou

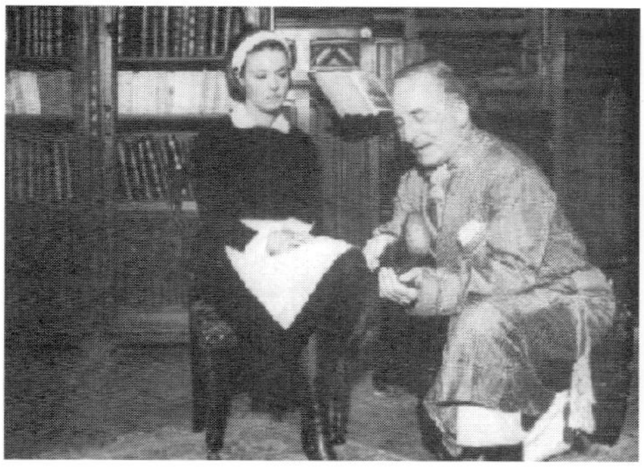

Diary Of A Chambermaid

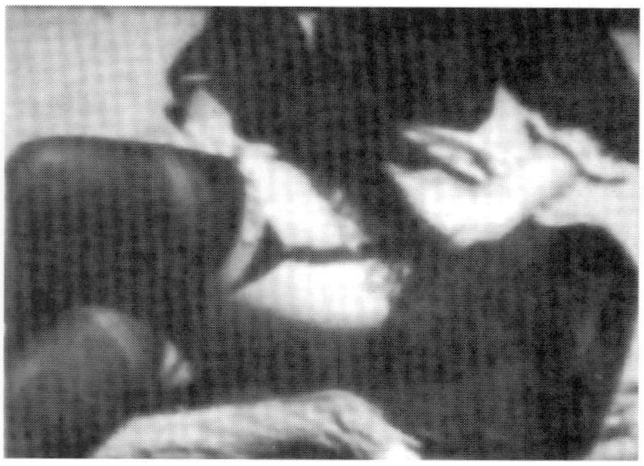

Simon Of The Desert

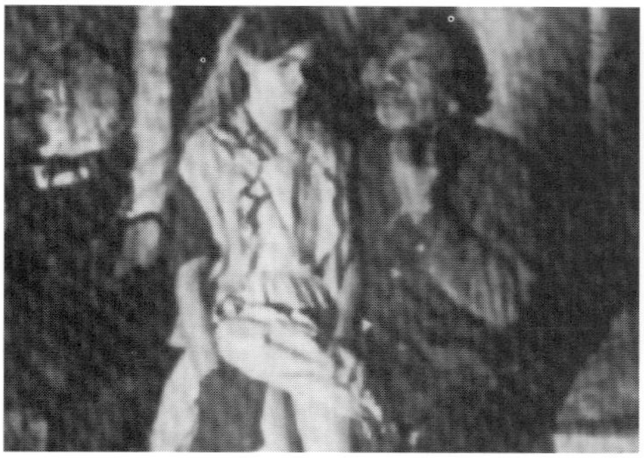

Los Olvidados

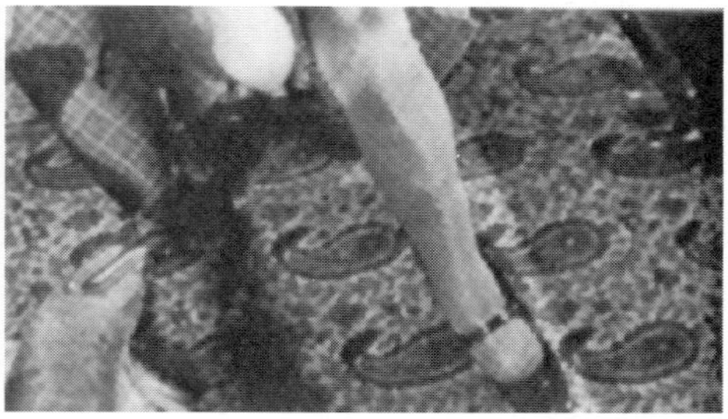

Tristana

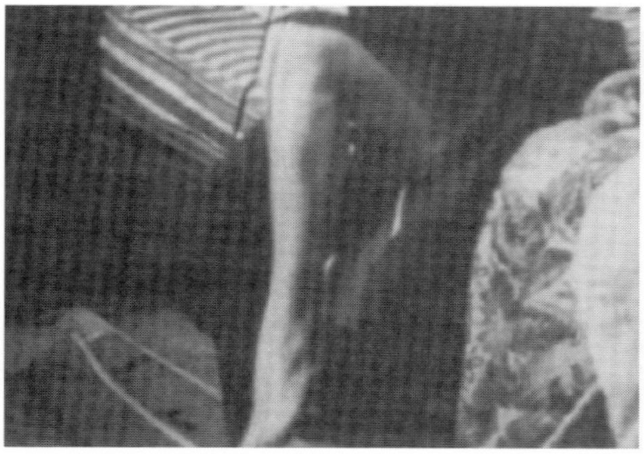

Viridiana

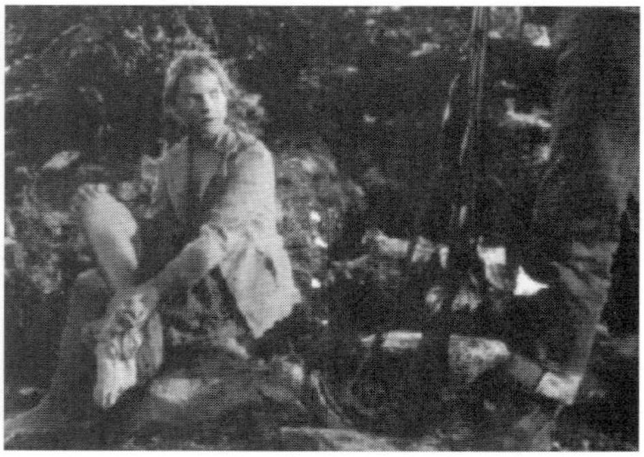

The Young One

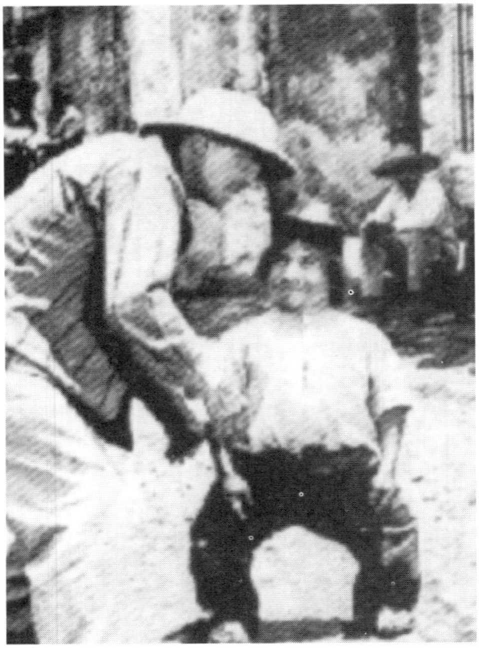

Nazarin

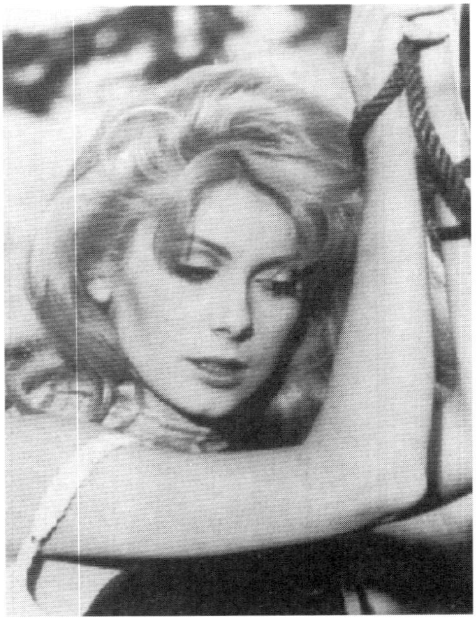

Belle De Jour

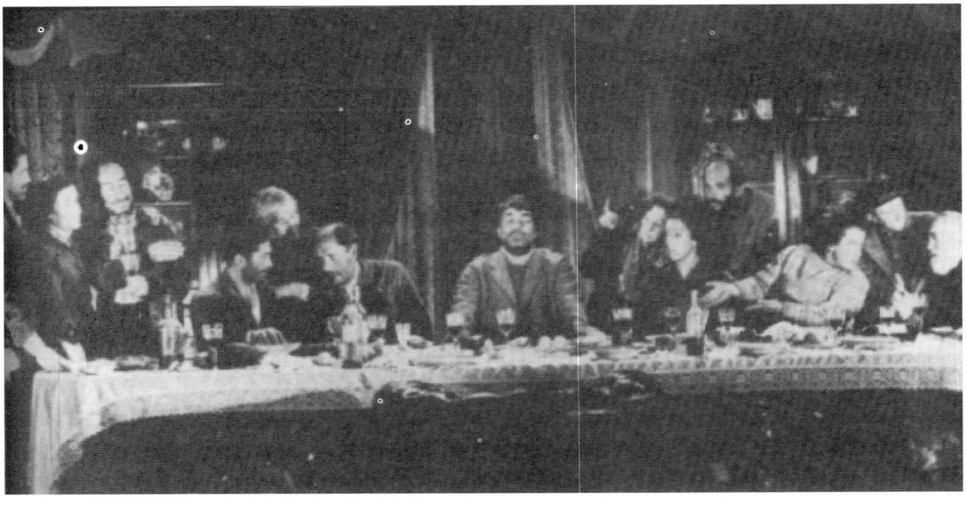

Viridiana

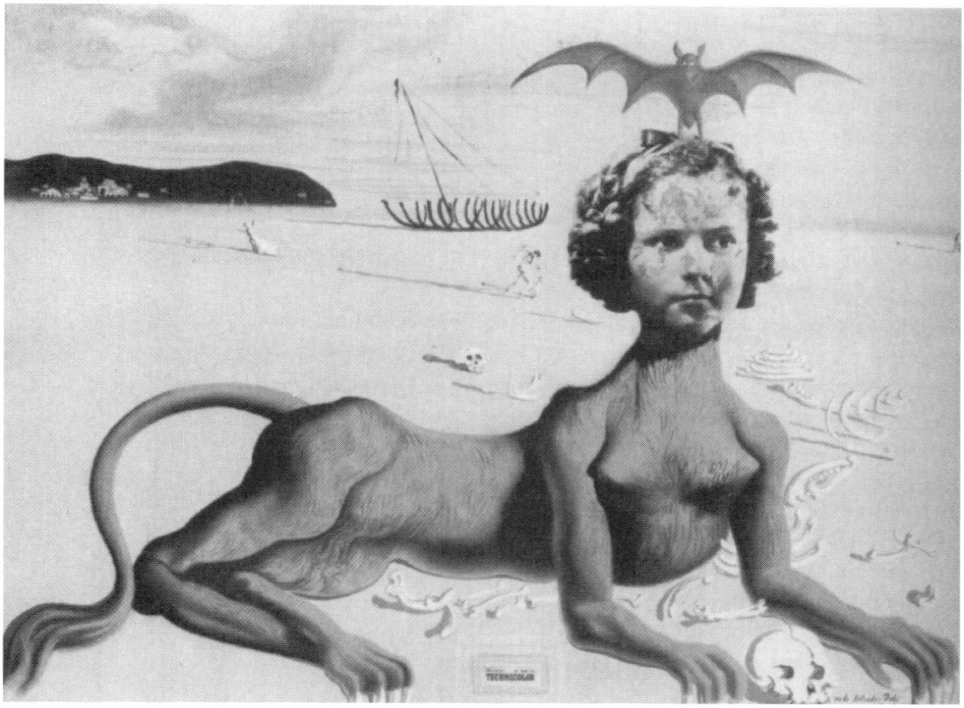

Salvador Dali; *Shirley Temple, The Youngest Sacred Monster Of Contemporary Cinema*

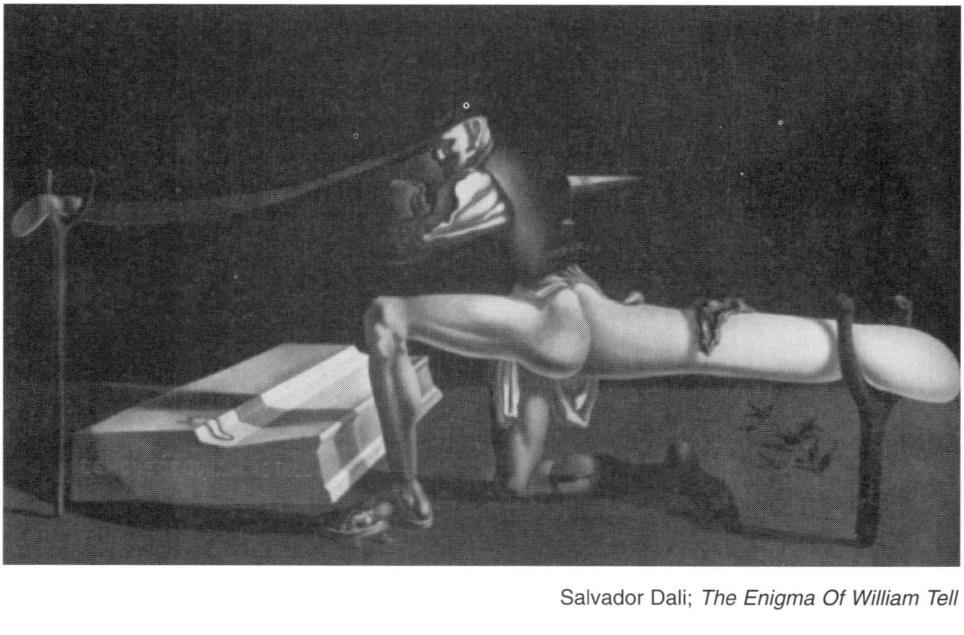

Salvador Dali; *The Enigma Of William Tell*

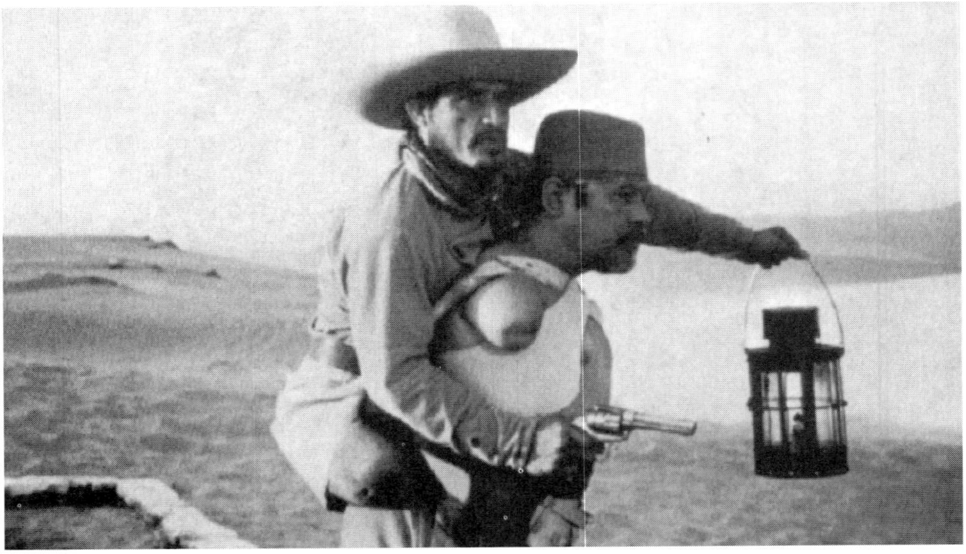

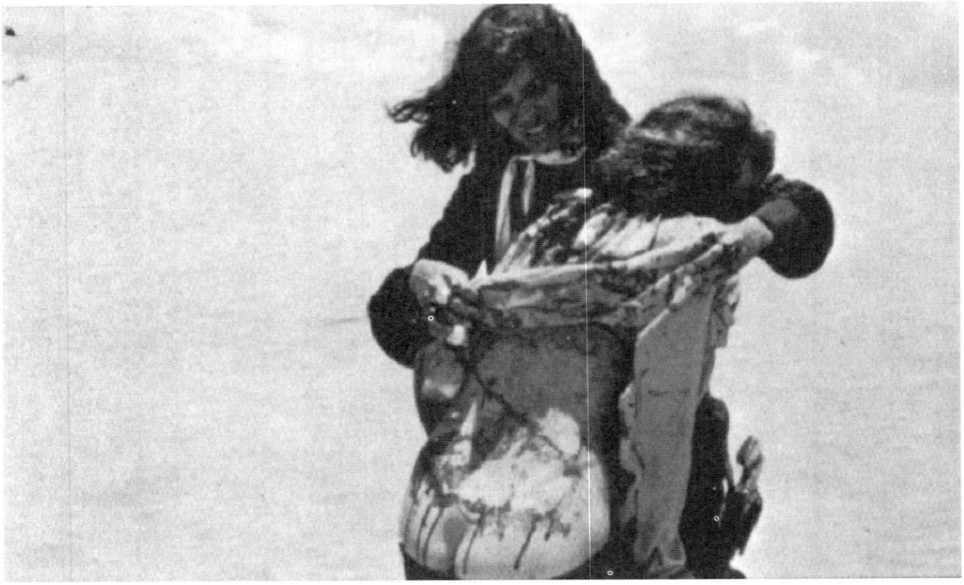

El Topo

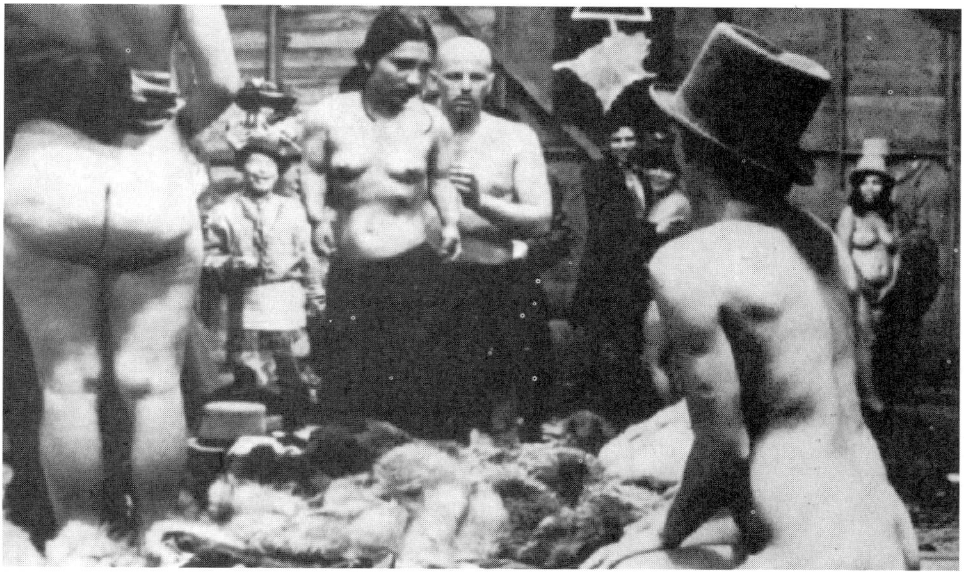

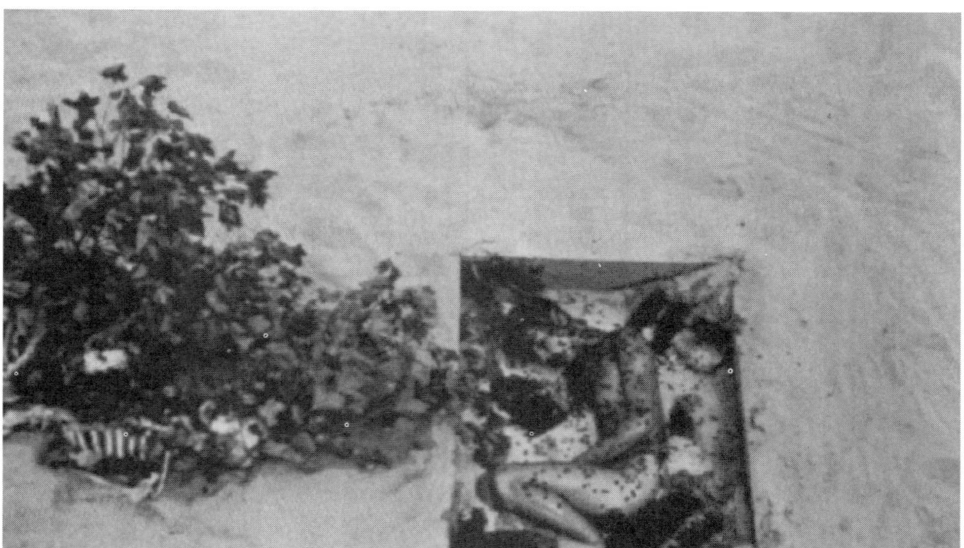

El Topo

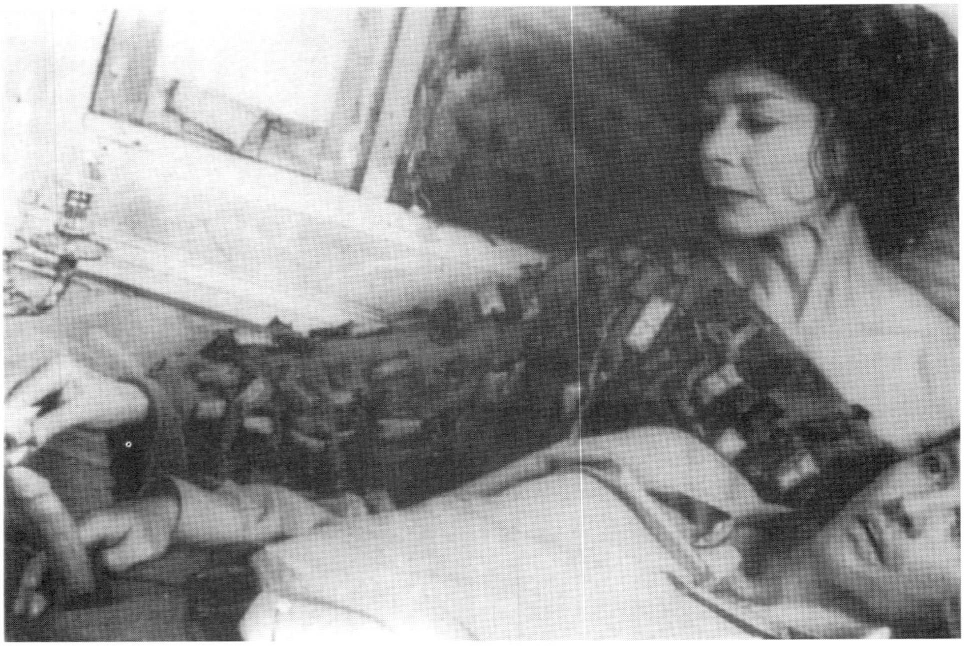

J'Irai Comme Un Cheval Fou

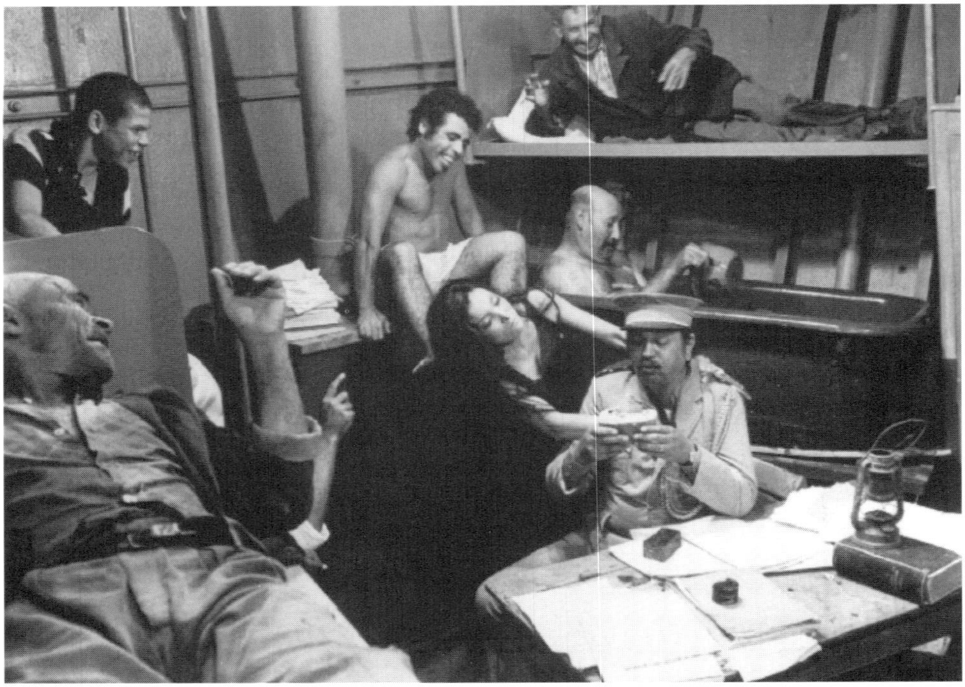

Viva La Muerte

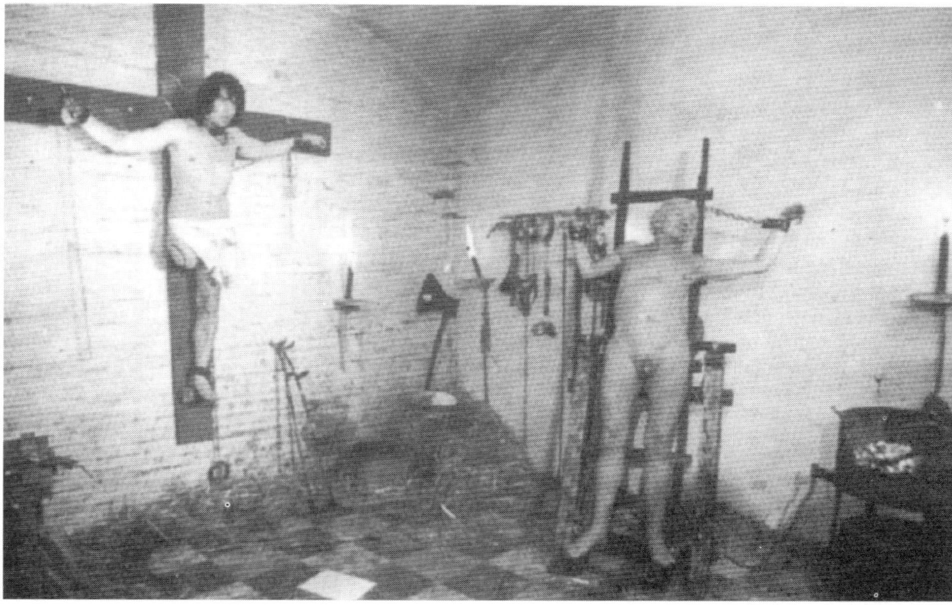

Dorothea

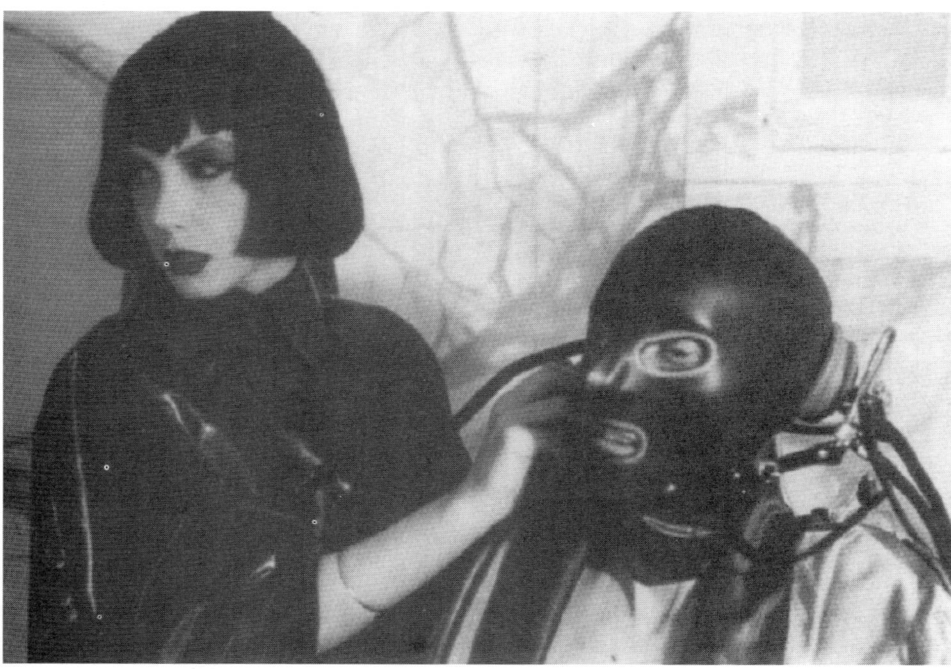

Maîtresse

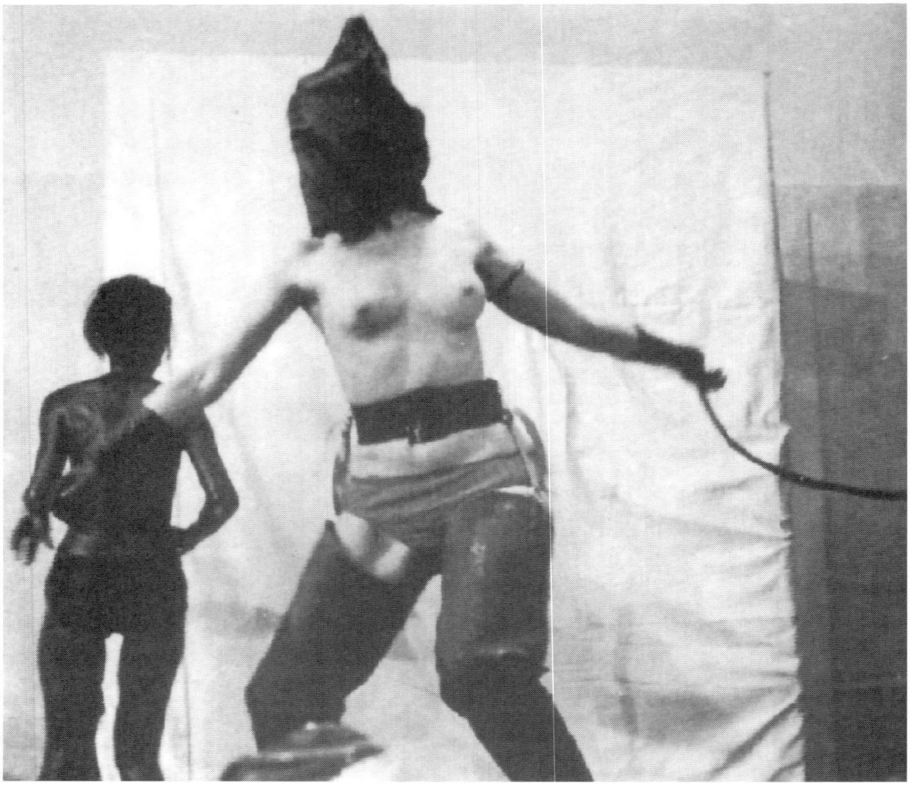

A Jodorowsky happening

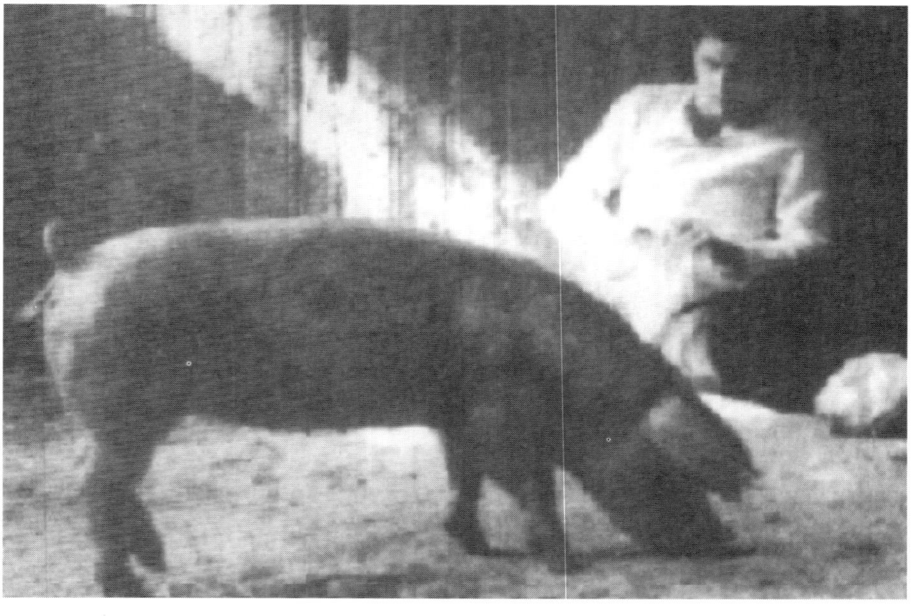

The Pig-Fucking Movie

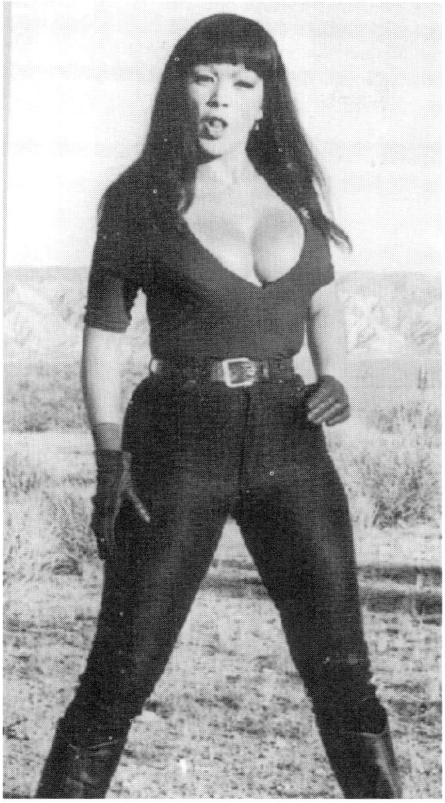

Tura Satana

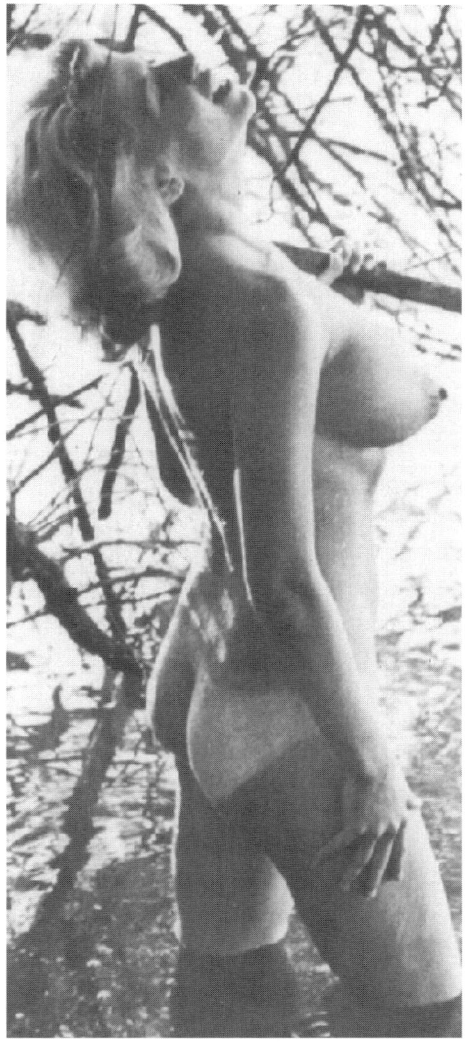

Lorna

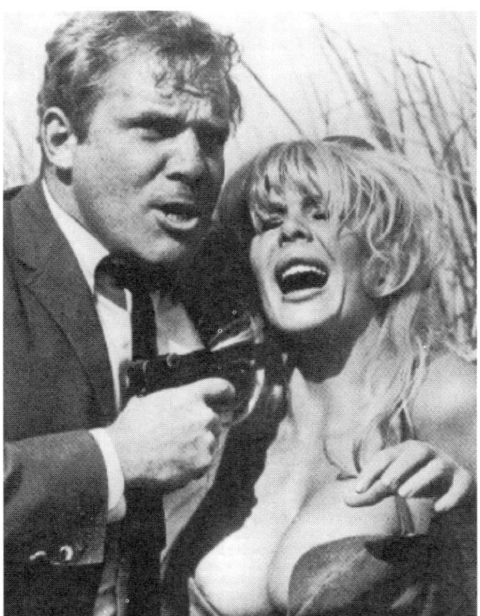

Common Law Cabin

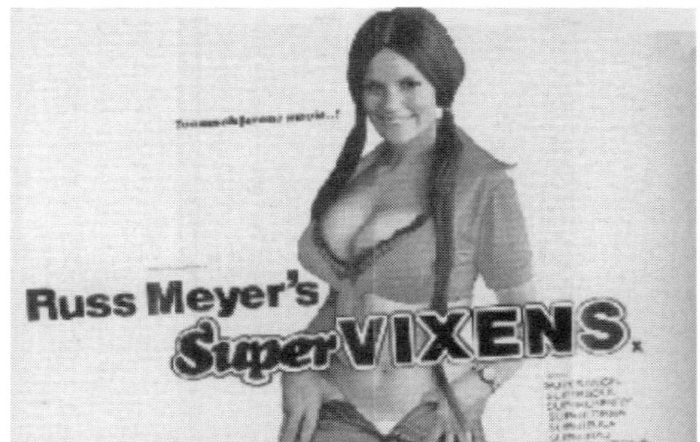

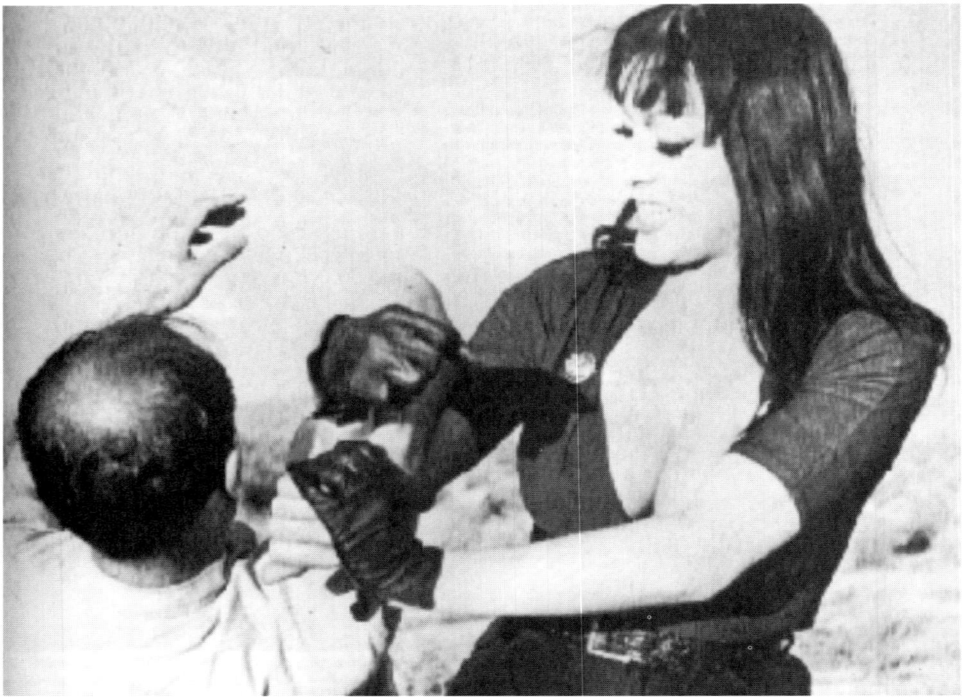

Faster, Pussycat! Kill! Kill!

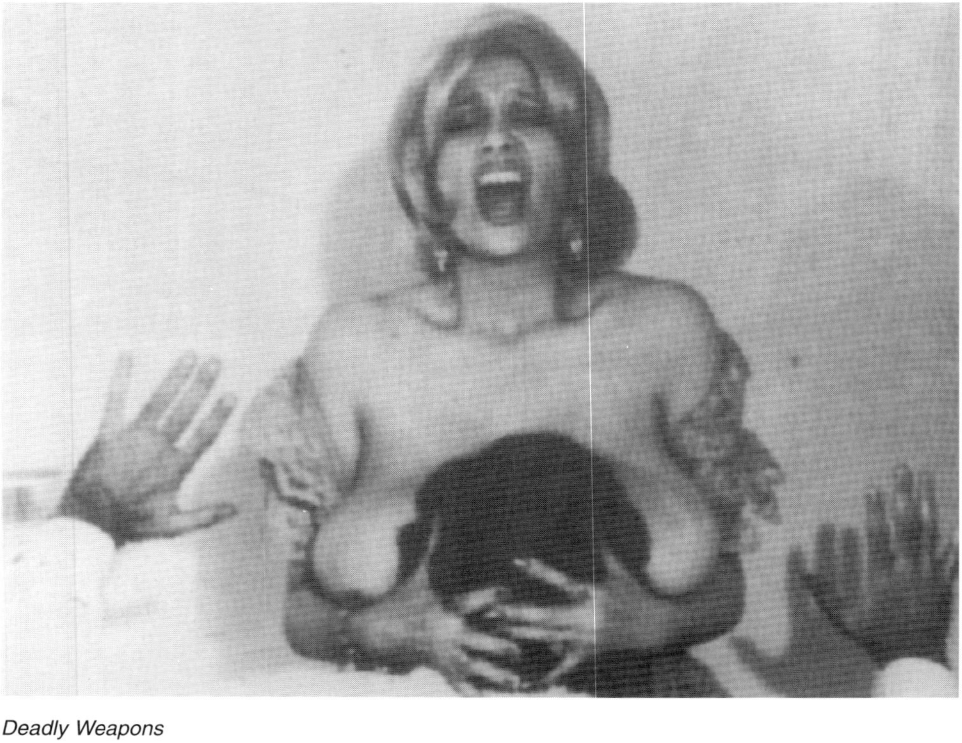

Deadly Weapons

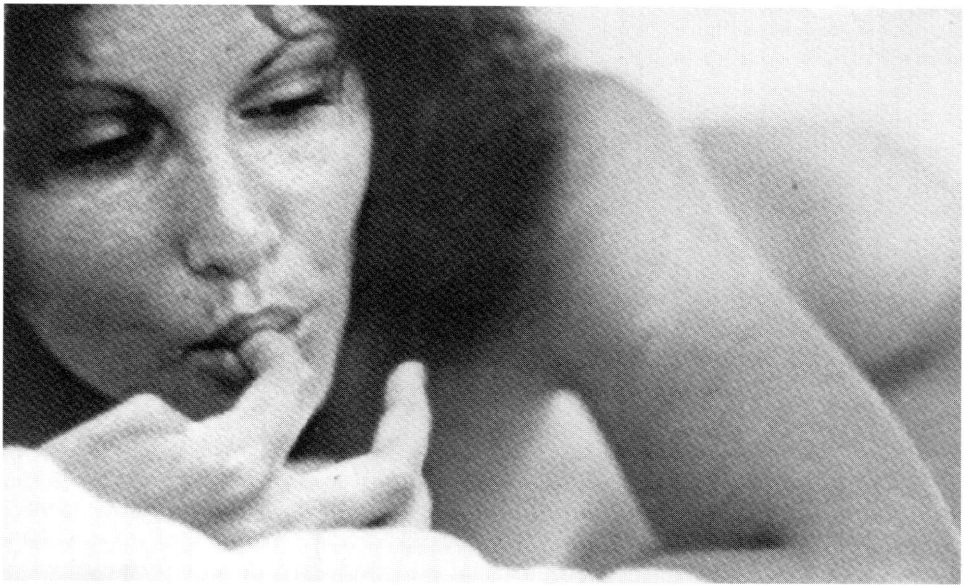

Deep Throat

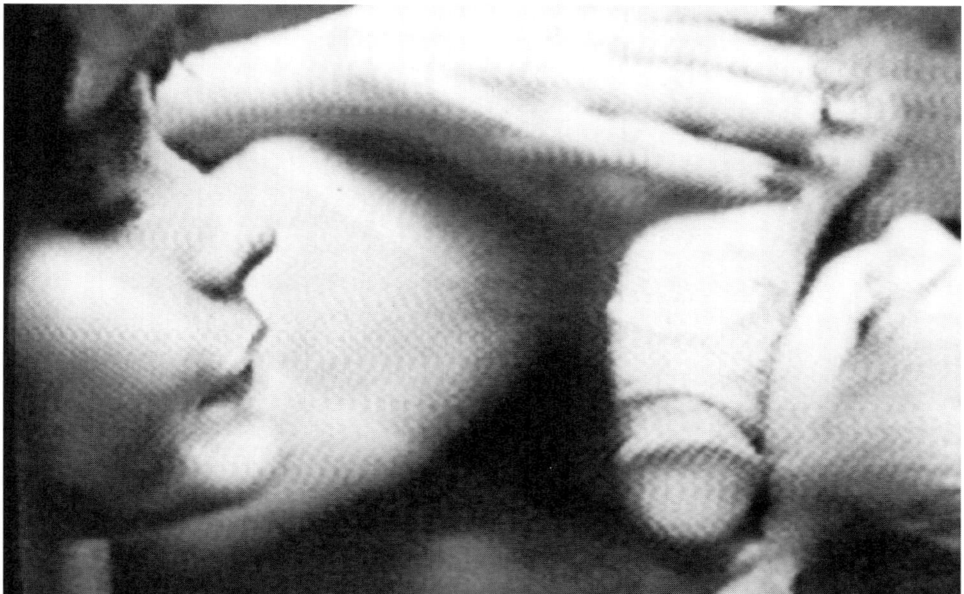

Johnny Holmes

THE SNAKE PIT

The porno cinema, like horror cinema, has been around in one form or another since the very invention of moving pictures; in the 1960s, the specifically voyeuristic nature of bizarre cinema was isolated and magnified in a new strain of demi-commercial film which in many ways presented a hybrid of freak, geek and peek: the Mondo movie. 'Mondo' – deriving from the Italian film *Mondo Cane* (Gualtiero Jacopetti, 1962) – was coined to describe a type of film which had in fact been around in a milder form for many years. True-life documentary, essentially voyeuristic, focusing in particular on strange or exotic people and rites from all corners of the globe. *Mondo Cane*'s impact resulted in the genre being firmly recognised, named and established; from then on it was a race to see who could come up with the most outrageous/offensive subject matter in a long series of films stretching into the '80s. Where *Mondo Cane* had been content with showing the likes of a woman giving suck to a pig, *Mondo Cane 2* (Jacopetti & Franco Prosperi, 1963) showed a (reportedly fake) act of self-immolation. *Kwaheri* (Thor Brooks, David Chudnow, 1964) boasted pygmy sex orgies, *Secret Paris* circus freaks, *Mondo Bizarro* (R L Frost, 1966) a human pin-cushion, *Secret Africa* (Guido Guerrasio, 1969) native 'geeks' eating live maggots and other insects, *Mondo Magic* (Alfredo & Angelo Castiglioni, 1974) scenes of jumping natives with over-sized genitals, *This Violent World* (Antonio Climati, Mario Morra, 1978) a fakir impaling his body and genitals with needles, *Bizarre Rituals: Dances Sacred And Profane* (Charles Gatewood, 1985) various other body modifications, *Let Me Die A Woman* (Doris Wishman, 1976) transsexual surgery, *Sex By Advertisement* (Joel M Reed, 1969) a marriage broker preying on physically disabled clients, *Shocking Asia 2* (Emerson Fox, 1985) 'dancing girls' pulling razor-blades from their vaginas, *Noi E Amore* (Antonio D'Agostino) various scenes of bestiality and urolagnia. Between them, these films also showed in graphic detail various types of human surgery, from primitive circumcision (both male and female) and trepanning, to modern male-female sex-change operations (testicles removed, penis skinned, slit in two and inverted, pelvic cavity cleared with power drills) and autopsy footage, which once more demonstrate how exposure to documentary mutilation has in a sense rendered tame the worst excesses of the imaginative cinema.

At the same time another left-field movement, the American Underground cinema, was reaching its zenith of creativity; and, thanks largely to Andy Warhol, receiving more and more widespread exposure. With its traditional themes of explicit sexuality, the recording of private acts and performances, and use of (often eccentric) non-actors, the underground film is also marked by a strong element of voyeurism. Kenneth Anger's masterpiece, *Inauguration Of The Pleasure Dome* (1954), shows an ornate ritual wherein the celebrants – comprised of his friends, including Anaïs Nin and Samson de Brier – dress as demigods or demons, consume a psychedelic potion and experience 'magick' revelations. Jack Smith's infamous *Flaming Creatures* (1962) records a garish, authentic transvestite orgy which culminates in cunnilingual rape. Ken Jacobs' *Blonde Cobra* (1962) is a candid, often grotesque portrait of film-maker Smith; Ron Rice's *Chumlum* (1963) features the outrageous Tiny Tim; Frederick Wiseman's shattering *Titicut Follies* (1967) is a frank account of inmates in a hospital for the criminally insane (another sector of humanity brutalized and marginalized as 'freaks'); Stan Brakhage's *Flesh Of Morning* (1957) is a candid document of himself masturbating, while the unflinching human autopsy footage of his later *The Act Of Seeing With One's Own Eyes* (1972) serves to remind us that no matter how deformed the exterior, we are all the same on the inside.

Warhol, whose earlier films such as *Sleep* (1963) and *Blow Job* (1964) are flat, unembellished documents of usually private moments of human experience, went on to incorporate a more overtly 'freakish' element into such works as the monumental *Chelsea Girls* (1967), *Flesh* (1968) and *Lonesome Cowboys* (1969). These films are marked by the appearance of Warhol's bizarre Factory retinue, a parade of narcissistic, posturing drag queens, junkies and misfits which included the likes of Candy Darling, Viva, Holly Woodlawn, Taylor Mead, Ingrid Superstar, Mario Montez, Ondine, and even anorexic Edie Sedgwick, so etiolated she could have worked sideshows as the human skeleton.

In Austria, the live performance work of the Vienna Action Group – including artists such as Günter Brus, Otto Muehl and Rudolf Schwarzkogler – and the activities of the Destruction In Art Symposium, led to the eventual production of films such as Kurt Kren's *6/64 – Mama Und Papa, 10/65 – Selbstverstümmelung* ('Self-mutilation'), and *Reel III 6/67*. Like Otto Muehl's own *Sodoma* (1969), these are largely visual recordings of copulation, masturbation, fellatio, defecation, urination, bondage, self-mutilation, animal-killing, coprophilia and general self-negation. The following notes are typical of Muehl's directions:

"Pour out 5 litres of milk into your chamber, all garbage cans, all fags collected in a month, 3 litres of salad oil, 5 kg of wheat flour, cast 50 eggs on it, then wallow with Cora 5 minutes like a steam-roller across the chamber; then get up, tie some boards to Alexandra's body, throw all Austrian newspapers over her, shovel up the filth around her with your hands and clap it on the papers, lift up Alexandra's body and let it fall down. It will be a sight like after bombing. Hang Doris upside down and let her piss into the air, piss into the cunt once, Libi did menstruate then, therefore we took a colour film."

This body of film was the culmination of 'actions' mirrored by other taboo-breaking events like Hermann Nitsch's ongoing Orgies And Mysteries Theatre (formed in 1957) and Carolee Schneemann's *Meat Joy* (Paris, 1964). The difference between bathing in raw offal and biting live prey, between these films and, say, *Born To Raise Hell*, lies purely in context and, some would even say, in the eye of the beholder.[4]

The rise of mondo, porno and underground/extreme art film in many ways led to the liberalising of commercial cinema to the extent where 'anything goes' – engendering the proliferation and acceptance of the 'trash' movie: the day of the geek. Early, mainstream geeks like Jerry Lewis (grown man acts like retarded infant to raise cheap laughs) would pale beneath the onslaught of 'social freaks' soon to willingly parade themselves and perform various acts of self-degradation before the cameras; these were the new human garbage, the cinematic equivalent of the chicken-biters of yore.

Doyen of the trash film, whose influences doubtless descend from all three of the above genres (via Herschell G. Lewis and Russ Meyer), is the Baltimore-based John Waters. Consisting of such dubious works as *Mondo Trasho* (1969), *Multiple Maniacs* (1970), *Pink Flamingoes* (1973) and *Female Trouble* (1974), Waters' pre-'80s oeuvre is populated almost exclusively by geeks; from transvestite, dogshit-devouring disco diva Divine and grotesque slobbering fat ladies Edie Massey and Jean Hill, down to 'bit-part' players like the stooge with the singing anus in *Pink Flamingoes*. The atrocities in that film alone would fill a dozen other Z-movie storylines: rape, murder, multiple perverted sex acts, a cannibal barbecue, exhibitionism, fetishism, various acts of cruelty, verbal obscenities, and last but far from least the climactic coprophilia scene where Divine eats a handful of steaming faeces straight from a poodle's backside. All of this is presented in such a shamelessly amateurish style that there is little to involve the audience, and the film – like Waters' other '70s works – amounts to little more than a freakshow on celluloid. *Desperate Living* (1977) is the most downbeat of the bunch. This nightmare fairytale of Mortville, a refuge for freaks, geeks, outsiders, losers and transgressors, boasts superior production values, is relieved of the over-familiar Divine presence, and achieves a few moments of authentic darkness. The scene where a female transsexual hacks through the gross, corpse-coloured flesh of her recently-grafted penis has an odd grimness, and tends to linger even after the images of 'ordinary' madness and mayhem have faded. It is probably Waters' least-liked film for these very reasons.

The only film to seriously rival Waters in the '70s trash stakes was Curt McDowell's *Thundercrack* (1976), scripted by and starring George Kuchar, whose own earlier films like *Hold Me While I'm Naked* (1966), *Eclipse Of The Sun Virgin* (1967) and *The Mammal Palace* (1969) were another great influence on trash cinema. Kuchar's *A Woman Distressed* (1962) was inspired by the thalidomide scandal and is a sick comedy about women giving birth to deformed babies. *Thundercrack* is set in an old, storm-bound house, peopled by human oddities and grotesques (including a young man with inhumanly swollen genitals) who in the course of its action get to explicitly practice pretty much every sexual perversion imaginable – even homosexual bestiality. An honourable mention in this area must also go to Ted V. Mikels' production *The Worm Eaters* (1977), whose title tells all; the film's director, Herb Robins, stars as a club-footed worm-breeder, with a supporting cast of unknown geeks who gladly devour live worms on screen. Artist Joe Coleman's notorious stage act, in which he ate live mice, was captured for posterity by Tommy Turner and David Wojnarowicz in their *Where Evil Dwells* (1985). Also noteworthy is *Exorcismo Negro* (1974), in which a geek actress chews the head off a live chicken.

With the dawn of the '80s, John Waters moved away from the total, obscene trash of his early works towards a more palatable form of American kitsch. Few stepped up to take his crown, and while the underground movement persisted with works from the likes of Eric Mitchell, Amos Poe, and Michael Oblowitz, a new concept in low-budget, voyeuristic film-making began to emerge out of the New York 'art-rock' scene: the so-called "cinema of transgression". Of all those involved in this short-lived upsurge, two artists in particular seem to epitomise its aspirations, achievements, and indeed its shortcomings – Nick Zedd, who christened the movement, and Richard Kern. While much of Kern's early output seems merely to involve herding his various musician/junkie friends in front of the camera and then filming them perform spontaneous acts of self-degradation (for example Lung Leg's desperately sad *Worm Movie*, in which she eats live worms), his *Fingered* (1985), starring Lydia Lunch and described by John Waters as "the ultimate date movie for psychos", is an extraordinarily charged piece of film-making, a short monochrome burst of intense sexual violence which impresses with its authentic taste of sleaze. Some of his later short work, in particular *The Evil Cameraman* (1990), displays a knowing appreciation of the voyeuristic dynamic, and his *Sewing Circle* (1992) also achieves a Sadeian intensity with its frank documentation of actress Kembra Pfahler having her vagina sewn up (for real) by two New York dominatrixes. Zedd, perpetrator of *Geek Maggot Bingo* (1983), pulls off some interesting effects in his later *War Is Menstrual Envy* (1992), but this segmented film is perhaps most notable, in the context of this chapter, for the section where a war veteran is slowly unbandaged by the topless Annie Sprinkle, revealing his awfully napalmed face and body.[5] Zedd's camera lingers on his dreadful disfigurements, affording us extreme close-ups of the desiccated, plasticized flesh in which it more resembles a lunar landscape than human torso. Then, in one of the more disturbing – though finally moving – sequences in cinema, Sprinkle starts to make love to the man, caressing his earless head, kissing his lipless mouth, licking the contours of his dry, ridged chest; he responds by attempting to suckle her enormous breasts, his charred, fingerless hands poignantly highlighted against her pliant white body. Possibly the only previously-known scenes which could compare to this – Alain Resnais' juxtaposition of the naked lovers and atomic burn victims in *Hiroshima Mon Amour* (1959) – pale by comparison. Although Zedd's and Sprinkle's intentions here are undoubtedly honourable, one feels that one could not – dare not – push the boundaries of this form of inevitably voyeuristic cinema any further.

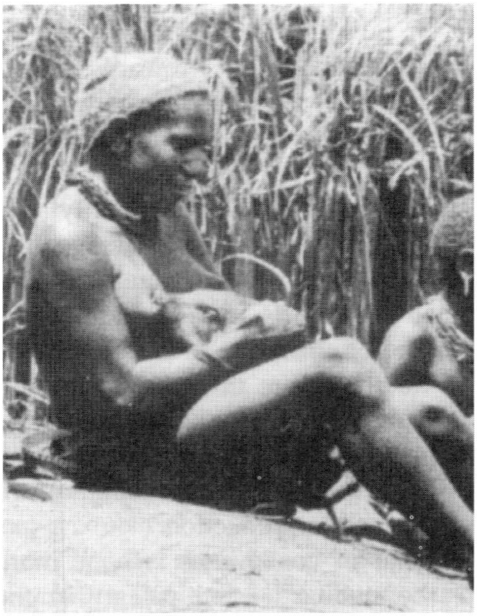

Mondo Cane

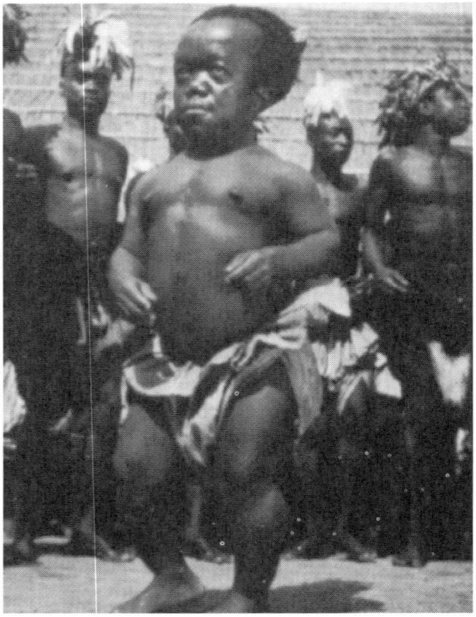

Congo – Savage Splendour

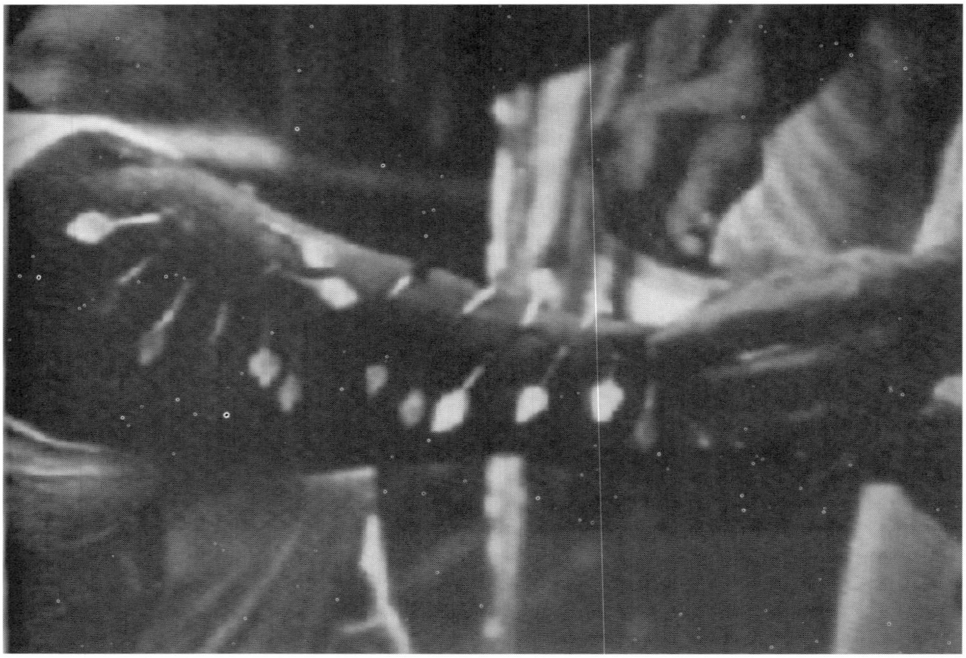

Mondo Infame

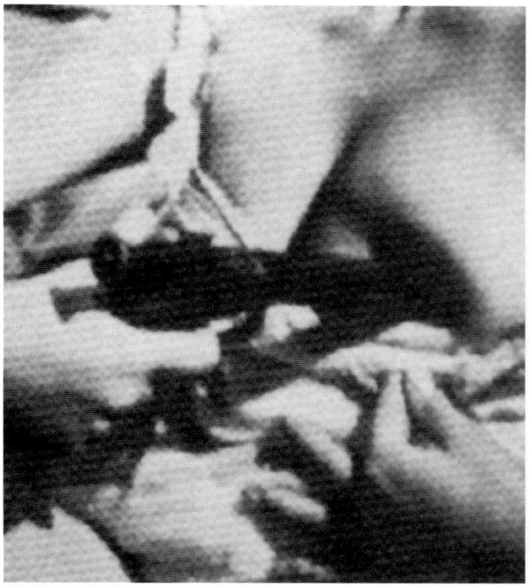

Forbidden World

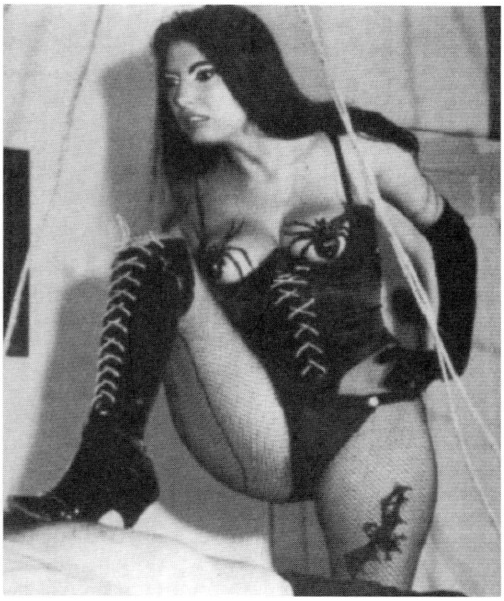

Mondo Keyhole

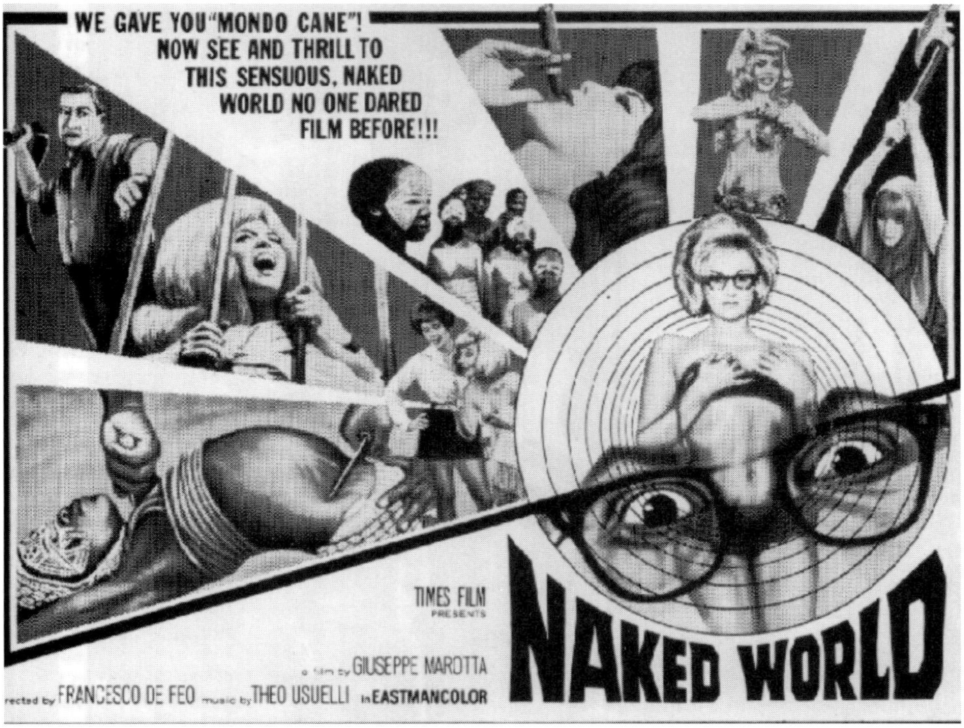

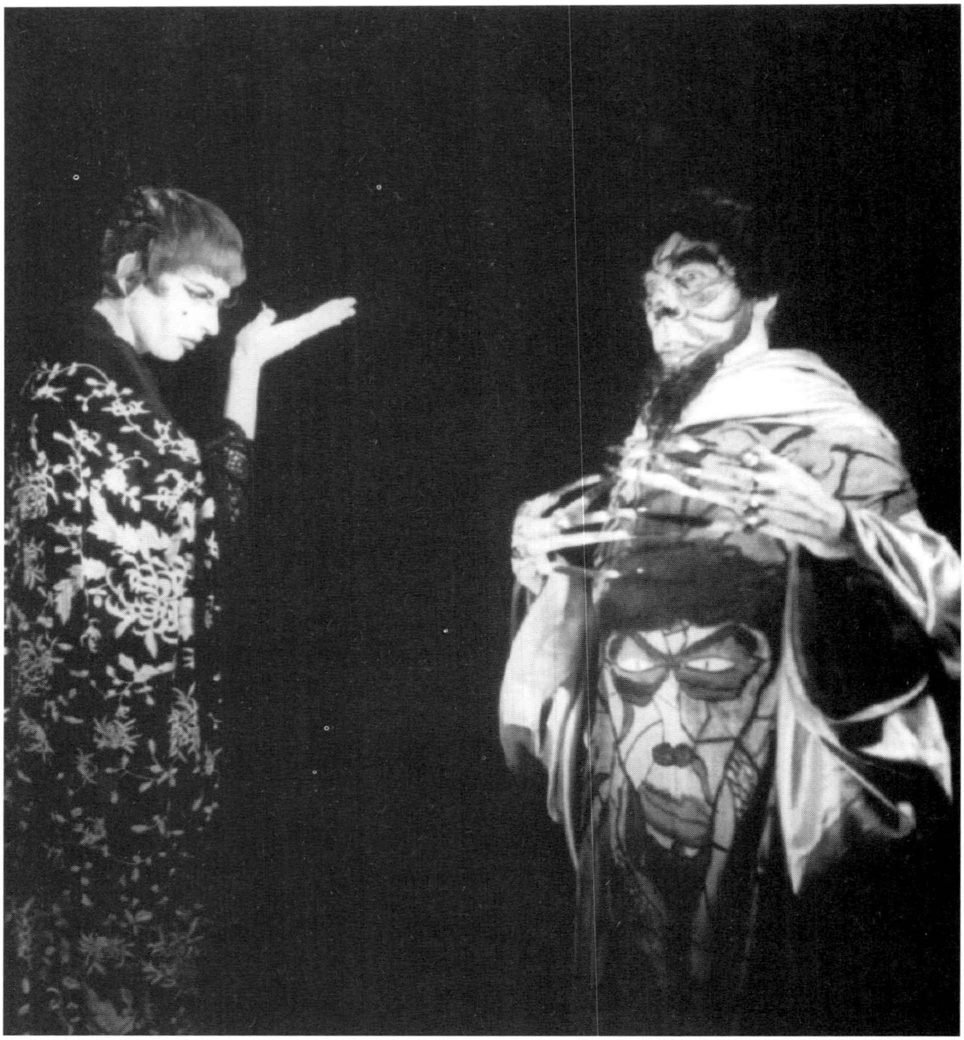

Inauguration Of The Pleasure Dome

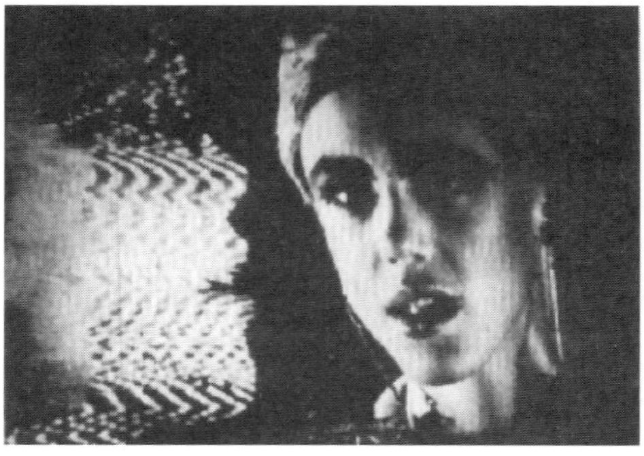

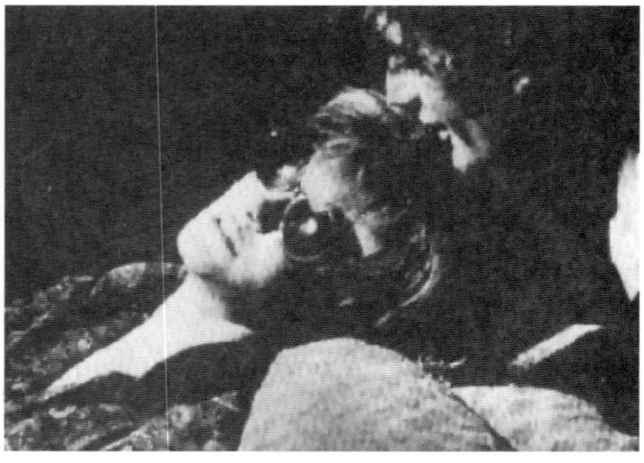

Chelsea Girls

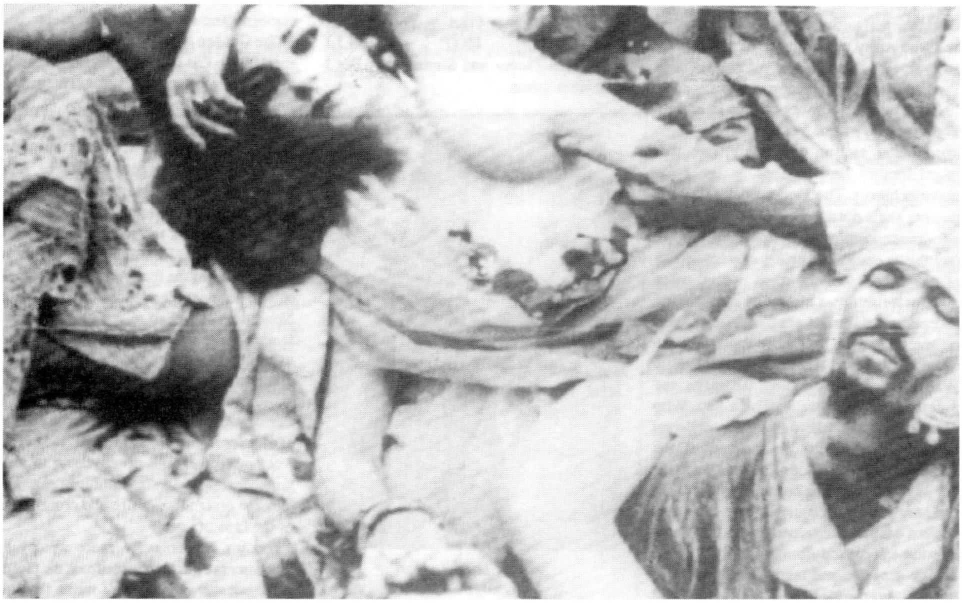

Flaming Creatures

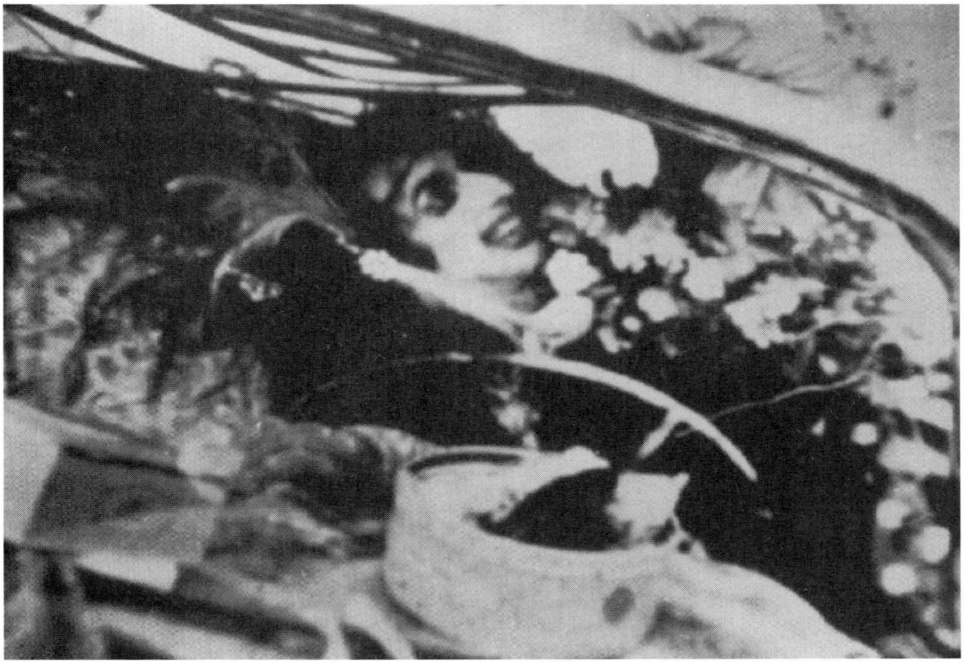

Tiny Tim; *Chumlum*

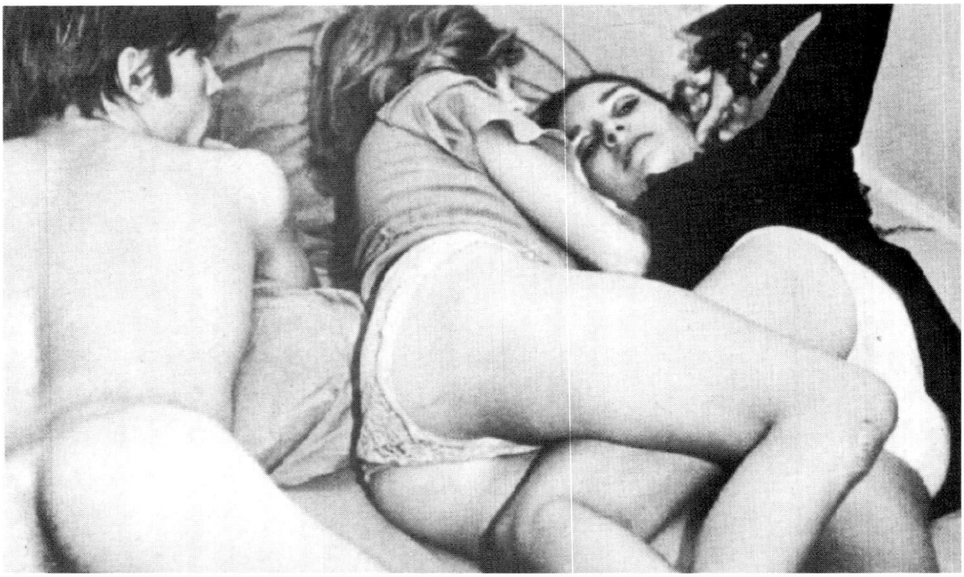

Flesh

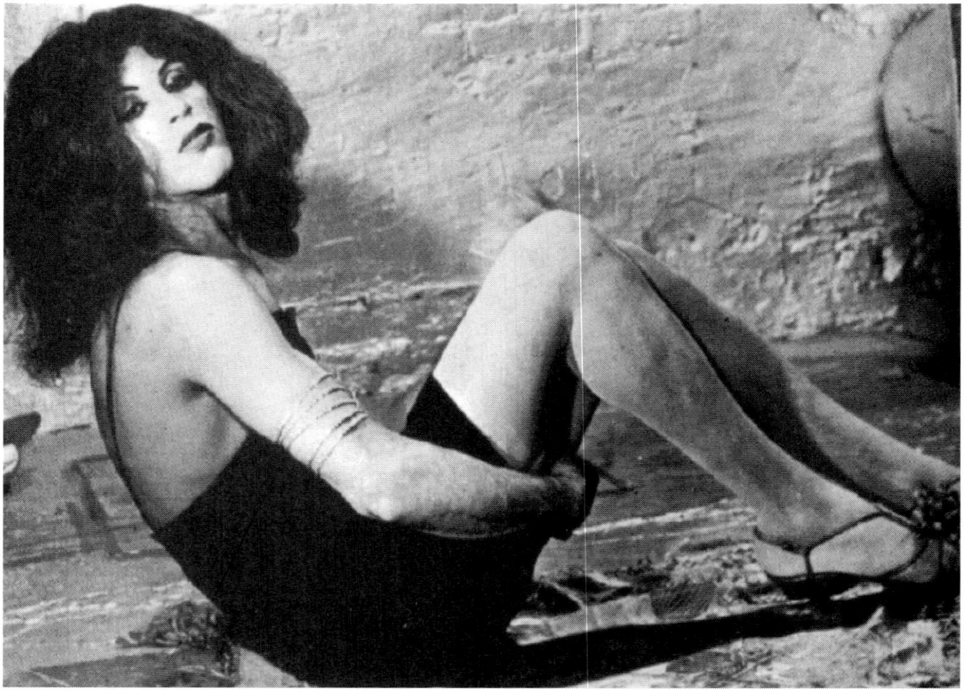

Mario Montez

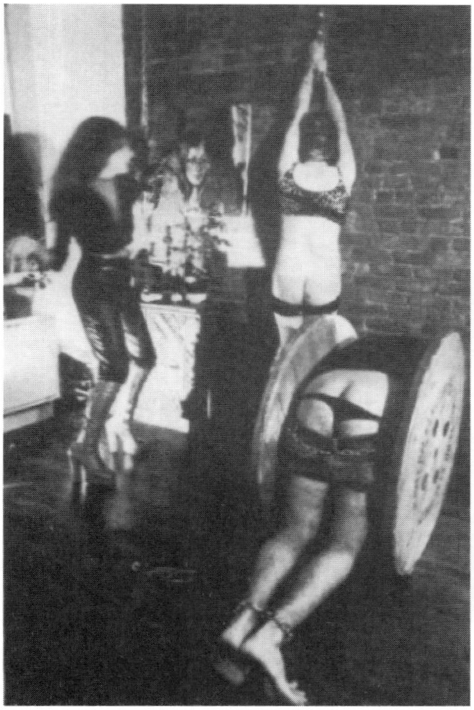

Sex O'Clock USA

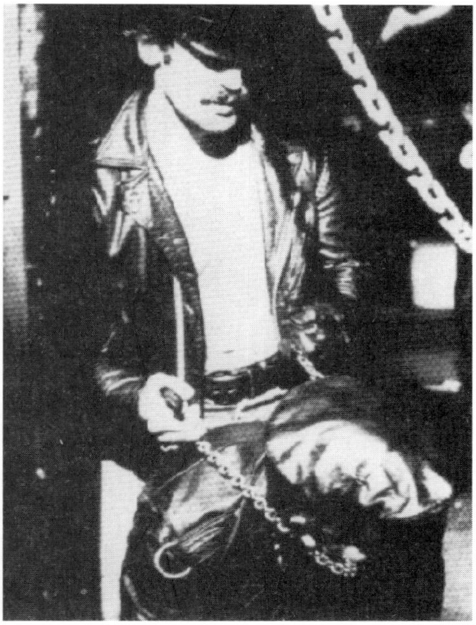

New York City Inferno

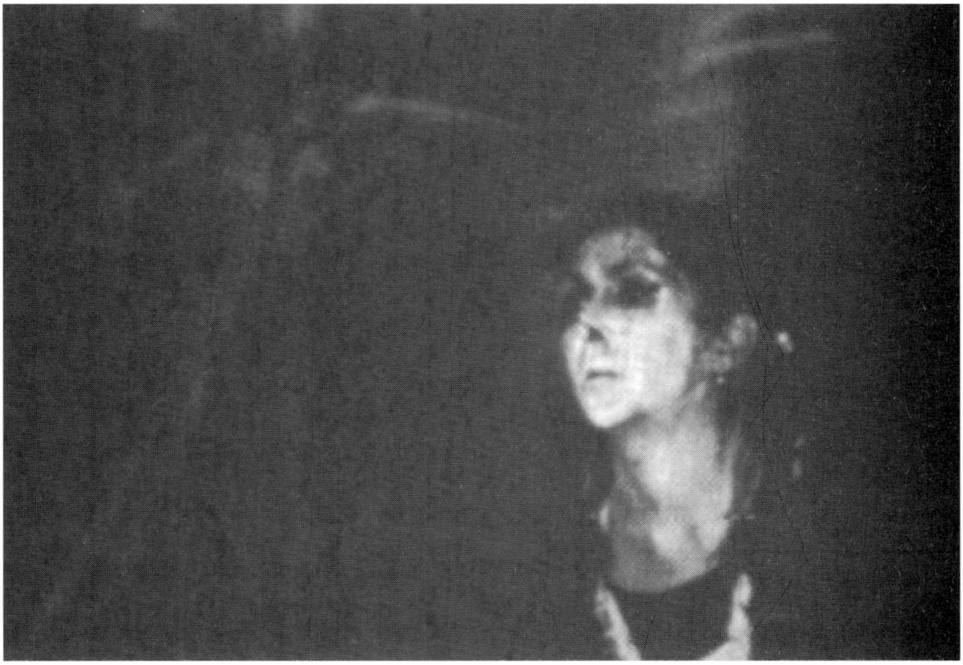

Meat Joy

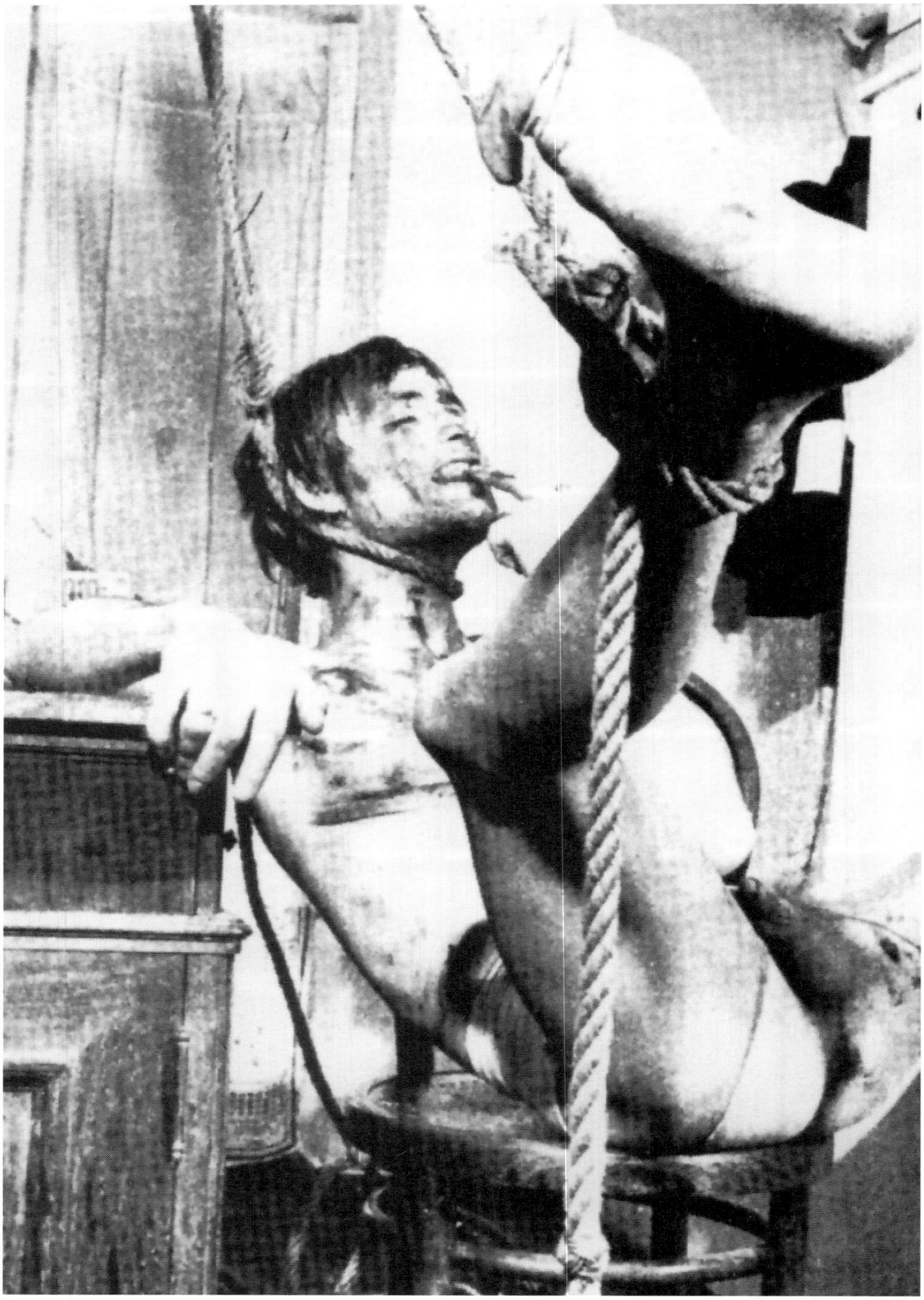

Günter Brus

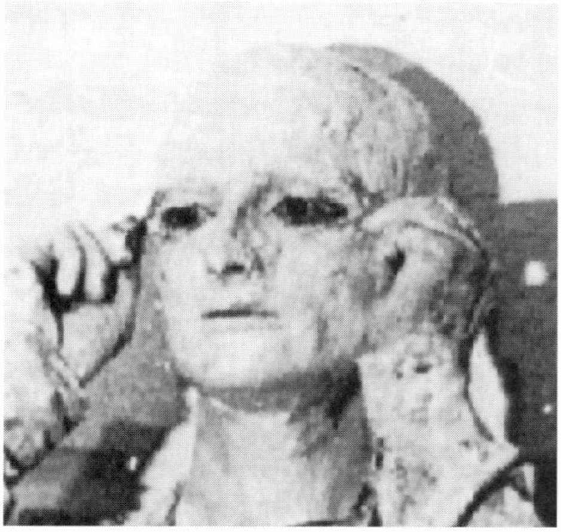

Selbstverstümmelung

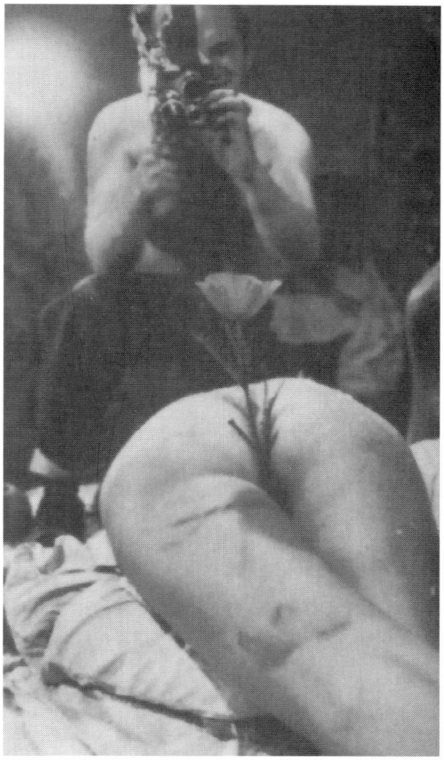

Kurt Kren

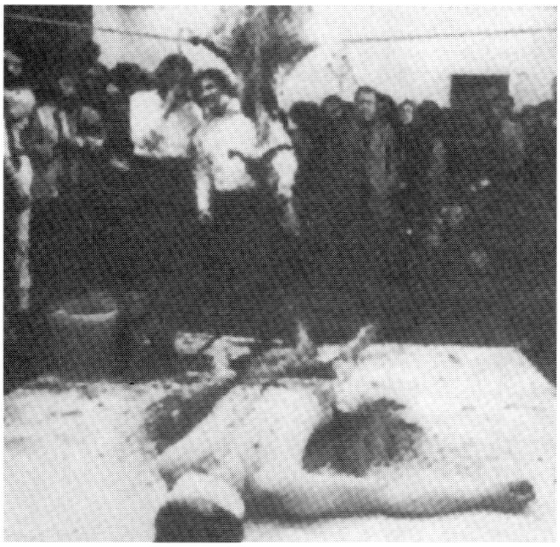

Hermann Nitsch

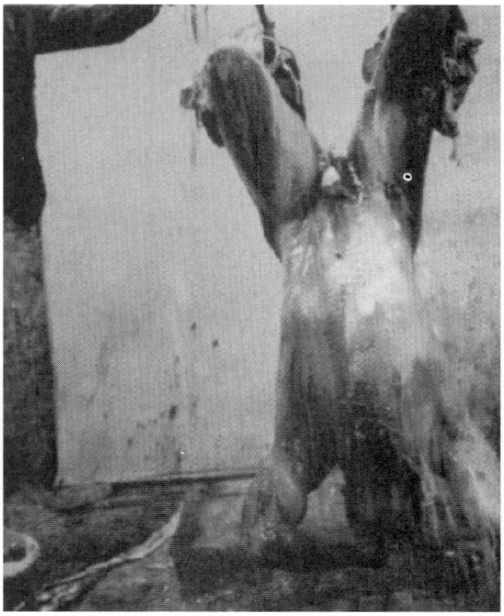

An Otto Muehl Materialaktion

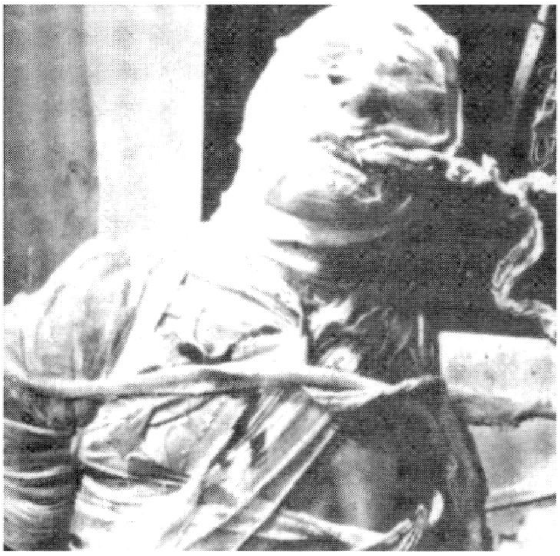

Rudolf Schwarzkogler

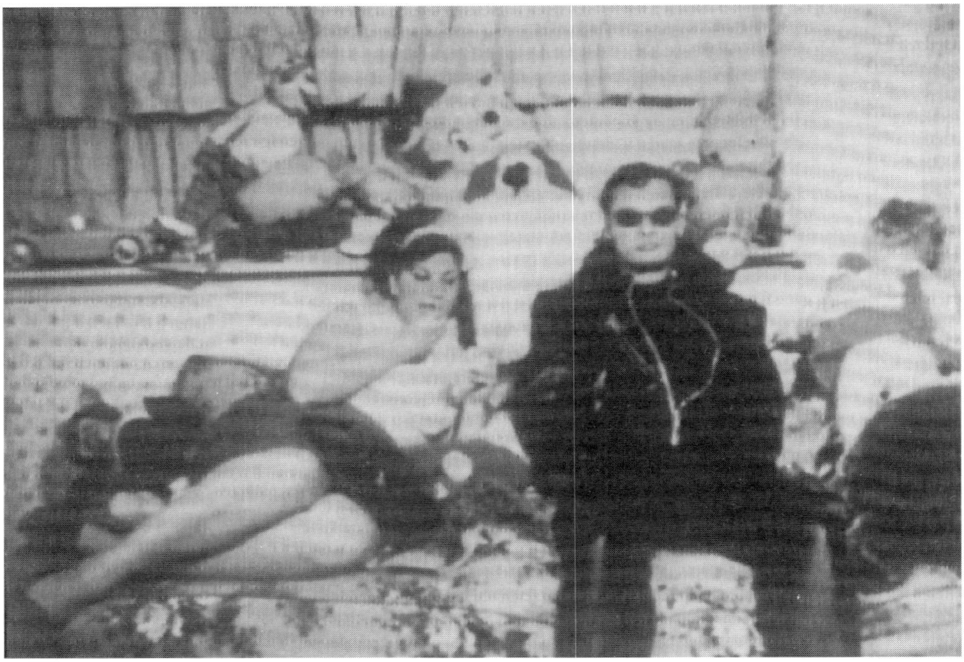

Eclipse Of The Sun Virgin

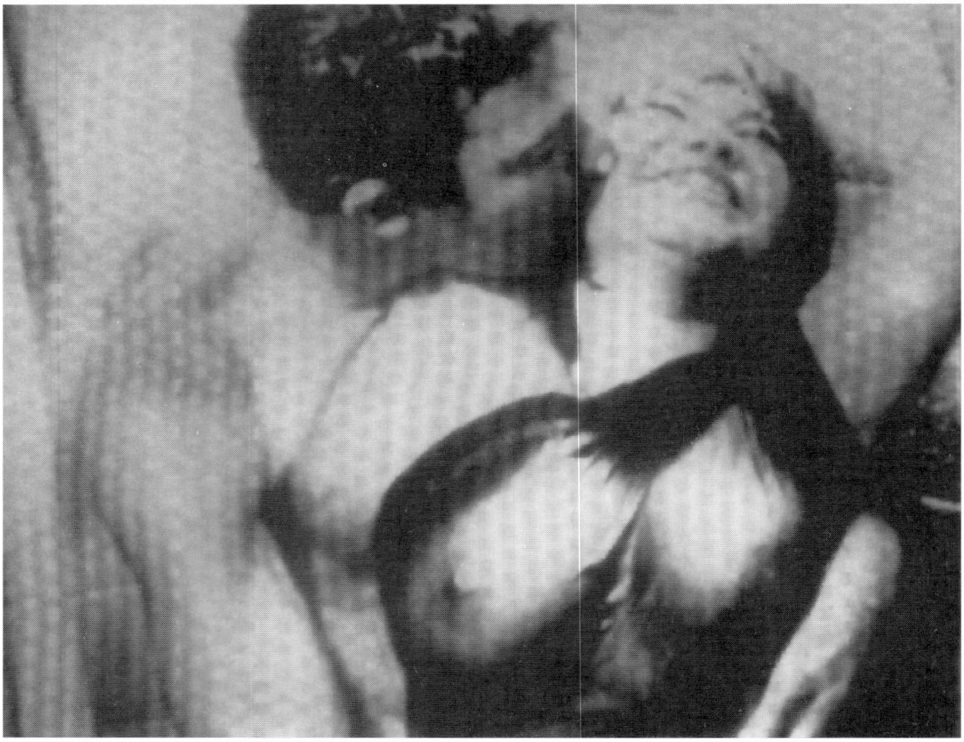

Hold Me While I'm Naked

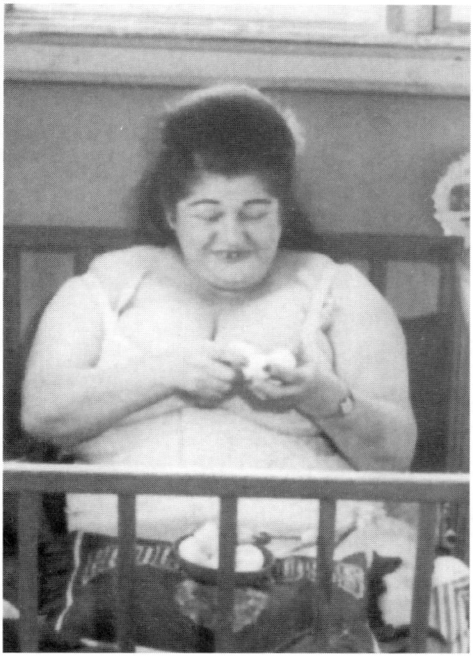

Pink Flamingoes

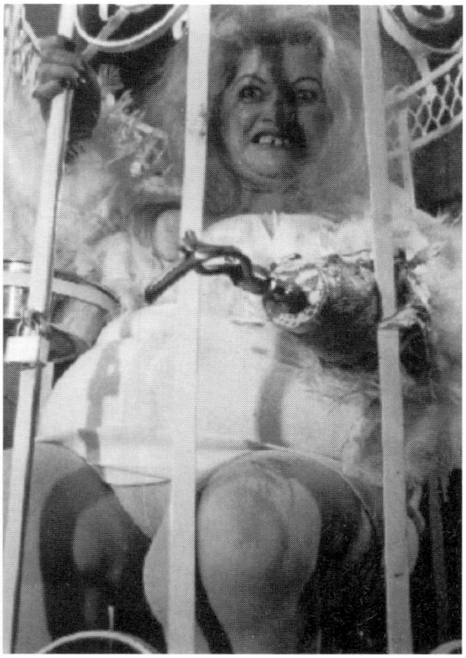

Female Trouble

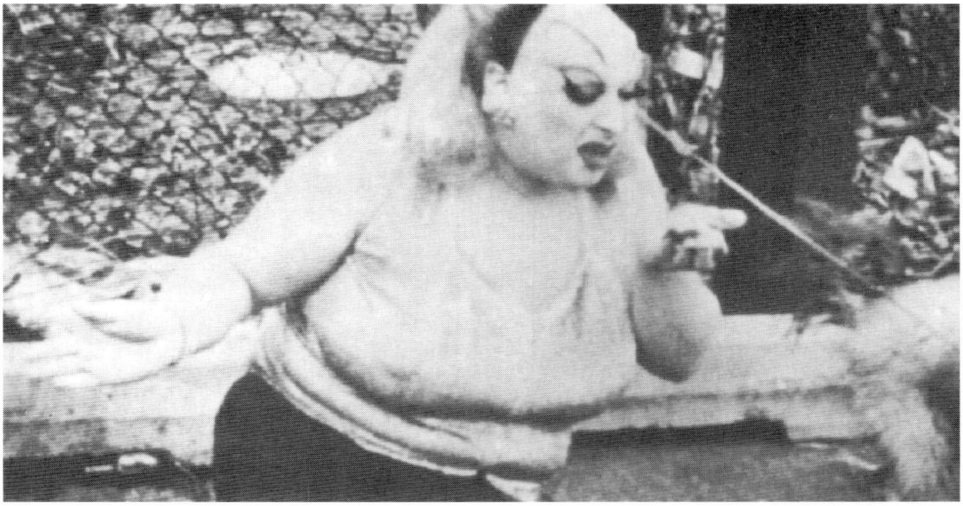

Divine; *Pink Flamingoes*

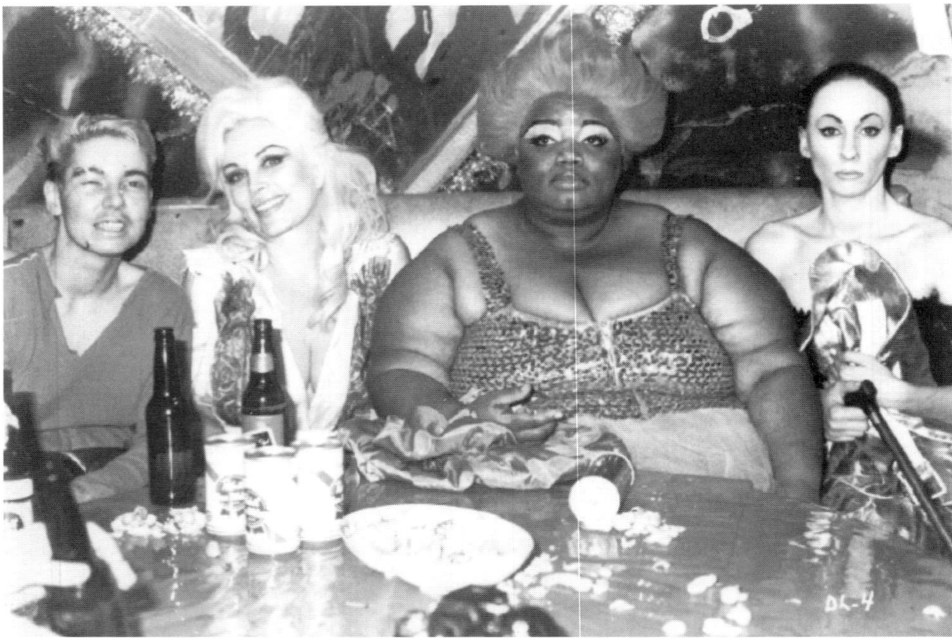

Desperate Living

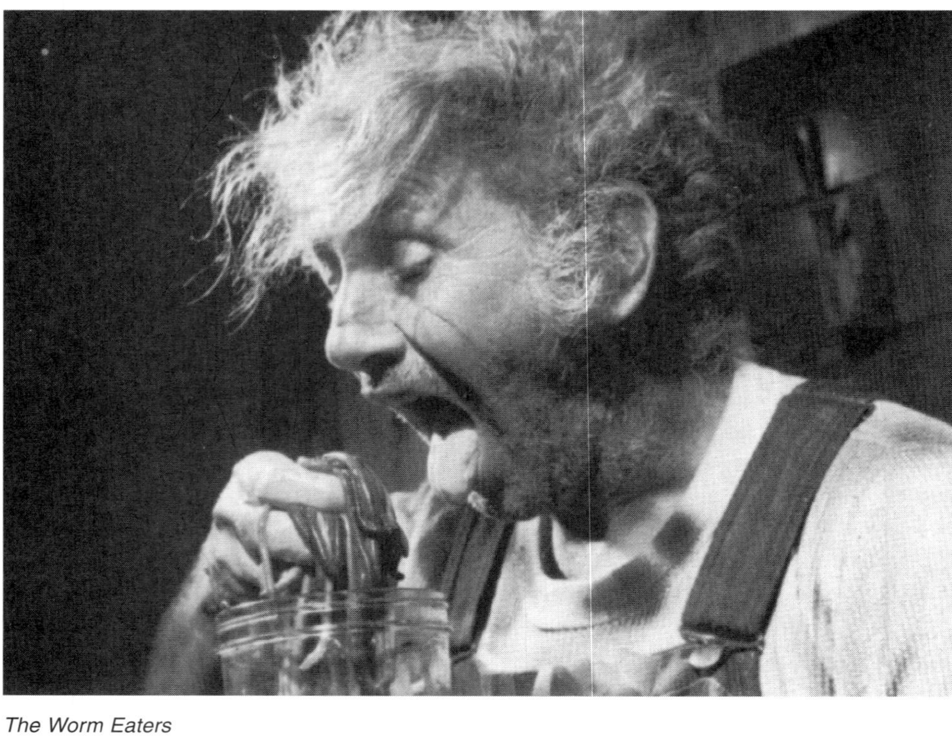

The Worm Eaters

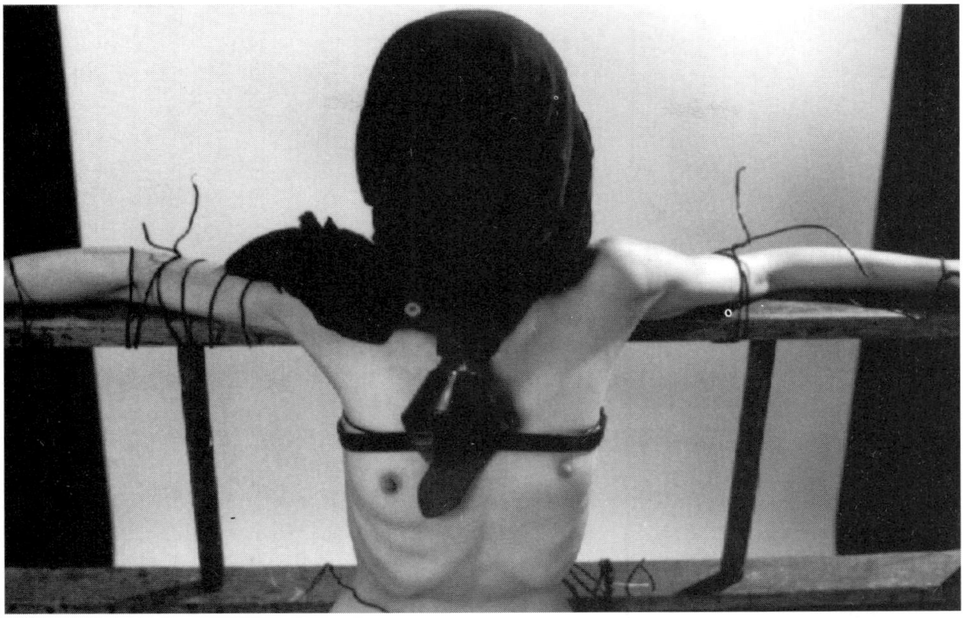

The Evil Cameraman

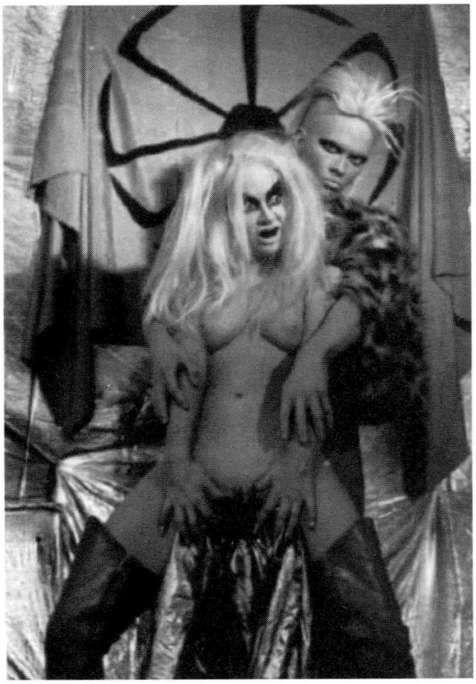

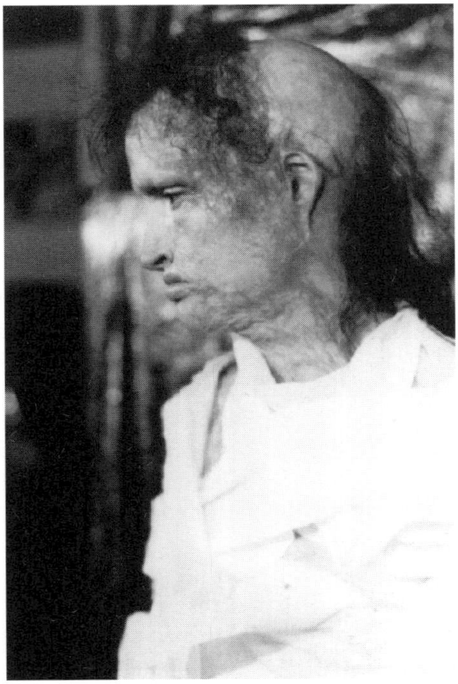

War Is Menstrual Envy

THE TORTURE GARDEN

The other perennial themes of bizarre cinema, as featured in *Freaks*, are the creation of human monsters through surgery, mutilation or disfigurement – usually presented with the maximum of sadistic relish – and people ostracized and driven to desperate acts of revenge or madness due to their 'otherness'. The cinema of mutilation can be traced as far back as *L'Homme Qui Rit* (1909), a silent version of Victor Hugo's novel about Gwymplaine, the nobleman whose mouth is surgically carved into a permanent, hideous rictus by *dacianos*, the outlaws who habitually perform such disfigurements to children to render them fit for begging or the freakshows. Better known is Paul Leni's version, *The Man Who Laughs* (1928), with Conrad Veidt as Gwynplaine, and a dark backdrop of torture and the gibbet, the fairground, and corruption in high places.

In *The Penalty* (1920), Lon Chaney portrayed a legless mobster who vows to cut off the legs of the daughter of the doctor who maimed him and graft them to his own stumps (a plot echoed in *King's Row* [1941], which boasted Ronald Reagan as a hapless amputee); Chaney had already portrayed Frog, a bogus cripple, in *The Miracle Man* (1919), and in 1923 he created the first of two icons of deformity and disfigurement for which he would always be remembered, appearing as the hunchbacked, one-eyed bell-ringer Quasimodo in Wallace Worsley's (otherwise unremarkable) version of *The Hunchback Of Notre Dame* by Victor Hugo. Chaney took his portrayal, as usual, to the point of masochism, trussing himself painfully in a body-harness for the duration of filming.[6] Then, in 1925, he played the title role in Rupert Julien's *The Phantom Of The Opera*, derived from the novel by Gaston LeRoux. In this film Chaney's make-up made him look like a human skull, and the scene where his female captive unmasks him has seldom been outdone for sheer power or terror. The gothic decor and subterranean labyrinths of the Phantom's lair add a final touch of the outlandish. Both these classic tales of freaks have been re-interpreted many times since, but no-one has rivalled Chaney's performances in either.

In 1928, Luis Buñuel and Salvador Dalí presented their legendary *Un Chien Andalou*, which apart from its visions of eyeballs being sliced in two by a straight razor and stumps caressing faces, marks an early appearance of what would become another recurring symbol in bizarre cinema: the (inert) severed hand.[7] This crops up again in Buñuel's own *El Angel Exterminador*. But probably the most interesting instance of all remains *Dementia* (aka *Daughter Of Horror*), directed in 1955 by John Parker. Apparently Parker's only film, it uses Expressionistic techniques to show the strange tale of a young madwoman. We see her wake up, meet a mysterious stranger, and through him get involved with an obese mobster (Z-movie doyen Bruno VeSota) who resembles her father – a violent man who she has already stabbed to death. She later kills the fat man in the same way, resorting to severing his dead hand when she realises it contains her pendant. We see her ditch the hand before the film leads us back to the first scene of the woman waking. We assume it has all been a dream, a simplistic explanation which is abruptly shattered when she opens her dresser drawer to reveal – the severed hand. A sinister dwarf newspaper vendor also appears (the ubiquitous Angelo Rossitto yet again), explicitly referring us back to the distorted arena of *Freaks*. A veritable catalogue of the uncanny filled with homicidal sexual abjection, human monsters, oneiric graveyard scenes and visions of phantom faces, *Dementia*'s drift is a Freudian shadow-key to the lock on a psychotic labyrinth. As trance-film (a rarefied division of bizarre cinema), *Dementia* effectively bridges the gap between Maya Deren's *Meshes Of The Afternoon* (1943) and Herk Hervey's *Carnival Of Souls* (1962), which in turn hark back to *The Cabinet Of Dr. Caligari* and anticipate *Eraserhead*.

1935 saw the release of two landmark films of sadistic surgical horror. Louis Frielander's *The Raven*, loosely inspired by Poe, features Bela Lugosi as Dr. Vollin, a deranged plastic surgeon with a house full of torture devices. Boris Karloff plays the escaped criminal who comes to Vollin for a new face and ends up being made into a mutilated, half-paralysed slave whose hideous features are endlessly displayed to him in a multi-mirrored room. More intriguing, and even more outlandish, is Karl Freund's *Mad Love*, a remake of *Orlacs Hände* (Robert Wiene, 1924). The story involves Orlac, a concert pianist (Colin Clive) who loses both his hands in a train wreck, and the surgeon Dr Gogol, who "cures deformed children and mutilated soldiers". Orlac is helped after his accident by Gogol (an amazing performance by Peter Lorre), who happens to be obsessed with the pianist's wife. She is leading lady in the Grand Guignol *Théâtre des Horreurs*, where the eldritch, bald and bug-eyed surgeon is a regular patron. Gogol reveals that he has in fact grafted the hands of a knife-throwing murderer, recently guillotined, onto Orlac's wrists, then tries to drive the latter insane by impersonating the 'resurrected' killer, complete with neck brace, goggles and metal hands. Gogol is a pathological freak, a sadist, a physical grotesque; in depicting his sibilant manias *Mad Love* manifests true delirium, a hysterical vision which manages to stay just this side of science fiction. Both films caused outrage in England, one prominent critic describing *The Raven* as *"quite the most unpleasant picture I have ever seen, exploiting cruelty for cruelty's sake"*.[8]

The next classic film of surgical horror did not appear until 1959, but it inspired a whole succession of similar entries centred around deranged doctors or plastic surgeons bent on skinning or disfiguring as many victims as possible in pursuit of their various ends. Georges Franju's *Les Yeux Sans Visage/Eyes Without A Face* remains far superior to its many successors, a black and white art film in which the director conjures poetry from the most grim subject matter. Dr Gessenier (Pierre Brasseur) is abducting young girls from whom to take skin grafts to restore the disfigured face of his daughter (played with exquisite melancholy by Edith Scob), who spends most of the film prowling their house behind an expressionless white mask. The scene of one these grafts being prepared, the skin peeled bloodily in clear close-up from the face of a 'donor', was shocking for its time and led to the film being heavily censored in Britain and America (where it was also ludicrously re-titled *Horror Chamber Of Dr Faustus*!). Finally, the daughter rebels and in a double murder first stabs her nurse (Alida Valli) and then abandons her father to the savage, vengeful jaws of his laboratory dogs. Between these three bloody moments, Franju (previously responsible for the unflinching documentary abattoir horrors of *Le Sang Des Bêtes* [1948]) shows contrasting scenes of sombre beauty. Whether the film, like *Le Sang Des Bêtes*, is ultimately meant as an anti-vivisectionist tract, is open to debate; what is clear is that Franju has bequeathed us a unique, transcendent work.

The plotline – if not the artistry – of Franju's film was pretty much retraced in later efforts such as *Gritos En La Noche/The Awful Dr. Orlof* (1962), which marked the start of Jess Franco's prolific career in exploitation pictures; Elio Scardamaglia's *Murder Clinic* (1966); Robert Hartford-Davis' *Corruption* (1968), with Peter Cushing decapitating prostitutes to provide gland implants for his disfigured fiancée (Sue Lloyd); Michael Pataki's *Mansion Of The Doomed* (1976), an early Charles Band production in which Richard Basehart plays the doctor removing eyes to transplant to his blind daughter; John Grissmer's *False Face* (1976); and Claude Mulot's *La Rose Escorchée/Ravaged* (1969). This last film is made even more bizarre by lesbian sex scenes and the presence of a pair of over-sexed dwarf servants dressed in animal skins. Franco returned to the theme in 1989 with *Les Predateurs De La Nuit/Faceless*, a remake of his earlier *Dr. Orlof* notable only for featuring not only Caroline Munro and Helmut Berger, but also Anton Diffring, who played the murderous plastic surgeon in *Circus Of Horrors*.

Directed by Sidney Hayers for Anglo-Amalgamated, *Circus Of Horrors* (1960) was one of several British films made at around the same time which all dealt to varying degrees with mutilation, murder and voyeurism. Hayers' film is the most specifically concerned with surgical cruelty. Dr Schuller (Diffring), a demented plastic surgeon, is on the run after being implicated in the torture of a patient/lover. Posing as a circus-owner, he finds the ideal cover for his practices, peopling his show with the ugliest people he can find, whom he re-models and presents in his Temple Of Beauty. Then, one by one, they try to leave him and soon meet with fatal accidents beneath the Big Top. The sensational murders, coupled with the freak arena of the circus, convey much of the public's voyeuristic appetites; while Schuller's scenes with his patients – lovingly caressing scar tissue, twisted flesh or bloody bandages – have a genuinely perverse quality.

Michael Powell's *Peeping Tom* (1960) features Karl Boehm as Mark, a photographer obsessed with physical flaws and scars. He is also psychopathic, and kills his models while he is filming them by means of a an extending spike affixed to his camera tripod. It turns out that Mark was the victim of similar experiments by his father, who filmed him relentlessly and subjected him to fright and suffering in order to record his reactions. With its unusually complex structure and layers of symbolism, *Peeping Tom* is without doubt the ultimate statement on the voyeuristic nature of the whole cinematic experience. The viewer not only watches films within films, but is made to experience the very act of film-making – and murder – subjectively while still acutely aware that he is being manipulated into this complicity by his relationship with the film-makers (Mark/Mark's father/Powell). Mark's choice of victims (tarts, models, actresses) are all girls routinely scrutinized and objectified in their 'glamorous' careers; by means of a large mirror mounted on his camera, Mark conveys the ultimate irony, forcing them to watch their own death throes as he impales them. He finally falls for a plain girl (Anna Massey), but her blind mother – the only one immune from this inwardly-collapsing gaze maze – is suspicious of him and engineers his downfall. The film was universally reviled upon release, a disaster for Powell (who to top things off plays the part of Mark's father in the 'home movies'), and it virtually ended his career. Like *Freaks*, *Peeping Tom* has since been rehabilitated; the only other British film-maker to rival its concentric accumulation of vicarious sadism has been Michael Reeves, with the vicious pulp psychosis and immolations of *The Sorcerers* (1967).

Also of interest here is *Horrors Of The Black Museum* (Arthur Crabtree, 1958), which concerns a journalist (Michael Gough) who commits a series of bloody murders to satisfy his readers. His increasingly sadistic methods include the use of 'trick' binoculars which gouge out the user's eyes with spring-loaded spikes, and a guillotine/bed device which decapitates a voluptuous prostitute. Less ingenious is another British entry, Robert Day's *Corridors Of Blood* (1958), which with its basic storyline of a surgeon (Boris Karloff) experimenting on various patients without anaesthetic, seems little more than an excuse to depict successive acts of mutilation.

There would not be another British film in this vein to challenge the complexity of *Peeping Tom* until 1986, when Peter Greenaway produced *A Zedd And Two Noughts*. This typically multi-layered film is the story of two Siamese twins, Oliver and Oswald, who were separated ('amputated' from each other) in infancy but have remained spiritually indivisible. Both zoologists, they lose their wives in a bizarre car crash caused when a swan escapes from the zoo. Oliver, unable to bear the thought of his wife (who we learn was ten weeks pregnant) rotting in her coffin, becomes obsessed with the notion of decomposition and cycles of life, commencing a series of photographic studies on decay in female animal corpses which culminates with the slaughter of a captive zebra. Meanwhile both twins become enamoured of Alba, the woman who was driving the car, and make love to her both separately and together in her hospital bed, despite (or because of) the fact that she has had a leg amputated. They are also involved with a hooker who services amputees and mental cripples alike in a zoo manger, and who is also ten weeks pregnant. Finally Alba, unable to bear life with one 'lonely' leg, undergoes a second amputation at the hands of her scheming surgeon (who also performs similar operations on the zoo animals) – but not before she has conceived twin children by the brothers. Soon rejected by her in favour of a male amputee lover, Oliver and Oswald dream of being stitched together again by the surgeon, and of procuring the hooker as the final specimen in their experiment, before committing suicide under their own camera's gaze.

A Zed And Two Noughts is a startling meditation on loss and regeneration, framed by obsessive notions of pairing and symmetry, which encompasses extreme sexual fetishism (amputation, bestiality, scopophilia) before its timelapsed reduction of all life forms to a single entity. People and animals, hospitals and zoos become interchangeable, and human thought/aspiration itself is revealed as the ultimate perversion.

Two Japanese films are also worthy of mention in this area; Hiroshi Teshigahara's *Tanin No Kao/The Face Of Another* (1967), from the novel by Kobo Abe, is the warped tale of a hideously burned man who disguises his face in flesh-like plastic in order to make love to his wife in the guise of another. At the same time, a girl terribly burnt at Hiroshima kills herself after allowing her brother to caress her scars and make love to her. Teruo Ishii's *Kyofu Nikei Ningen/Horror Of The Deformed* (1969) tells the equally *outré* story of a deranged, disfigured man plotting to abduct babies and render them as ugly as he is.

Back in America, William Castle's *Mr. Sardonicus* (1961) was pretty much a re-run of *The Man Who Laughs*, with Guy Rolfe as the man with the fixed grin, while Hy Averback's *Chamber Of Horrors* (1966) was more unusual, made as a TV pilot but deemed too extreme for home viewing. Patrick O'Neal stars as Cravatte, a homicidal maniac who escapes custody by chopping off his own hand, and then has his stump fitted with a special appliance which can be equipped with the various hooks and blades he uses to mutilate his victims. John Frankenheimer's *Seconds* (1966) was a more serious entry, starring Rock Hudson as the businessman who attempts to regain his youth by means of radical plastic surgery and pays an inevitable price.

Self-mutilation and religious masochism predominate in John Huston's *Wise Blood* (1979), a truly bizarre working of Flannery O'Connor's classic novel of American gothic. Brad Dourif plays Hazel Motes, obsessed with the sluttish jail-bait daughter of blind preacher Asa Hawkes (Harry Dean Stanton). Motes forms a rival church, whose figurehead becomes a mummified freak taken from the museum by a local retard, and takes to binding himself in barbed wire; when Hawkes is exposed as a grift, Motes proves himself superior by putting out his own eyes with quicklime.

The most recent entry into the field of 'custom-made' freaks is *Boxing Helena* (1993), directed by Jennifer Lynch (fittingly, daughter of David). In this story of obsession and possession, a surgeon (Julian Sands) performs an unnecessary quadruple limb amputation on his girlfriend (Sherilyn Fenn) when she comes to his operating-table after a road accident, turning her into a basket-case who can (literally) never leave him. Whereas Lynch Sr. could possibly have redeemed this questionable storyline, there is little to elevate his daughter's debut above exploitation level; suffice to say it failed to start a fresh trend.

Finally, a handful of film-makers have brought into plain view the ultimate mutilation, the secret fear which sufflates the uncanny. Self-castration, or submission to castration by a lover, represents the final victory of Thanatos over Eros. Where Tod Browning could only suggest this in his tortured tales of damned flesh, more recent films have graphically illustrated the act: in Marco Ferreri's *La Dernière Femme* (1976) Gérard Depardieu emasculates himself with an electric carving knife; Pierre Lampe is castrated by *La Fée Sanguinaire* (Roland Lethem, 1969); and in Nagisa Oshima's masterpiece *Ai No Corrida* (1975), a woman strangles her lover to death during orgasm and then severs his genitals, which she carries around with her for several days.[9]

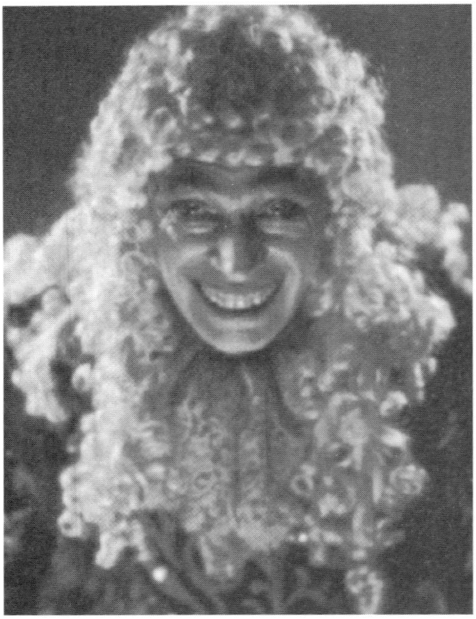

The Man Who Laughs

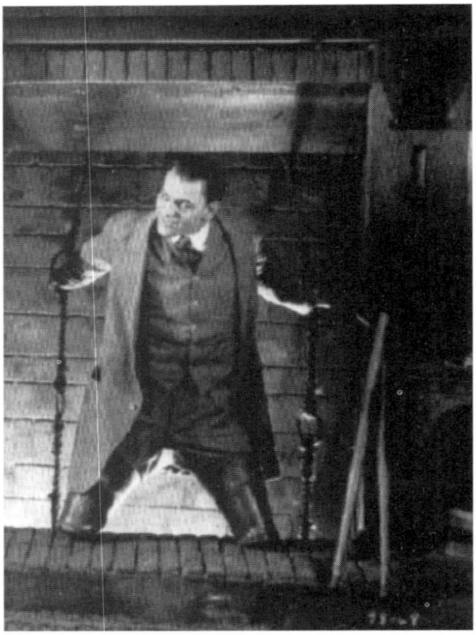

The Penalty

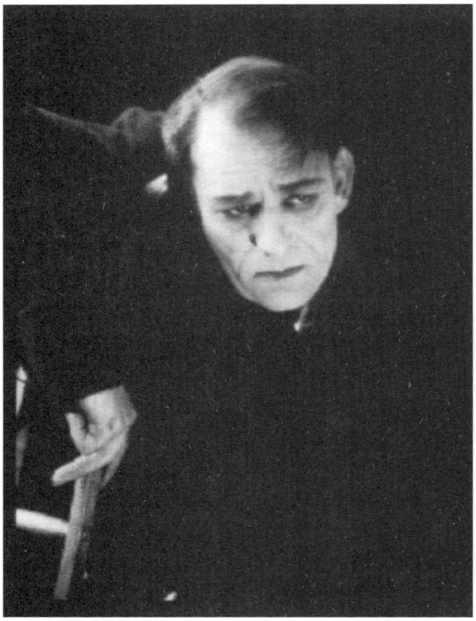

The Blackbird

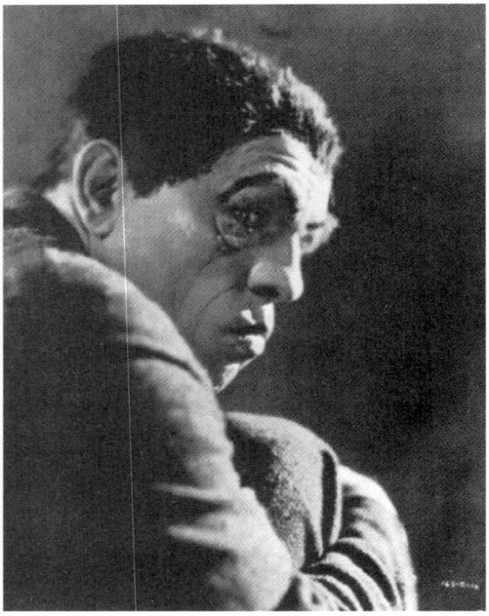

A Blind Bargain

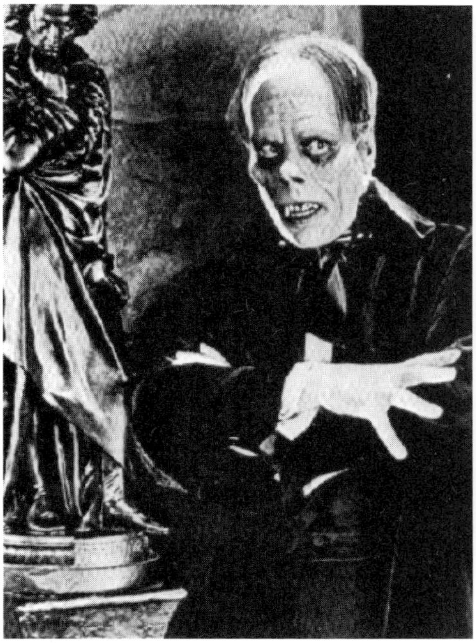

The Phantom Of The Opera

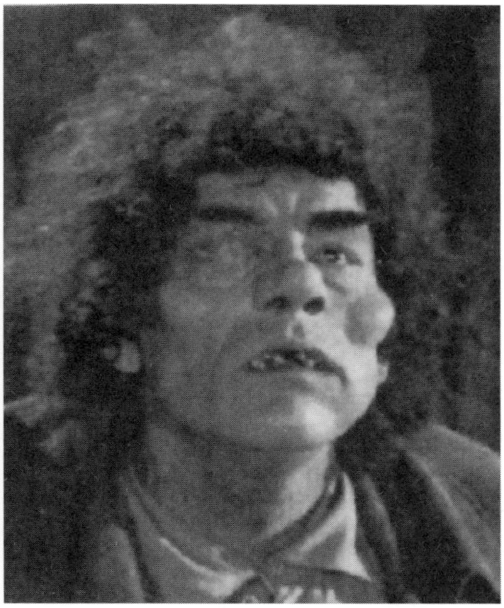

The Hunchback Of Notre Dame

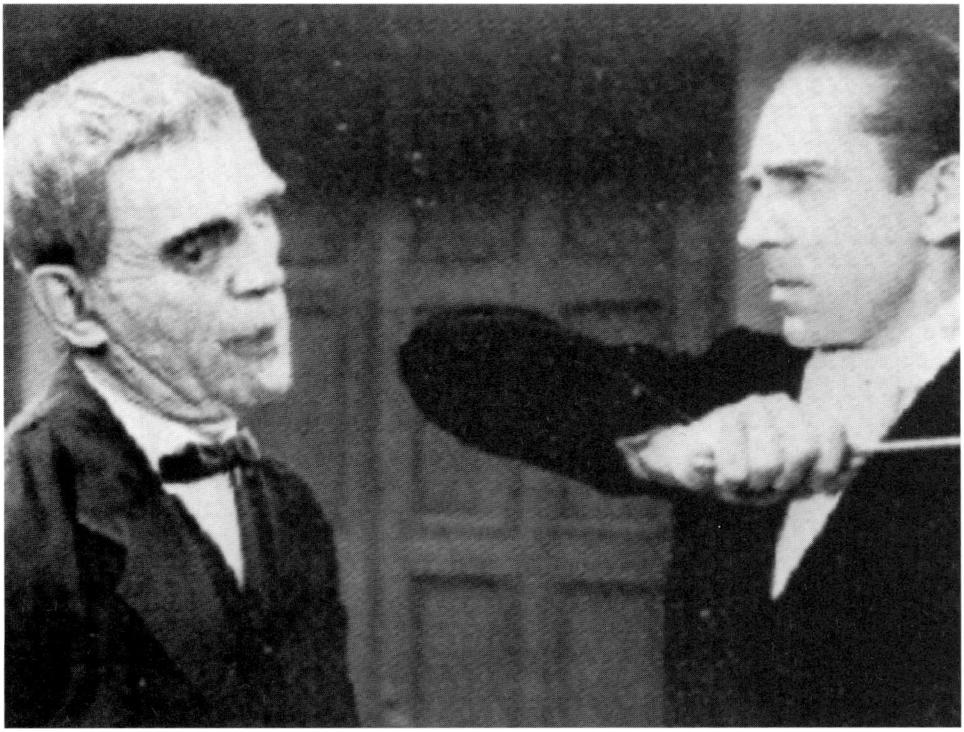

The Raven

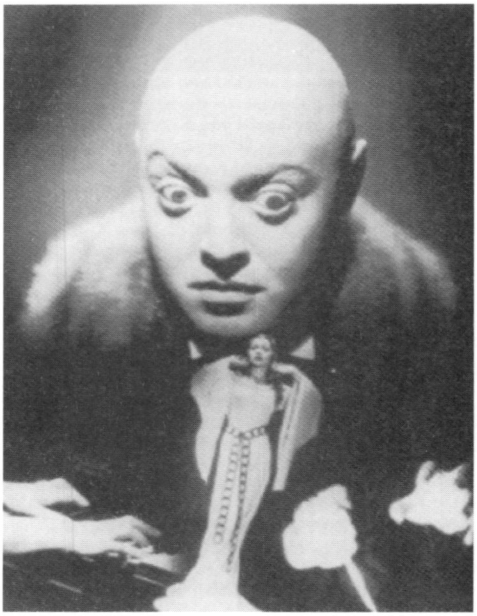

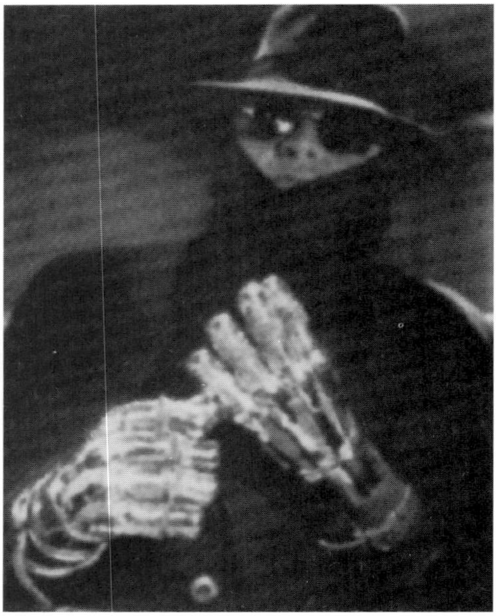

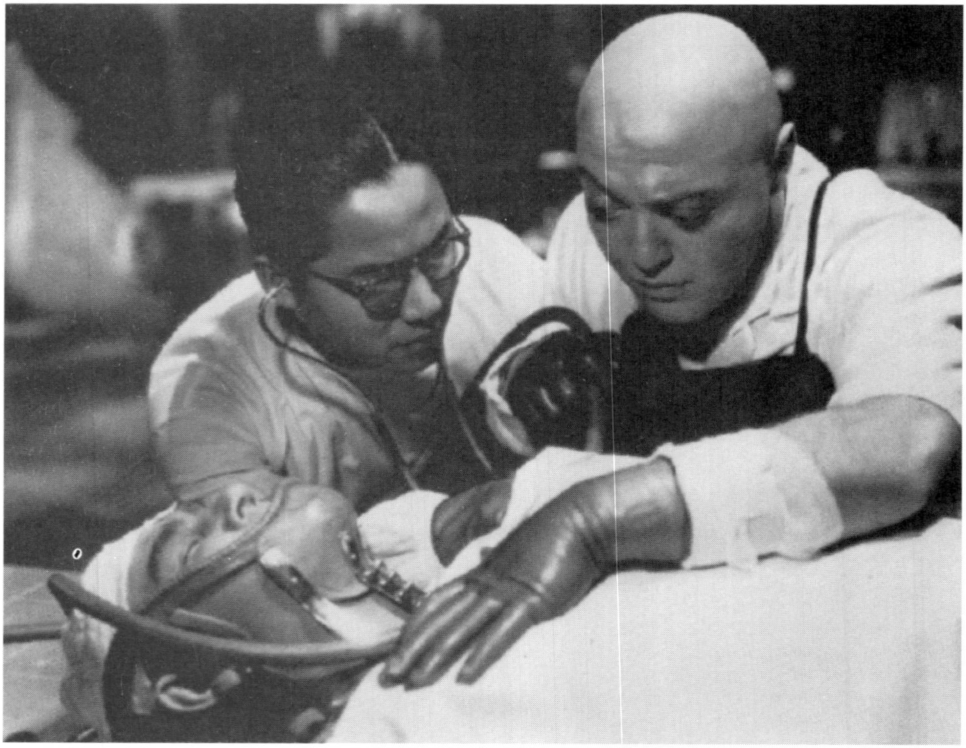

Mad Love

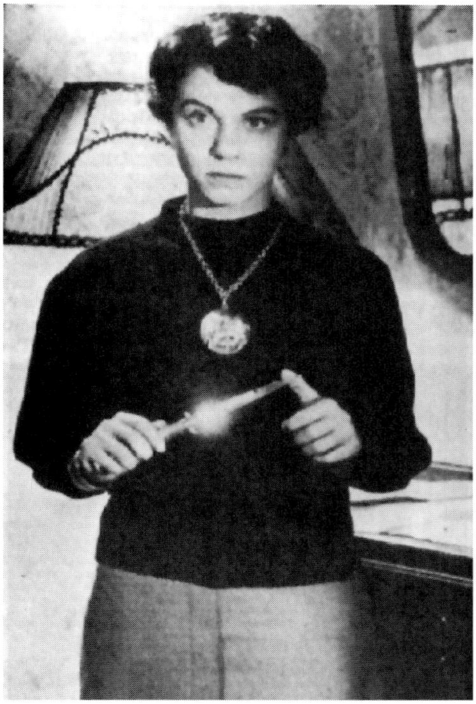

Dementia

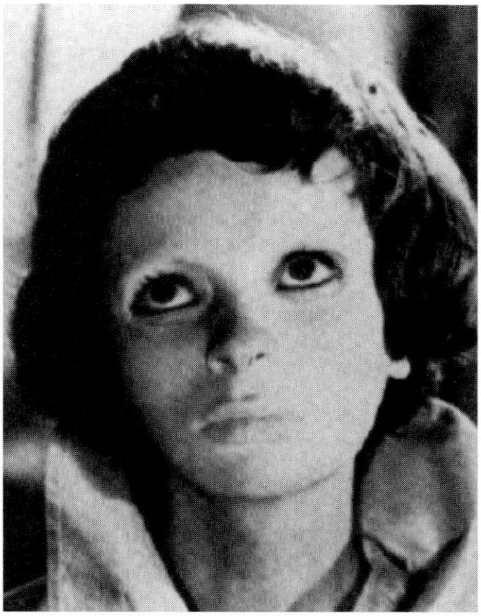

Les Yeux Sans Visage

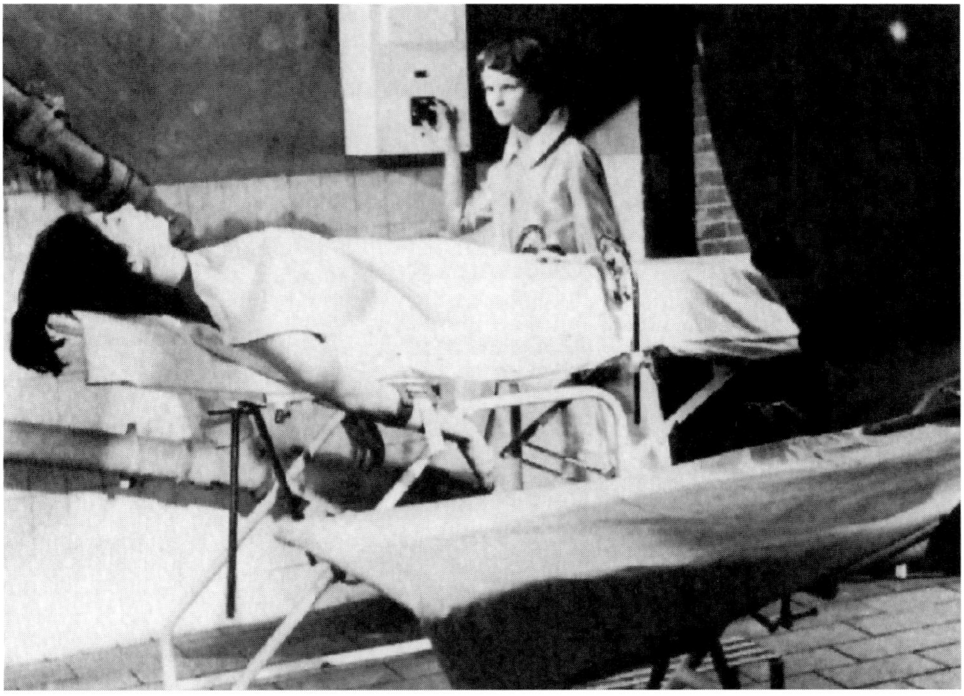

Les Yeux Sans Visage

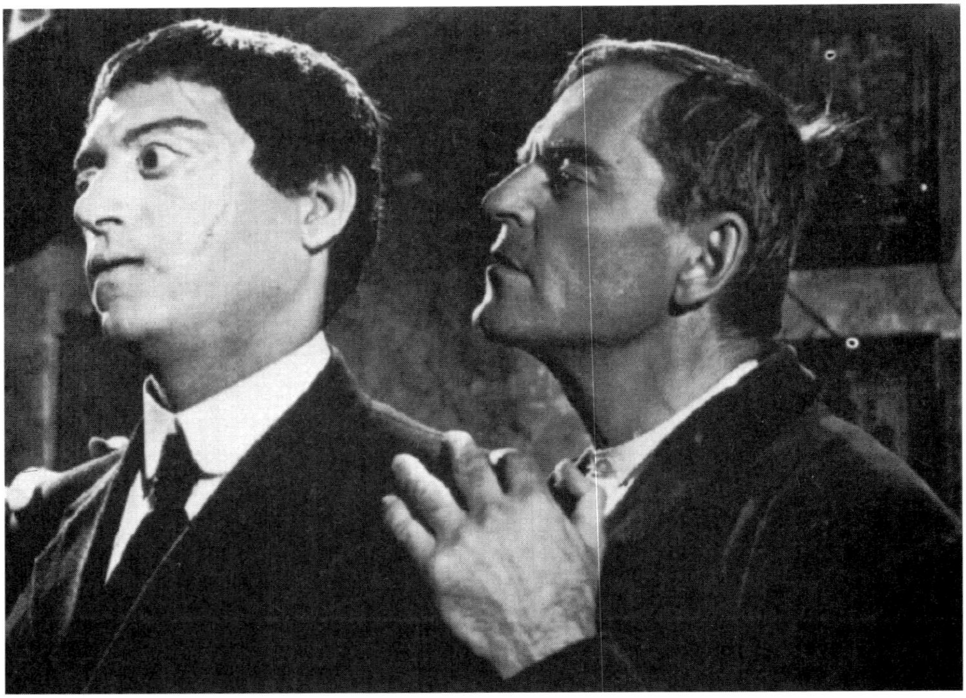

Gritos En La Noche

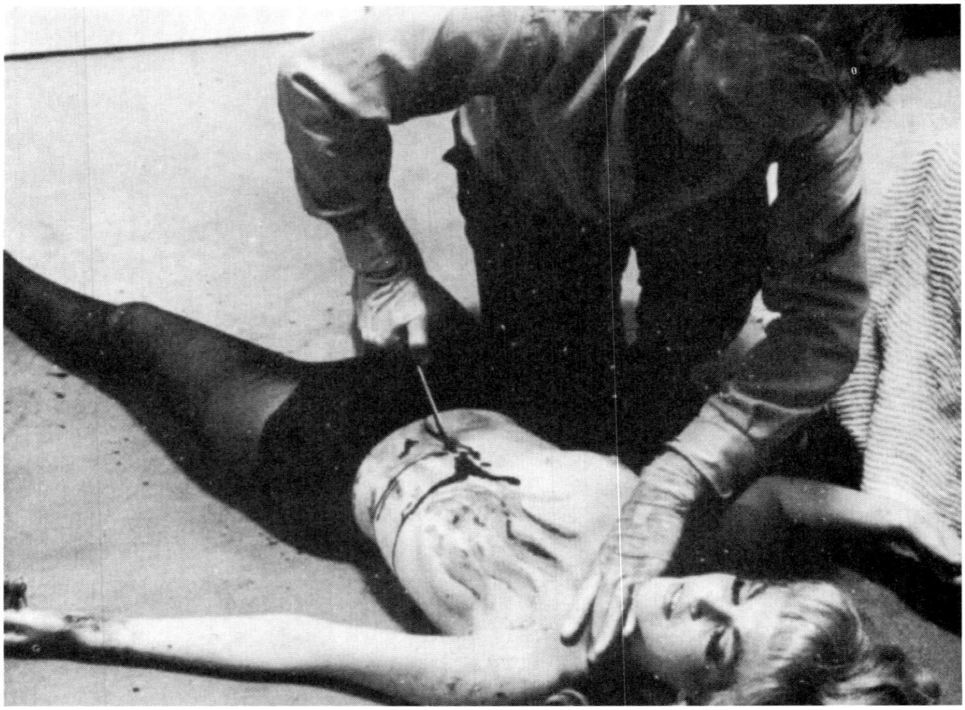

Corruption

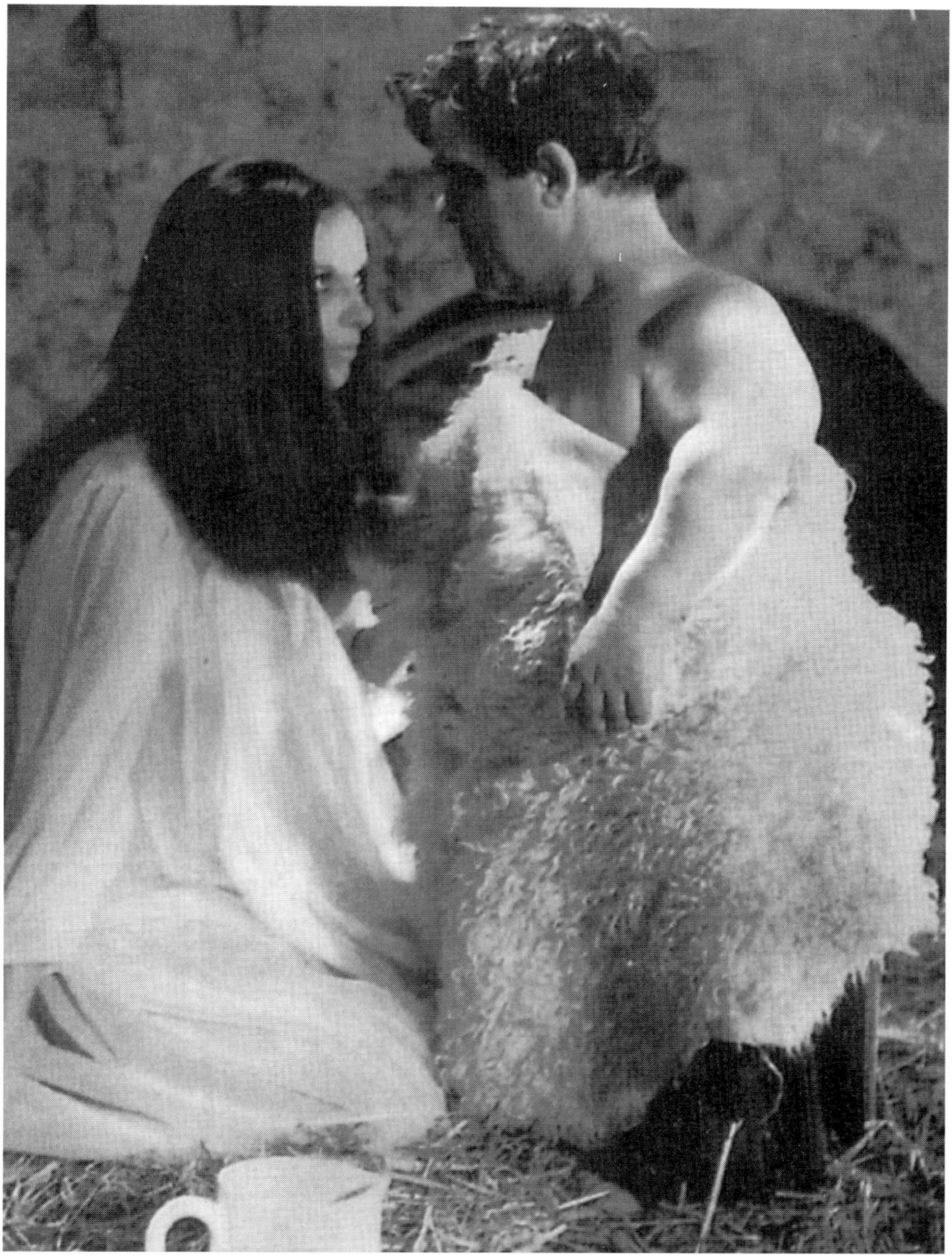

La Rose Escorchée

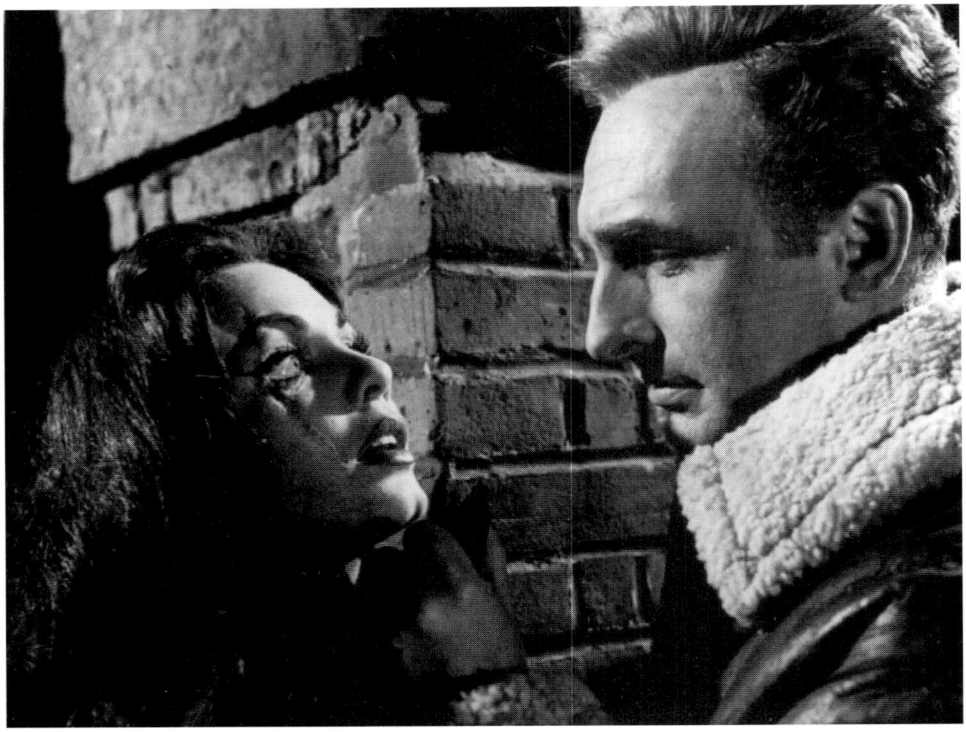

Circus Of Horrors

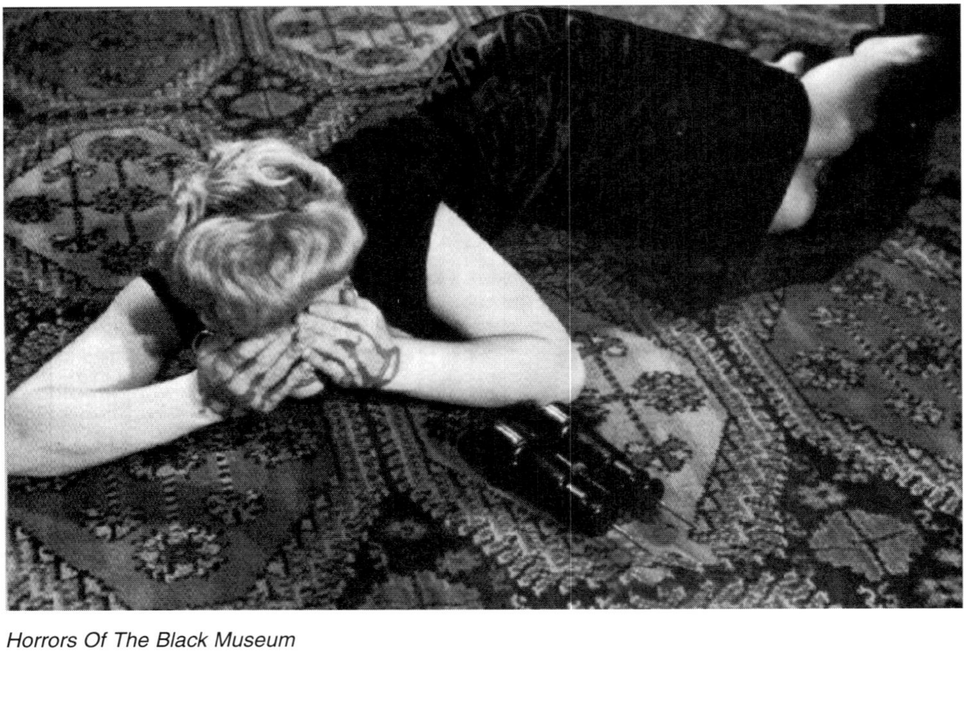

Horrors Of The Black Museum

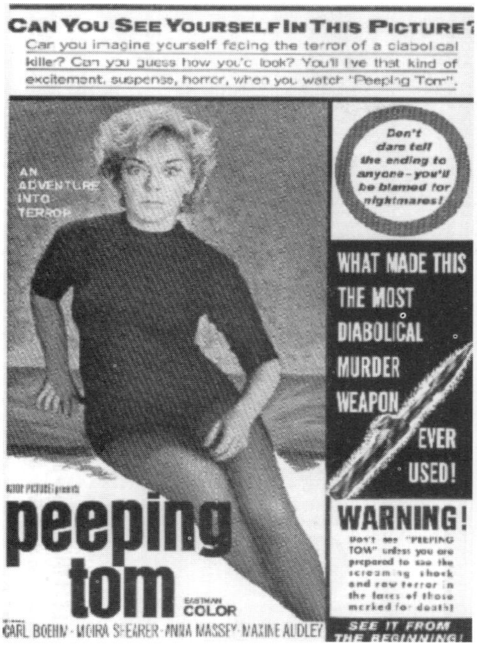
CAN YOU SEE YOURSELF IN THIS PICTURE?
Can you imagine yourself facing the terror of a diabolical killer? Can you guess how you'd look? You'll live that kind of excitement, suspense, horror, when you watch "Peeping Tom".
AN ADVENTURE INTO TERROR
Don't dare tell the ending to anyone – you'll be blamed for nightmares!
WHAT MADE THIS THE MOST DIABOLICAL MURDER WEAPON EVER USED!
WARNING!
Don't see "PEEPING TOM" unless you are prepared to see the screaming shock and raw terror in the faces of those marked for death!
peeping tom
COLOR
CARL BOEHM · MOIRA SHEARER · ANNA MASSEY · MAXINE AUDLEY
SEE IT FROM THE BEGINNING!

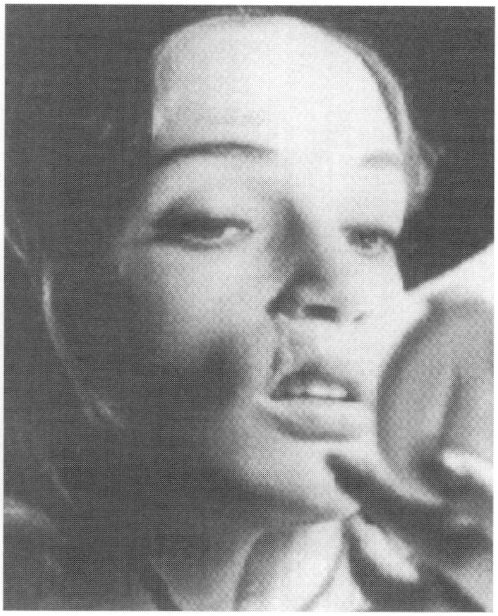

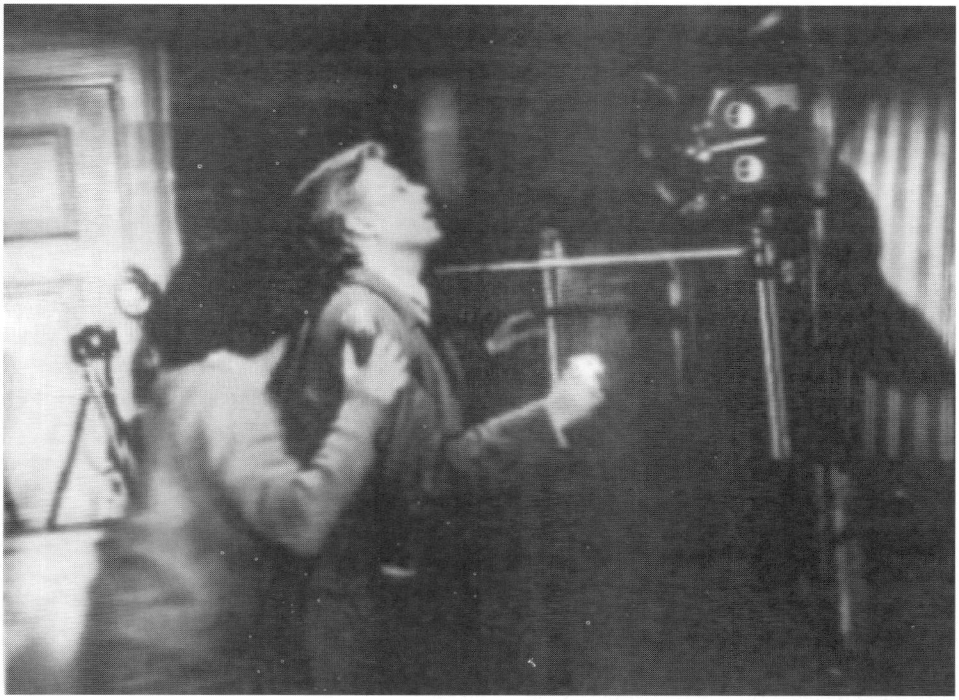

Peeping Tom

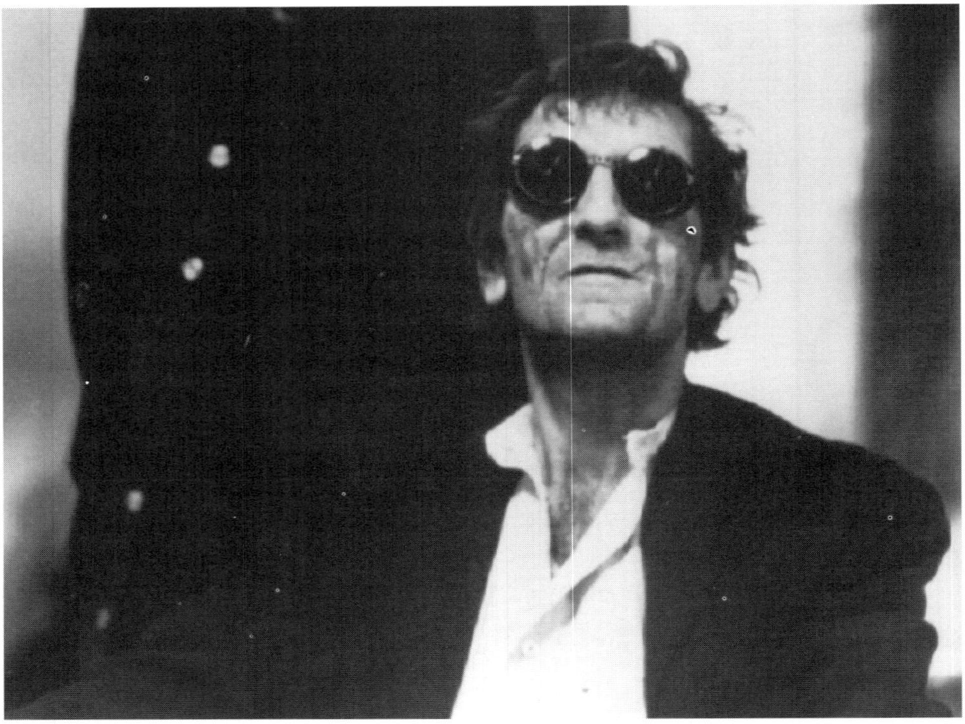

Wise Blood

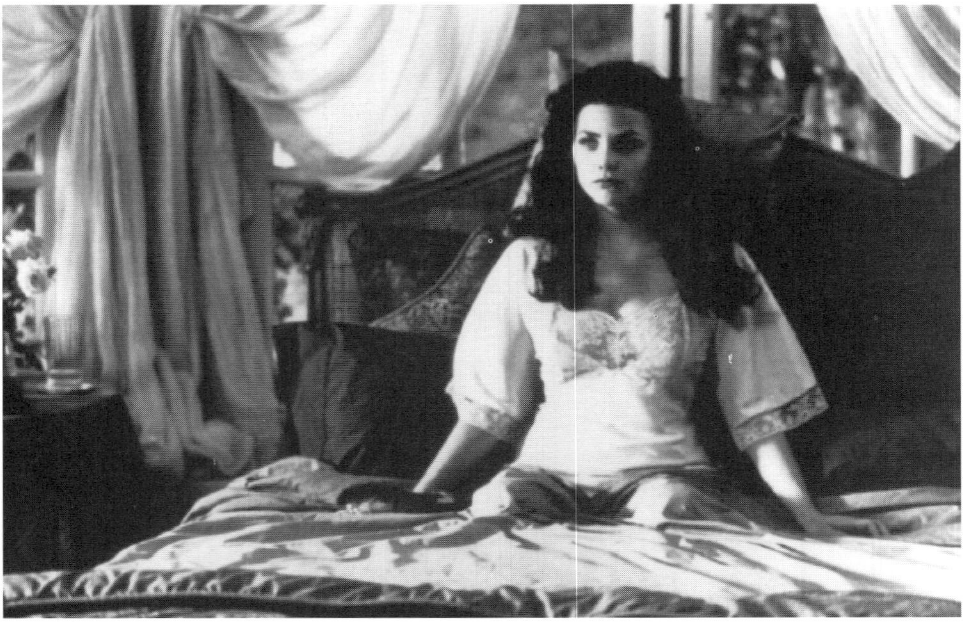

Boxing Helena

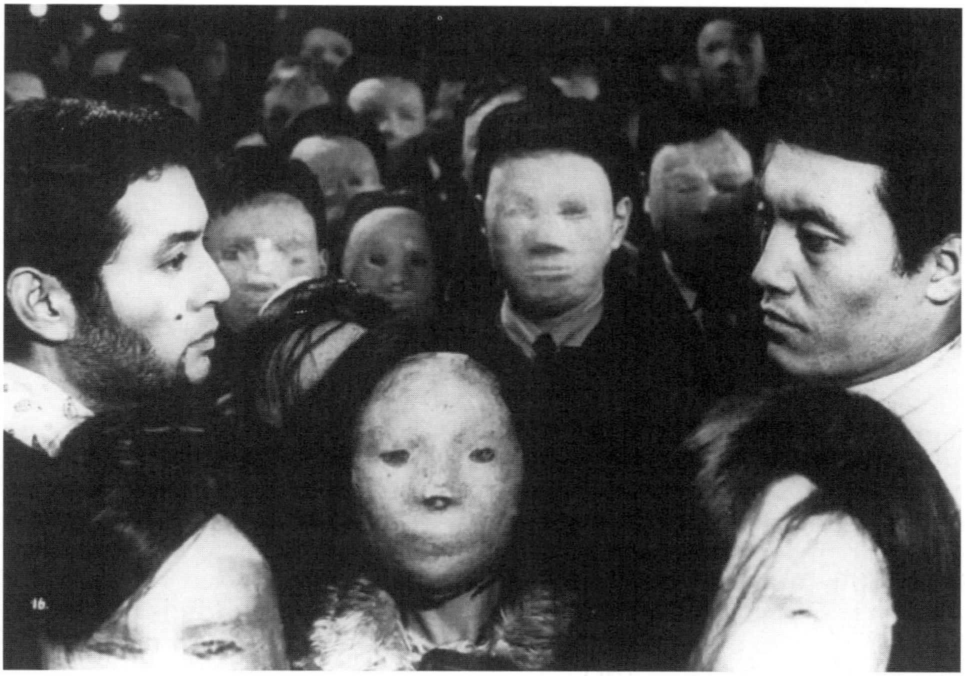

Tanin No Kao

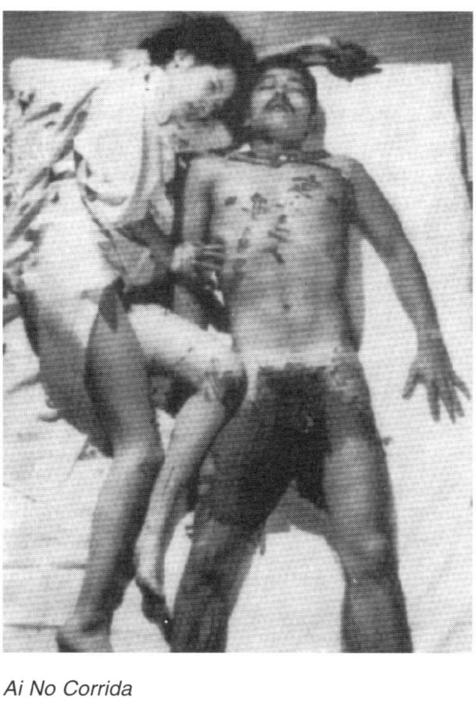

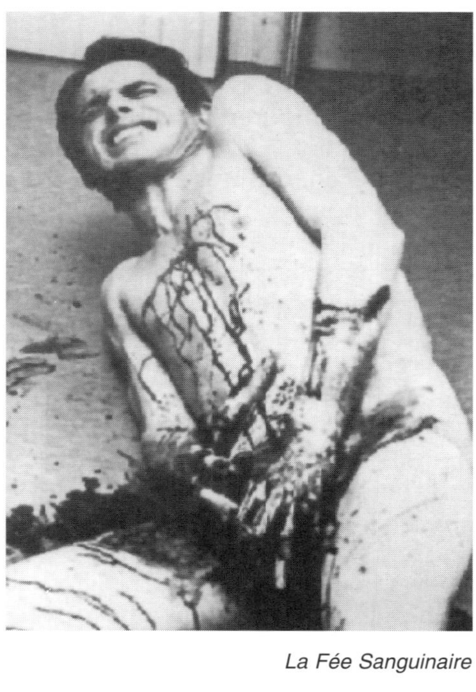

La Fée Sanguinaire

Ai No Corrida

MIRRORS OF EVIL

Tod Browning's *Freaks* was one of the first films to present a 'family' of human anomalies and outsiders as a grotesque mirror image of the 'normal' nuclear family or society. Like many subsequent films, Browning pursues this theme to the point where it is the 'normal' people who seem twisted, immoral, monstrous. The same year, James Whale directed his classic of screaming gothic *The Old Dark House*, and the tradition of the 'anti-family' in bizarre cinema was established. Based on the novel *Benighted* by J. B. Priestly, *The Old Dark House* is catalogue of grotesqueries arranged around a simple situationist plotline: five travellers – played by Melvyn Douglas, Charles Laughton, Raymond Massey, Gloria Stuart and Lillian Bond – seek refuge from a violent thunderstorm in an old, crumbling mansion, and come face to face with the eccentric Femm family during a night of strange events and confrontations. Ernest Thesiger plays the deranged Horace Femm, and Eva Moore his hag sister, who head the household; their pyromaniac brother is portrayed by Brember Wills, and their 102-year-old father by a woman, an old crone of uncertain identity (despite being listed cryptically in the cast as 'John Dudgeon'); Boris Karloff completes this weird retinue as Morgan, the mute, hideously-disfigured butler. Nothing much happens in the film, which lasts a brief 70 minutes, but Whale wrings every last drop of midnight black humour from his scenario; Horace Femm's dour proclamations, his sister's histrionics, the shaking pyromaniac in a constant search for matches, and the hideous, asexual ululations of the bed-ridden yet homicidal father, punctuated by the butler's wordless, unexplained comings and goings. The photography is superb, the soundtrack of wind, rain, thunder, slamming doors, creaking floorboards and flapping shutters unrelenting (there is no musical score). The climax comes with a conflagration, when Wills finally gets his hands on the matches.

With *The Old Dark House*, James Whale simultaneously parodied, and created the apotheosis of, the 'old/haunted house' movie, while his juxtaposition of the five visitors/five residents reflects human duality and questions notions of 'normal' behaviour; the whole experience tinged with sinister, even malevolent humour.

For some reason, Hammer Films commissioned William Castle to produce a pathetic, best-forgotten remake in 1962; Curt McDowell's *Thundercrack* (1976) comes on like a perverse porno version.

Inspired by the book inspired by the case of Ed Gein, the mother-fixated cannibal necrophile, Alfred Hitchcock in 1960 produced perhaps the most famous and discussed of all bizarre films, *Psycho*. Where Gein had adorned himself in a suit and mask of maternal human skin to dance by moonlight, Hitchcock's insane protagonist Norman Bates (Anthony Perkins) was content to stuff his mother's body and keep it preserved in a top bedroom. The real trouble starts when Bates, blasted by Oedipal guilt, imagines she is still alive and issuing directives to slay young women to whom he is attracted. Finally her personality engulfs him, and in an end-scene reminiscent of the ventriloquist's dummy segment of *Dead Of Night* (1945) we see Bates possessed, a two-in-one being or psychic hermaphrodite heteradelphian, a living testament to familial sickness. More than 20 years later two insignificant sequels appeared: *Psycho II* (1983) and *Psycho III* (1986). Both are best forgotten in comparison to the original.

The spirit of *The Old Dark House* was invoked, some thirty years later, by a truly outlandish offering, Jack Hill's *Spider Baby* (1964). Here we meet the Merrye family, another demented, inbred brood this time suffering from their own indigenous illness, Merrye's Syndrome. The chief symptom of this affliction appears to be mental regression to the level of infancy, accompanied by homicidal urges and cannibalism. The family consists of Elizabeth (Beverly Washburn), a grown women who dresses and behaves like an eleven-year-old; Virginia (Jill Banner), the Spider Baby of the title who believes she is a spider and eats flies; and Ralph (Sid Haig), a bald sub-infantile freak. They are watched over by faithful chaffeur Bruno, played by Lon Chaney Jr (who also sings the title tune). When two distant relatives turn up with their lawyer to try and claim the family mansion for themselves, the scene is set for a grotesque display replete with greed, mental and physical disintegration, cannibalism, rape and murder, which is nonetheless saved, by dint of its primitive sensibilities, from being cynically gratuitous. More seriously deranged and dangerous than the Femm family, though still with an edge of profoundly black humour to their antics, the Merryes seem to anticipate the ultimate degenerates of Tobe Hooper's *Texas Chainsaw Massacre*.

Family madness has featured in many other notable bizarre films. The most famous of all twisted sisters appeared in Robert Aldrich's *Whatever Happened To Baby Jane* (1962), an over-the-top *grand guignol* piece with Bette Davis and Joan Crawford offering hideous self-parodies as the sisters who hate each other to the point of murder. This theme of demented siblings had been treated earlier in *Three Bad Sisters* (1956), in which one girl kills herself after being disfigured by her hateful sister. Brian de Palma later came up with *Sisters* (aka *Blood Sisters*, 1973), a clever story utilising split-screen techniques in which the surviving Siamese twin from a failed separation switches between her own personality and that of her dead sister to become a murderess. David Cronenberg's *Dead Ringers* (1988) was a typically strange, though sober, addition to this field, echoing Peter Greenaway's *A Zedd And Two Noughts* in its tale of two identical twins (played by Jeremy Irons) who indulge in identity-swapping and descend into a psychotic state, signified by the creation of hellish gynaecological instruments which could only be employed on the most freakish of human monsters. In *The Bad Seed* (1956), Patty McCormack played the evil child who kills anyone threatening to come between her and her idiot mother.

Post-atomic angst and the shadow of thalidomide – two examples of the results of unchecked patriarchy – can be seen as strong factors in a cinematic trend which took the 'anti-family' one step further: the fantasy of the 'demon baby'. Though most films in this area were strictly tales of the supernatural,[10] perhaps the most horrifying 'baby' of them all appears in a classic of bizarre cinema which, though often hallucinatory, operates in an all-too-plausible post-industrial zone. *Eraserhead* (1977) marked the debut of a director who would go on to work almost exclusively in or around this genre: David Lynch. The film, shot in stark monochrome, is a relentless exhibition of deformity and alienation, set in a grinding, claustrophobic factory landscape. Henry, a rotund oaf (played by John "Jack" Nance), is invited to dinner by his girlfriend's parents. They are borderline psychotic, their house is a hovel, their daughter is repulsive and, much worse than that, mysteriously pregnant. She soon gives birth to a hideous baby, a wailing freak which resembles an animal foetus. Henry is soon left to tend to this diseased offspring by himself. Lynch introduces nightmares within nightmares, compounding the horror of this hopeless existence. While Henry fantasises about a chanteuse with cancerous facial deformities crushing sperm-like teratomas behind his radiator, the baby grows sick, vomiting blood and finally coming apart in a welter of fecal pus. *Eraserhead* confirms the hideous, ineluctable nature of reproduction, showing the universe itself as a septic womb in which there are untold legions of foetuses within poison foetuses vying for the transient sickness, the ceaseless freakshow that is life.

Meanwhile, America had produced a weird and lethal 'family' for real. Straight out of Death Valley, the Charles Manson family (consisting largely of patriarch Charlie and a veritable harem of unquestioning, murdering rich-bitch drop-outs) took centre-place in the American psyche from 1969-70 when they perpetrated the savage murders of Roman Polanski's pregnant wife Sharon Tate and several others. Film-makers were quick to exploit this notoriety, producing works (or even re-packaging existent movies) to invoke the Family, such as *Sweet Saviour* (1970), *The Deathmaster* (1972), *I Drink Your Blood* (1971), *The Night God Screamed* (1972), *Satan's Sadists* (1969), porn flicks *Love In A Commune* and *The Manson Massacre* (1971), *Cult Of The Damned* (aka *Angel, Angel, Down We Go*, 1969), *The Other Side Of Madness*, and last but not least Michael and Roberta Findlay's *Slaughter*, remarkable mainly because, when eventually released 5 years after shooting with a new ending tacked on and re-named *Snuff*, it almost single-handedly started the modern myth of 'snuff-movie' making (itself one of many heinous activities linked to Manson by gonzo journalist Ed Sanders in his true-life account *The Family*).

All of these efforts however, pale beside a film produced in 1973, when director Tobe Hooper looked beyond mere murder and free love and came up with the ultimate example of the grotesque, inbred, psychotic family unit. *The Texas Chainsaw Massacre*, one of the great unrelenting hell-films of all time, involves a cannibal family whose experience in the meat industry has led them beyond the pale to a preference for human cattle. The cook (Jim Siedow) has to look after Granpaw, the master slaughterman now so old he can barely grasp his killing-hammer, and the two idiot brothers Leatherface (Gunnar Hansen) and 'Hitcher' (Ed Neal). Inspired, like *Psycho*, by the Ed Gein case (as were *Deranged* [1974] and *Three On A Meathook* [1973]), the film shows the fate of a group of youngsters who fall prey to these demented butchers in the course of a day trip. Coming to a seemingly disused farmhouse, they investigate and discover a death zone of obscene beauty, furnished with human bones and skin. Often interpreted as a parody of the all-American way, Hooper's film in fact proudly presents the *perfect* American family, home and lifestyle, the only logical destination for denizens of an abattoir economy. The vague ecological concerns, albinos and inbreds of John Boorman's *Deliverance* (1972) are small beer compared to this.

Leatherface slaughters and meathooks his 'guests' like animals; of course, they offer no resistance (the reality of the death instinct). The sole surviving girl (Marilyn Burns) is reserved as main course in a cannibal banquet. She escapes only when Granpaw proves incapable of delivering the fatal blow. Possessed of lethal, hell-black humour which fails to leaven its atrocious impact, *The Texas Chainsaw Massacre* remains one of the most complete cinematic experiences; an unapologetic, authentic glimpse at the absolute beauty of a pure, unfettered aesthetic and philosophy rivalled only by Ford Coppola's purgatorial end-of-river inferno in *Apocalypse Now*.

The film has spawned two sequels (all three are still banned completely in England). *Texas Chainsaw Massacre 2* (Tobe Hooper, 1986) stars Dennis Hopper as saw-wielding preacher on the trail of his nephew's murderers, prepared to fight fire with fire. The film is funny and bloody in equal measure but the mixture never gels satisfactorily. Jeff Burr's *Leatherface: Texas Chainsaw Massacre 3* (1989) is nastier, a swamp-bound redneck evocation of 'free hate'.

Wes Craven's *The Hills Have Eyes* (1977) resembles a desert/Western version of the first *Chainsaw* movie, though far less convincing (there is an inference that the deranged cannibal family here may be radiation victims; worst of all, their prey fights back). An American family on vacation encounter the dune-dwelling psychos in a violent clash, resulting in the abduction of their baby as potential dinner. Sadly, the infant is retrieved and the cannibals killed in a 'happy' ending. Pluto, the most grotesque family member, is played by professional 'crazy', Michael Berryman. *The Hills Have Eyes, Part 2* (1984) was a pointless follow-up, though Craven's intermediary *Deadly Blessing* (1981) was notable for its homicidal Hittite hermaphrodite. Apart from in spoofs like the recent *Addams Family* films, the 'freak family' has since been largely neglected; it is difficult to imagine anyone ever bettering Hooper's original vision.

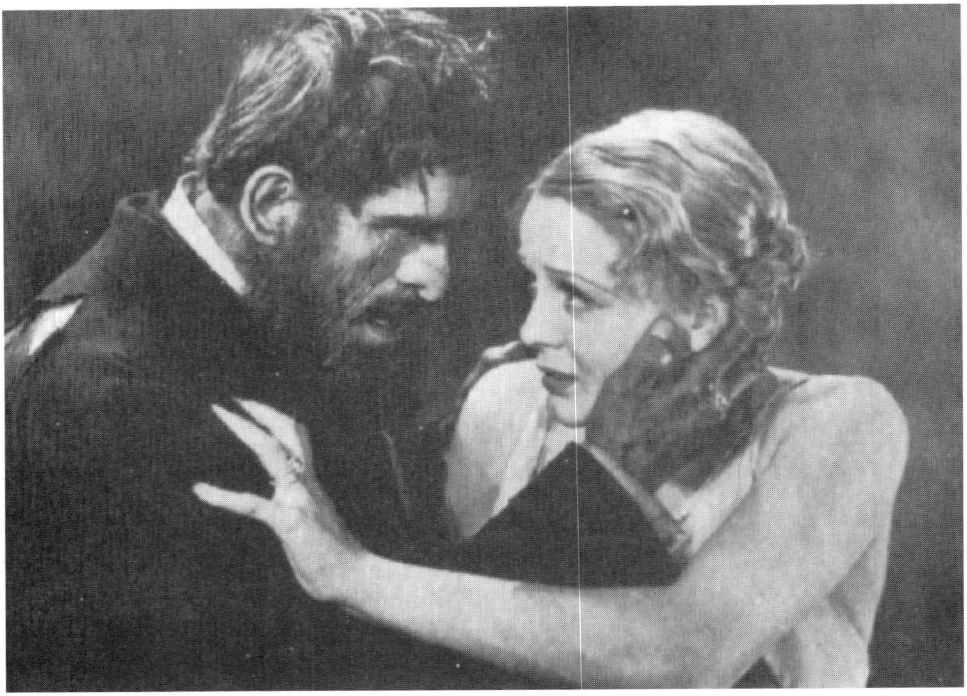

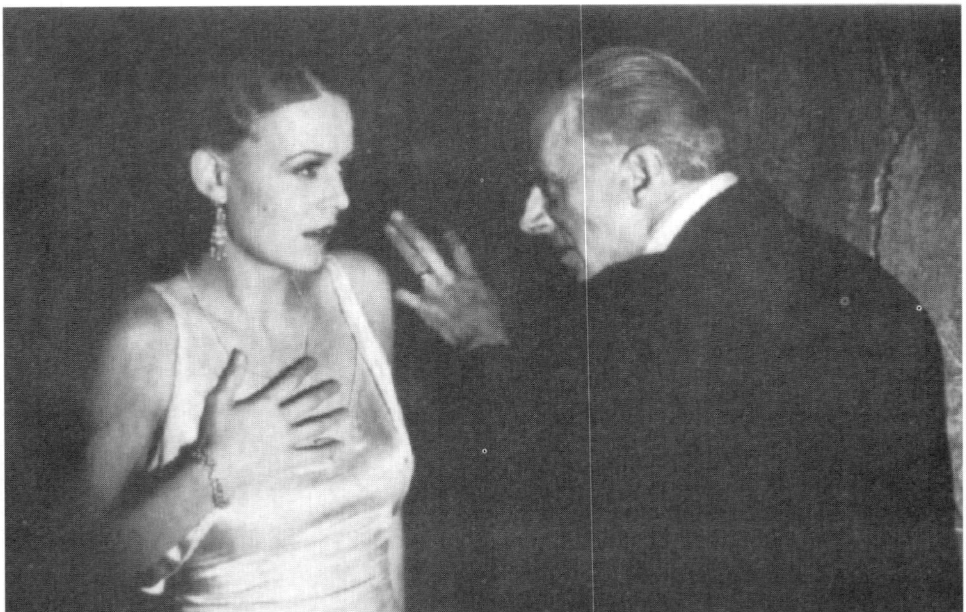

The Old Dark House

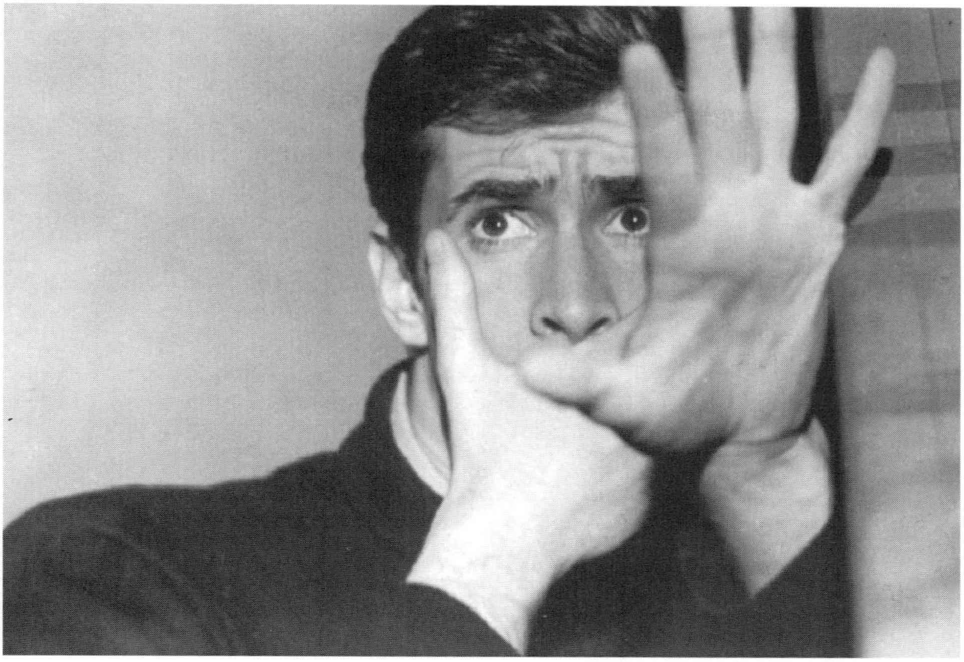

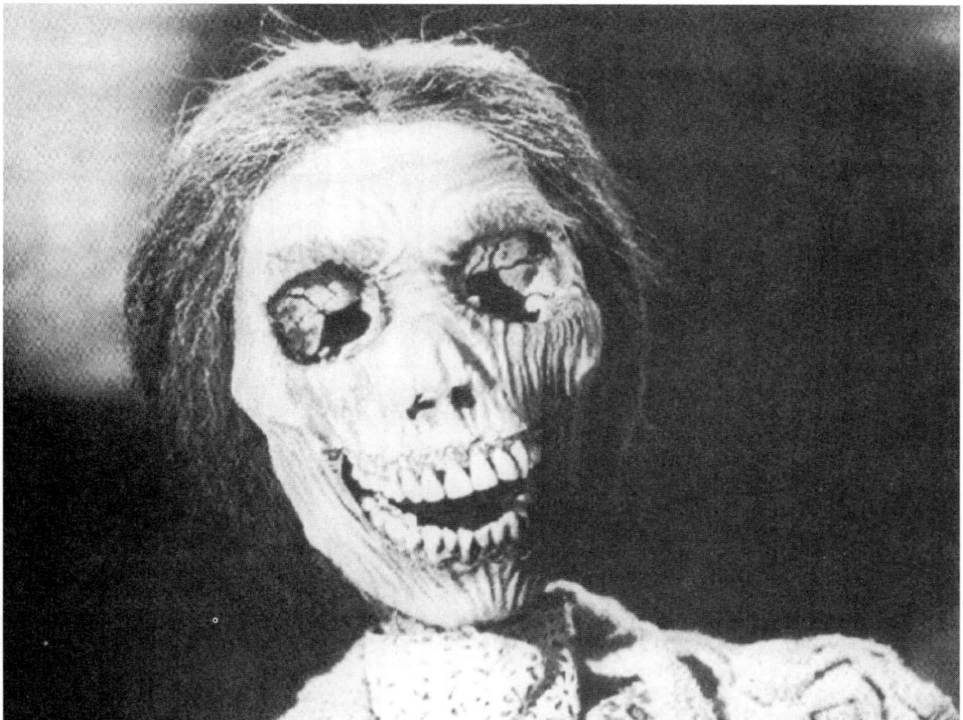

Psycho

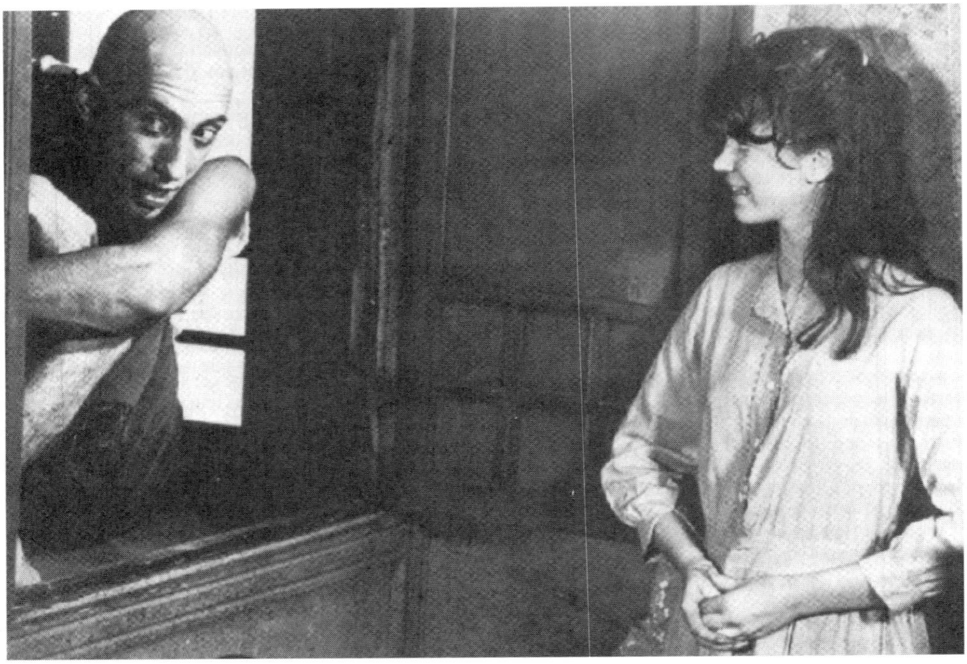

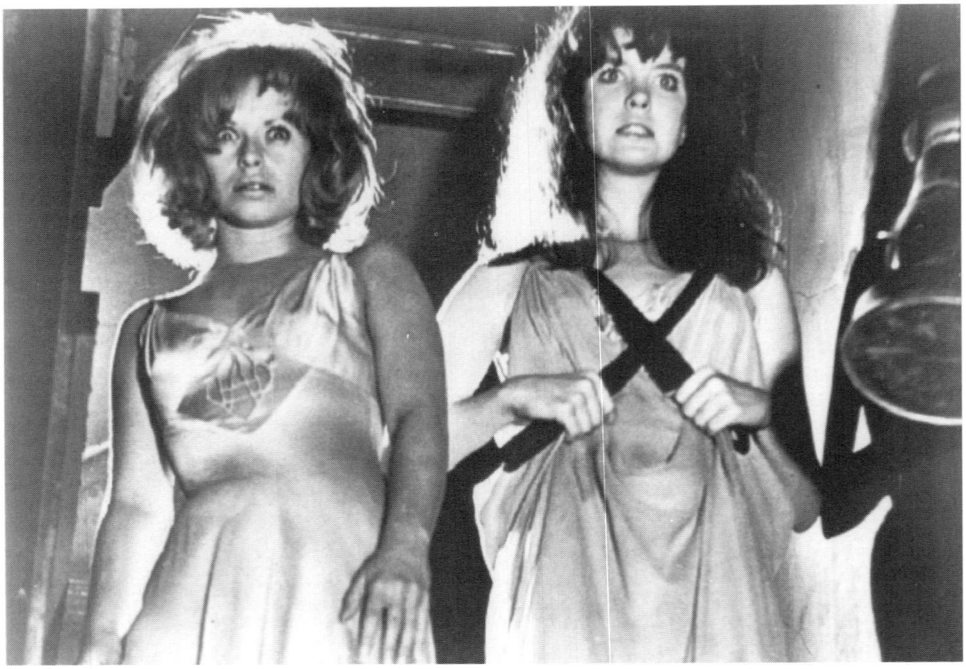

Spider Baby

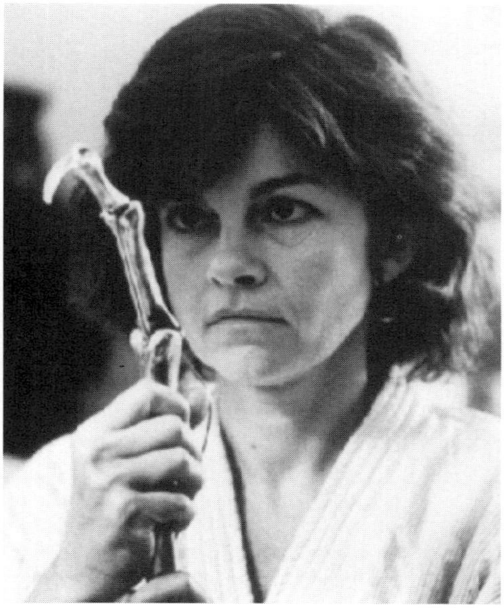

Dead Ringers

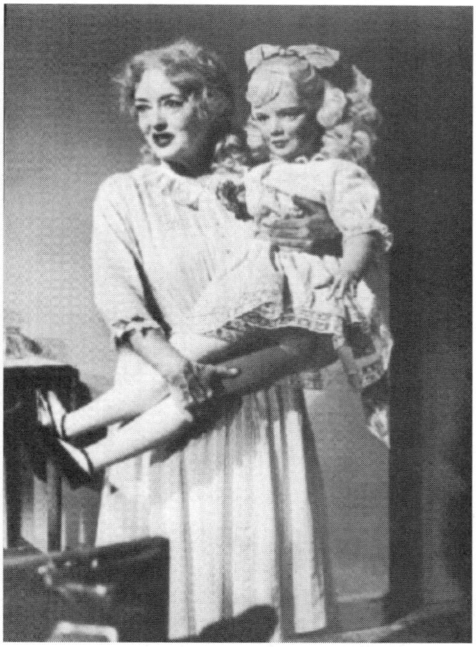

Whatever Happened To Baby Jane?

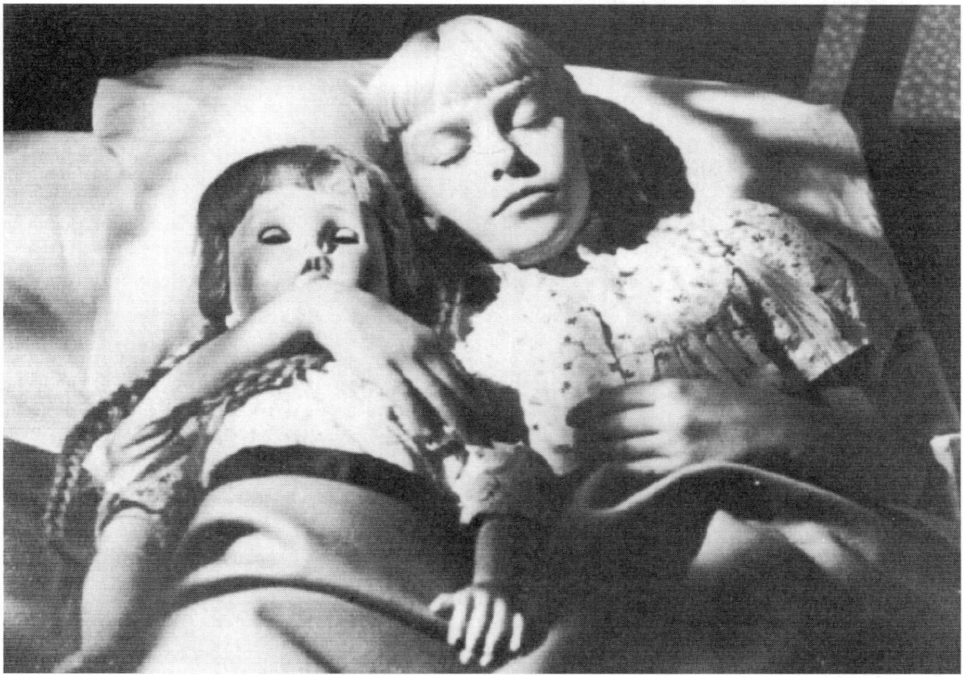

The Bad Seed

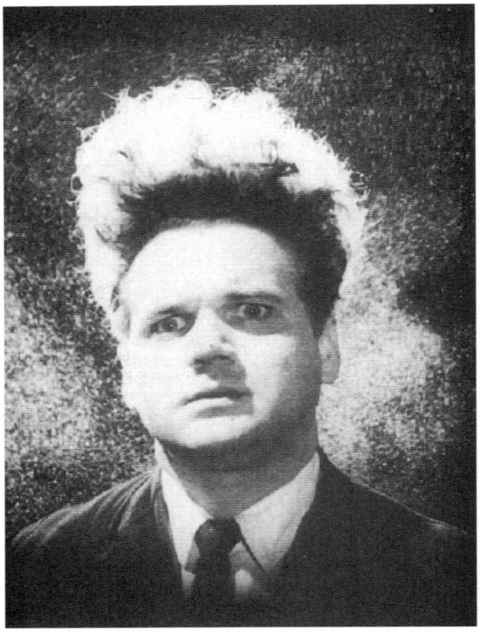

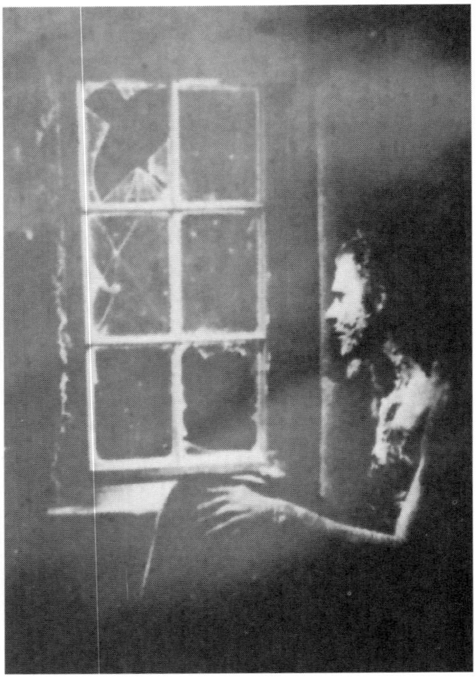

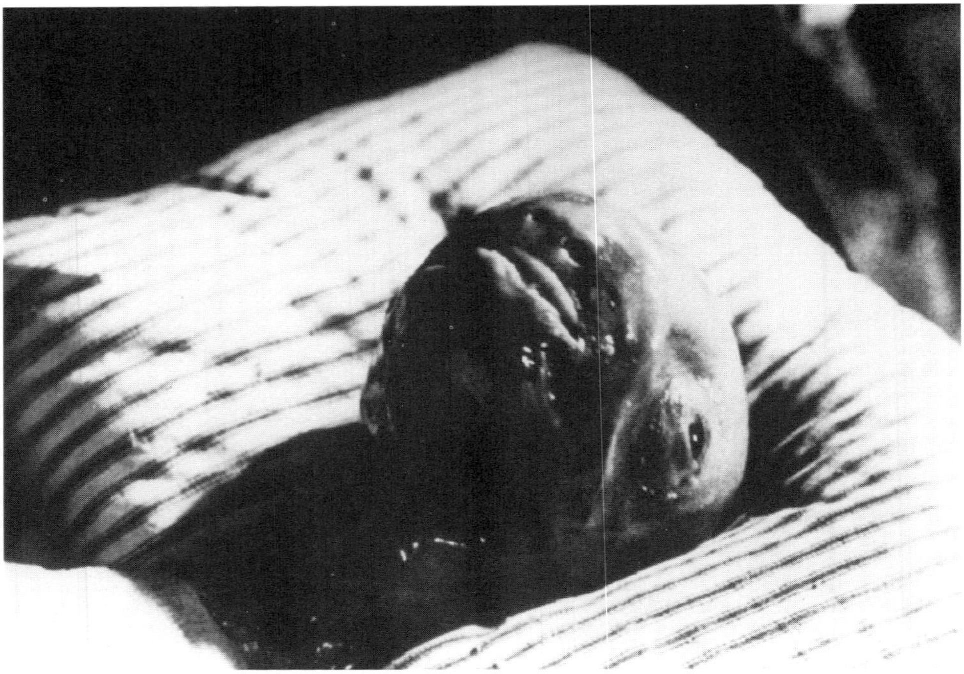

Eraserhead

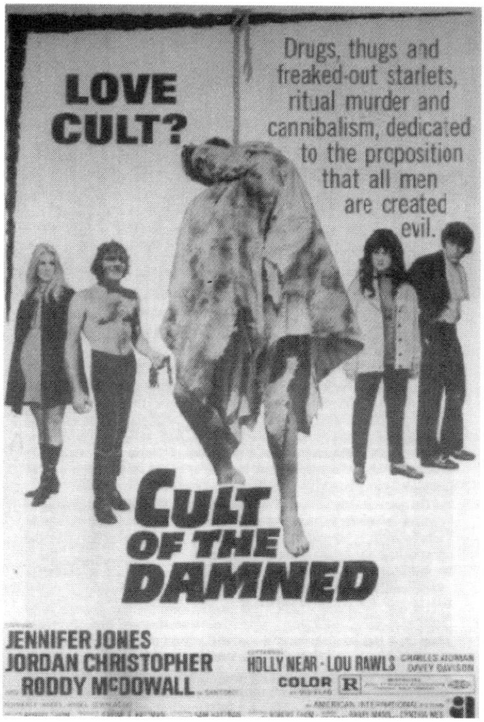
LOVE CULT?
Drugs, thugs and freaked-out starlets, ritual murder and cannibalism, dedicated to the proposition that all men are created evil.
CULT OF THE DAMNED
JENNIFER JONES
JORDAN CHRISTOPHER
RODDY McDOWALL
HOLLY NEAR · LOU RAWLS
COLOR

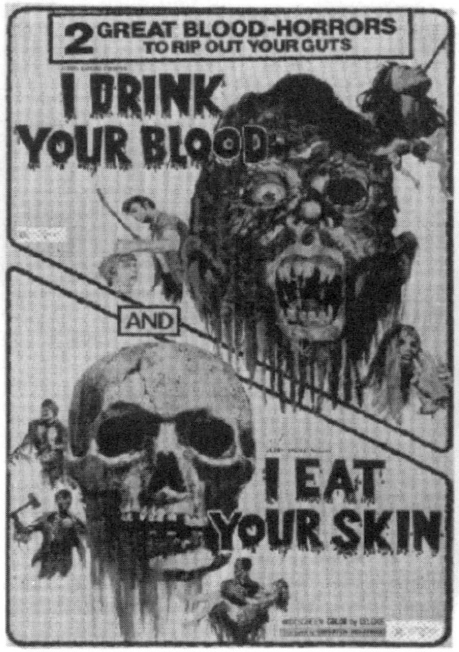
2 GREAT BLOOD-HORRORS
TO RIP OUT YOUR GUTS
I DRINK YOUR BLOOD
AND
I EAT YOUR SKIN

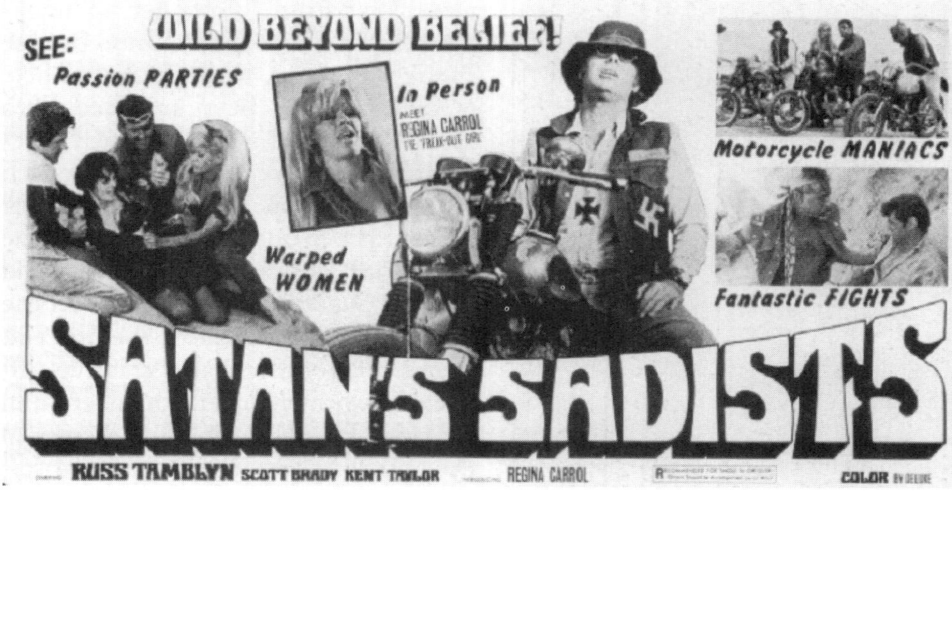
SEE:
WILD BEYOND BELIEF!
Passion PARTIES
In Person
REGINA CARROL
Warped WOMEN
Motorcycle MANIACS
Fantastic FIGHTS
SATAN'S SADISTS
RUSS TAMBLYN SCOTT BRADY KENT TAYLOR
REGINA CARROL
COLOR

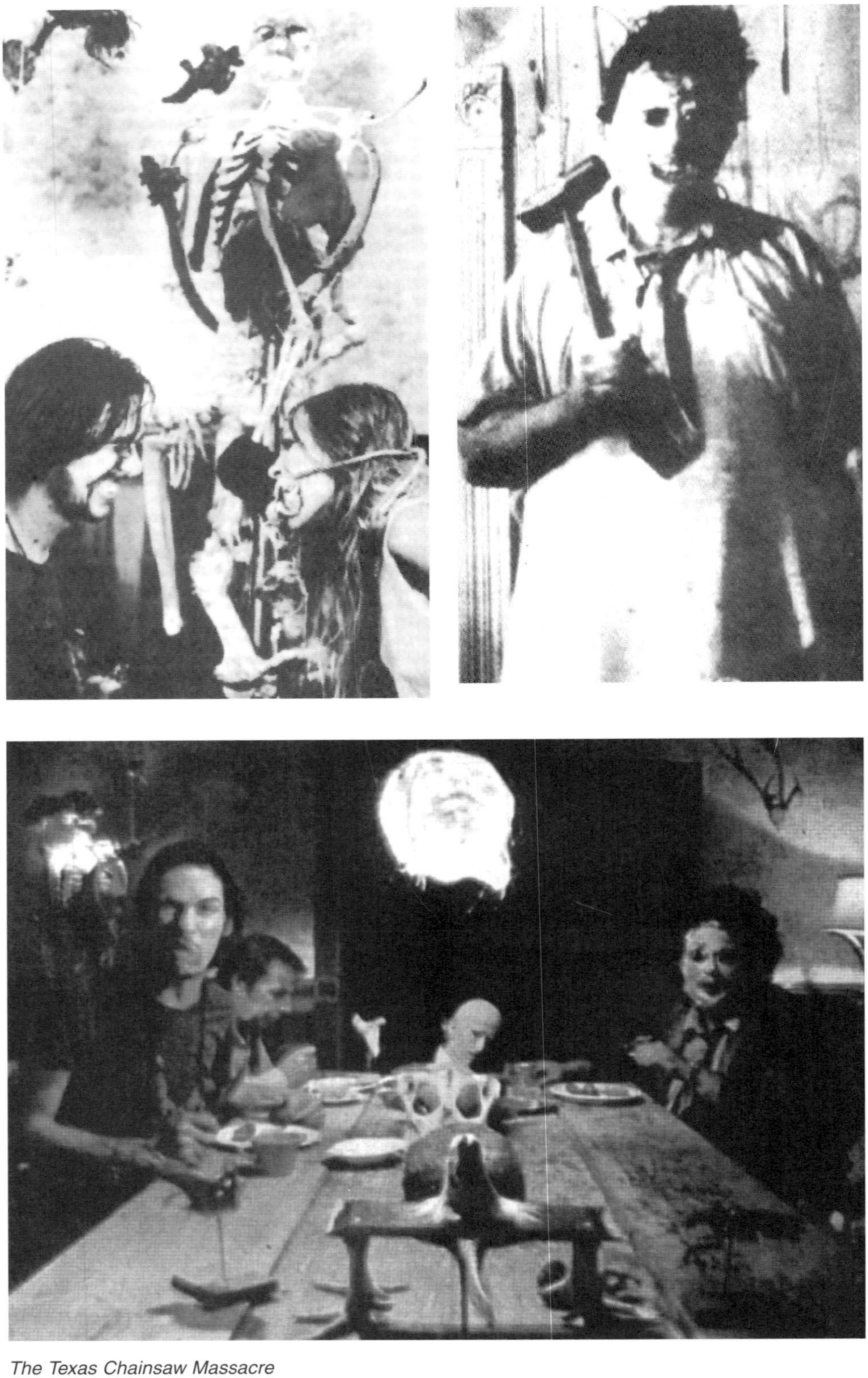

The Texas Chainsaw Massacre

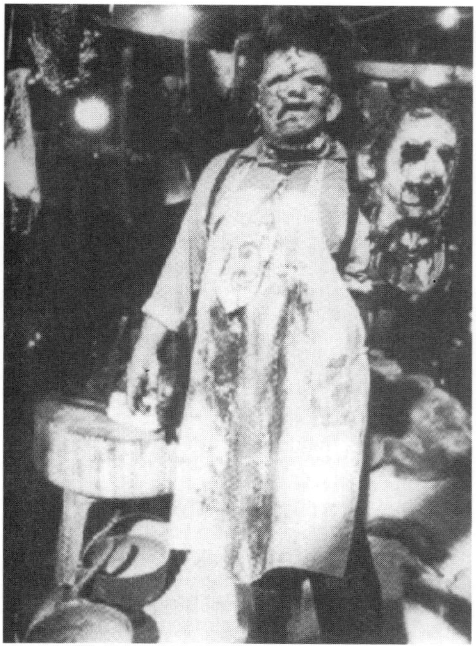

Texas Chainsaw 2

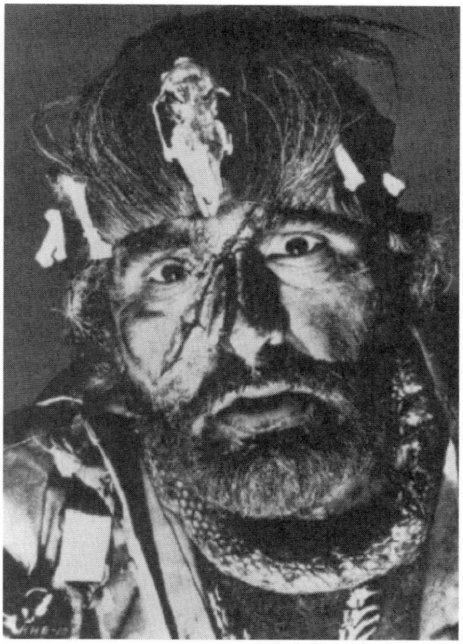

The Hills Have Eyes

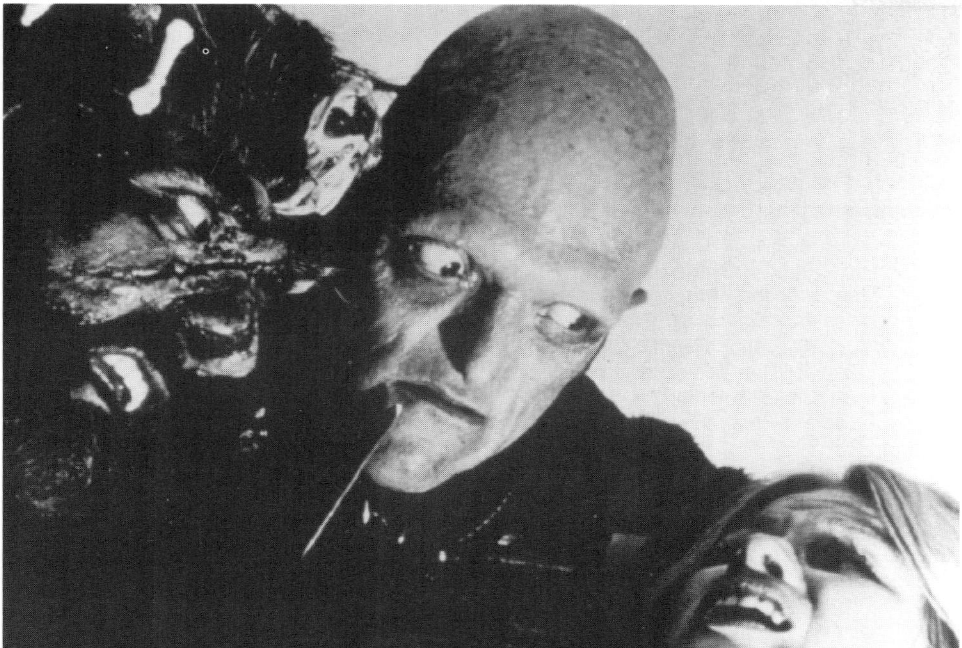

The Hills Have Eyes

NOTES

1 Dalí retained an interest in film, producing, amongst others, an unrealized scenario with Harpo Marx (!) entitled *Giraffes On Hunchback Salad* – despite this promising title, little is known of its proposed content. Agreeing to collaborate with Alfred Hitchcock on *Spellbound* (1945), Dalí's unique vision was again compromised. Upon arrival at the studio, he was dismayed to find that his scenario of fifteen grand pianos laden with statues and suspended above the heads of cut-out silhouettes had been transmuted to miniature model pianos hanging over some forty real-life dwarfs.

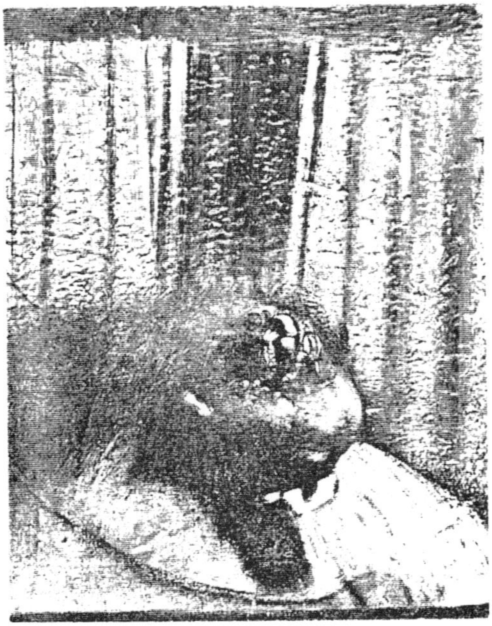

2 Only Francis Bacon, with works such as his *Three Studies For Figures At The Base Of A Crucifixion* (1944) and *Head I* (1948), has equalled Dalí for horrific expositions of the meltdown of human flesh under the extreme conditions (war, spiritual abjection, paranoia) of this century.

3 Inevitably, hardcore films such as *Freak Sex* (see the midget disappear between the fat lady's buttocks) have also appeared, as have efforts featuring obviously prosthetic freaks such as *Joined – The Siamese Twins* (1990), *Edward Penishands* (1991), *Cyrano* (man with a penis-nose, 1991) and *Long Dan Silver* (man with 24" penis, also 1991). The *Freaks Of Nature* series includes supposed hermaphrodites (more likely 'freaks of surgery') amongst its weird and wonderful participants.

4 The tradition of these performance 'actions' has been kept alive by such groups as Coum Transmissions (1969-76), and individuals as diverse as Joseph Beuys, Paul McCarthy, Chris Burden, Linda Montano, Stelarc, Kim Jones and André Stitt.

On video, noise/performance group SPK produced *Despair* (1981), featuring images of autopsies, pathological specimens and malformed embryos set to industrial music. It has since become commonplace for groups such as Psychic TV or the Butthole Surfers to use video backdrops of sex-change surgery or mutilation/suicide/murder.

Main transgressors on the pop front were Soft Cell with their *Sex Dwarf* video in 1982. Featuring a semi-naked dwarf running amok with a chainsaw, it was duly banned from the High Street.

5 The 'actor', known only as Ray, in fact incurred his burns in a severe camping accident. Annie Sprinkle was then his current lover in 'real life'.

6 After this, and Dwight Frye's portrayal of Colin Clive's twisted assistant in *Frankenstein* (1930), the hunchback quickly became a cliché figure in the horror genre; featuring in not only the various remakes of *Notre Dame*, but also in nearly all the Universal *Frankenstein* sequels, and recurring right through *Blood Of The Vampire* (1958) to the likes of Tigon's *Cry Of The Banshee* (1970), Hammer's *Captain Kronos* (1972) and, best of all, the Spanish Paul Naschy vehicle, *Hunchback Of The Morgue* (1972). Ken Russell's *The Devils* (1971) even had Vanessa Redgrave as a hunchbacked nun, who projects her blasphemous erotic fantasies onto the priest Urbain Grandier.

7 When 'alive', the severed hand becomes a crawling, almost arachnid motif in the supernatural horror film; featuring in such works as Robert Florey's *The Beast With Five Fingers* (1945, originally to have been directed by Buñuel), *The Crawling Hand* (1963), *Dr Terror's House Of Horrors* (Freddie Francis, 1964) and Oliver Stone's *The Hand* (1981), with Michael Caine.

8 Another German director working in America, Fritz Lang, later made a similar impact with a key

scene in *The Big Heat* (1953), in which a sadistic killer (Lee Marvin) hideously disfigures his girlfriend (Gloria Grahame) by hurling boiling coffee in her face.

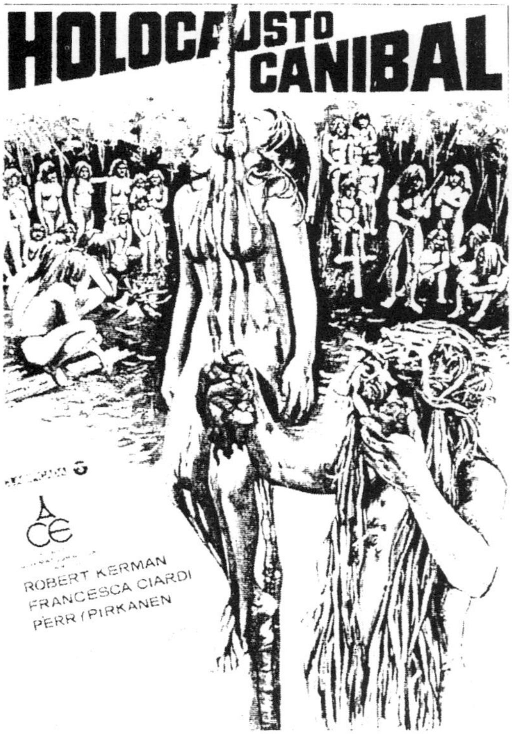

9 Exploitation films like *I Spit On Your Grave* and *Cannibal Holocaust* have also shown graphic castrations performed as acts of revenge or cruelty, but the element of sexual mania, the masochistic urge to endure life as a cripple in body as well as spirit which feeds the meta-narrative of Freak Film, is absent in such cases.

10 Probably the most significant initial entry in this field was Roman Polanski's *Rosemary's Baby* (1968), in which a young woman (Mia Farrow) is impregnated by Satan himself and bears his demi-human, goat-eyed child. Larry Cohen's *It's Alive!* (1974), was the definitive article with a cannibalistic baby causing bloody havoc from the very moment of birth. Cohen produced a less interesting sequel, *It Lives Again* (1978), but was beaten to it by Peter Sasdy, whose derivative *I Don't Want To Be Born* (1976) featured Joan Collins as the reluctant mother (cursed by a malevolent dwarf!) of an extremely nasty wombful. [Sasdy had previously displayed a distinct anti-familial attitude in the few films he directed for Hammer: in *Taste The Blood Of Dracula* (1970), Dracula punishes a group of businessmen by turning their daughters into parricidal, castrating angels of death; in *Countess Dracula* (1971), Elizabeth Bathory acts out the fairytale role of the cannibal mother who eats her young; and in *Hands Of The Ripper* (also 1971), Jack The Ripper's daughter displays her father's murderous talents at the very suggestion of sex.]

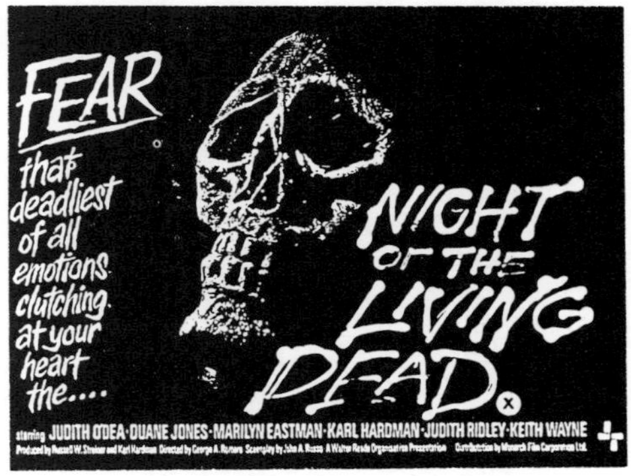

David Cronenberg was responsible for one of the more extreme interpretations of the 'devil child' phenomenon, *The Brood* (1979). This tells the story of a woman (Samantha Eggar) who, by means of a revolutionary technique called 'psychoplasmics', gives vent to her bad thoughts in the shape of malformed, homicidal children which incubate in sac-like growths all over her body. Adrzej Zulawski's *Possession* (1981) goes one step further, with Isabelle Adjani as the disturbed young woman who gives birth to a squamous, octopoid creature and goes on to fornicate with it. Offspring from Hell also appear in such films as George A. Romero's *Night Of The Living Dead* (1968), in which a mother is butchered and devoured by her zombie daughter; Bob Clark's *Deathdream* (1972), in which a mother's wish resurrects the murderous corpse of her son, killed in Vietnam; and, most notoriously, William Friedkin's *The Exorcist* (1974), in which an eleven year-old girl (Linda Blair) is possessed by the Sumerian demon Pazuzu, causing her to levitate, vomit over priests, speak in tongues (voice courtesy of Mercedes McCambridge), break a man's neck, and generally perform logic-defying physical contortions. The infamous scene in which the girl violently drives a crucifix in and out of her vagina, then grabs her mother by the hair and forces her to lap up the hymenal blood, is surely the ultimate screen moment of blasphemy, sexual perversion, and anti-Christian, anti-maternal hate.

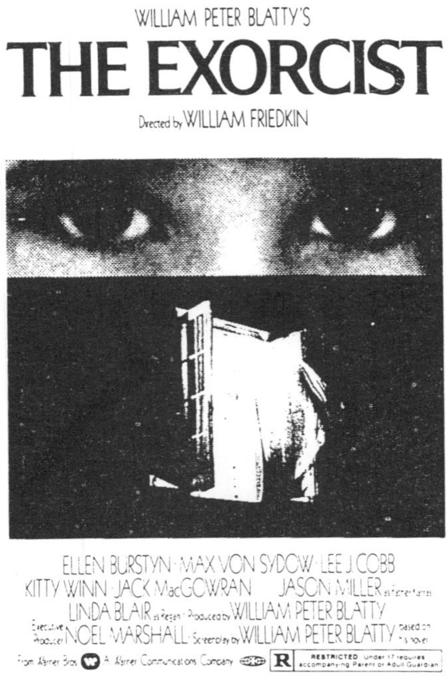

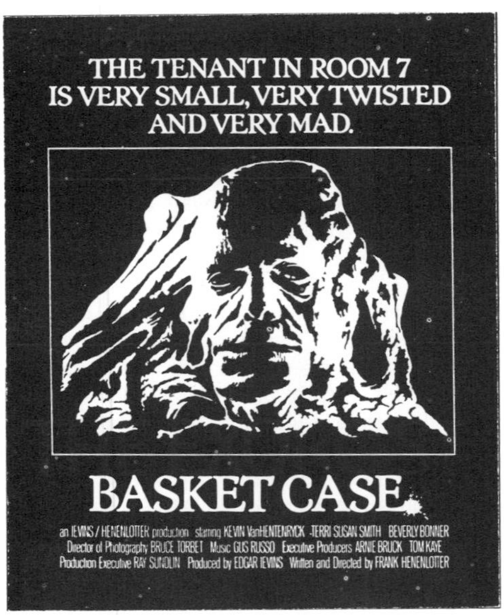
THE TENANT IN ROOM 7
IS VERY SMALL, VERY TWISTED
AND VERY MAD.
BASKET CASE

The idea of a deranged Siamese twin was exploited to the probable ultimate by Frank Hennenlotter's horror fantasy *Basket Case* (1981), in which a young man retains a telepathic link with Belial, the loathsomely malformed twin which was surgically severed from him at birth, and whom he now carries around in a basket. The story concerns Belial's bloody revenge against the doctors who performed the operation and left him for dead. Buddy Giovinazzo's Troma production *Combat Shock* (1985) features a vile mutant baby, the product of genes irradiated by Agent Orange. Finally, Ridley Scott's *Alien* (1979) gave us the rare spectacle of a man (John Hurt) 'giving birth', in this case to a flesh-eating predator which goes on to eat its 'adoptive family', the crew of a cavernous space-freighter.

FILMOGRAPHY

The following is a short, personal selection of movies which between them illustrate the whole spectrum of Freak Film.

Codes:
aka = also known as
prod = producer
dir = director
scr = scriptwriter
w = with
r = running time (where known)

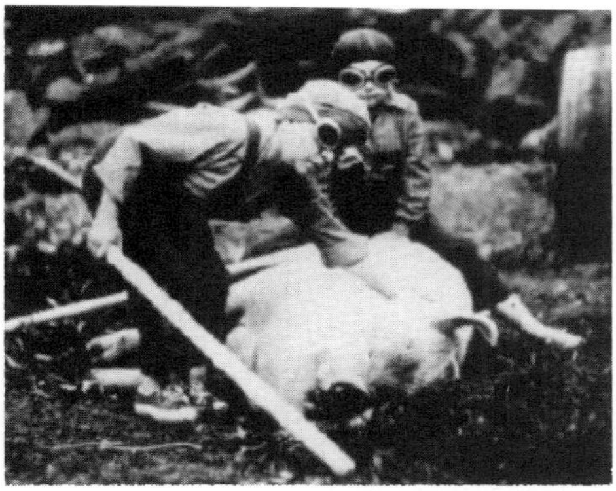

AUCH ZWERGE HABEN KLEIN ANGEFANGEN
(aka *Even Dwarfs Started Small*)
Germany, 1970
prod/dir/scr: Werner Herzog

BLOOD-SUCKING FREAKS
(aka *The Incredible Torture Show*)
Rochelle Productions, 1978
prod/dir/scr: Joel M Reed
w: Seamus O'Brien, Niles McMaster.

DAS KABINETT DES DR CALIGARI
(aka *The Cabinet Of Dr Caligari*)
Decla, 1919
prod: Erich Pommer *dir:* Robert Wiene *scr:* Carl Mayer, H Janowitz
w: Conrad Veidt, Werner Krauss, Lil Dagover.
r: 69 mins

CHAINED FOR LIFE
Classic Films, 1950
prod: George Moscov *dir:* Harry L Fraser *scr:* Nat Tanchuck
w: Violet And Daisy Hilton, Allen Jenkins.

UN CHIEN ANDALOU
(aka *An Andalusian Dog*)
France, 1928
prod/dir: Luis Buñuel *scr:* Buñuel, Salvador Dalí
w: Pierre Batcheff, Simone Mareuil, Luis Buñuel, Salvador Dalí.
r: 17 mins

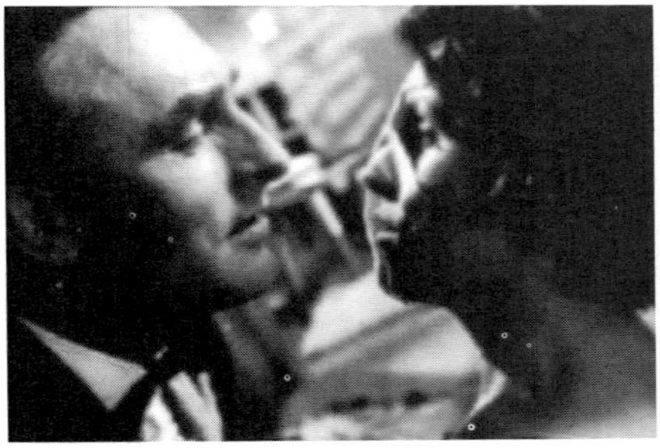

DESPERATE LIVING
New Line, 1977
prod/dir/scr: John Waters
w: Liz Renay, Mink Stole, Edith Massey, Jean Hill, Mary Vivian Pearce.
r: 90 mins

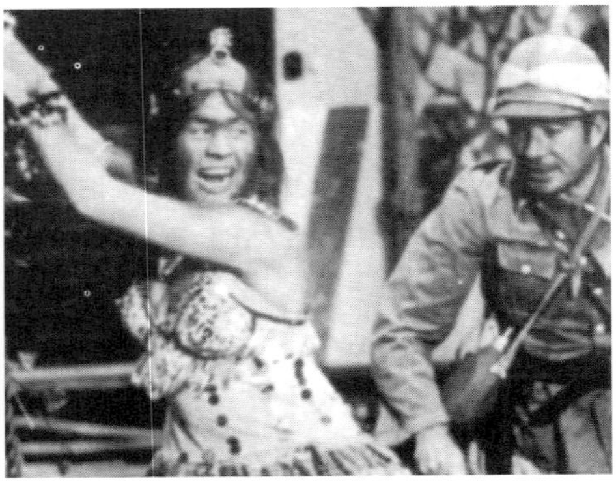

CIRCUS OF HORRORS
Anglo-Amalgamated/AIP, 1960
prod: Julian Wintle, Leslie Parkyn *dir:* Sidney Hayers *scr:* George Baxt
w: Anton Diffring, Yvonne Romain, Donald Pleasance.
r: 89 mins

DEMENTIA
(aka *Daughter Of Horror*)
Van Wolf-API, 1955
prod/dir/scr: John Parker
w: Adrienne Barrett, Bruno Ve Sota, Angelo Rossitto.
r: 55 mins

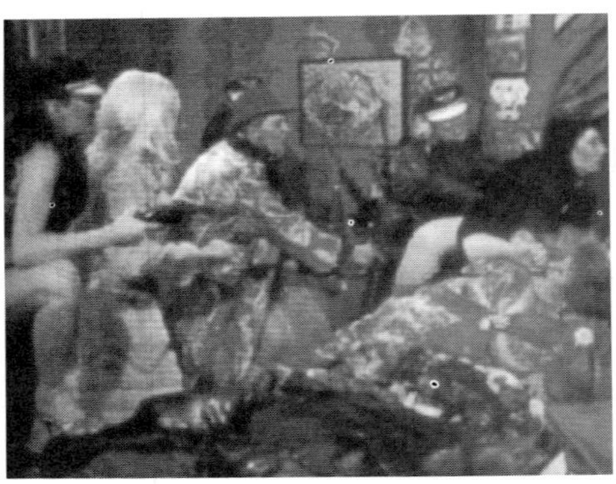

LA DONNA SCIMMIA
(aka *The Ape Woman*)
Embassy, 1963
prod: Carlo Ponti *dir:* Marco Ferreri *scr:* Ferreri, Rafael Azcona.
w: Annie Giradot, Ugo Tognazzi.
r: 97 mins

EL TOPO
(aka *The Mole*)
producciones Panicas, 1970
prod: Roberto Viskin *dir/scr:* Alejandro Jodorowsky
w: Alejandro Jodorowsky, Jacqueline Luis, Mara Lorenzio.
r: 123 mins

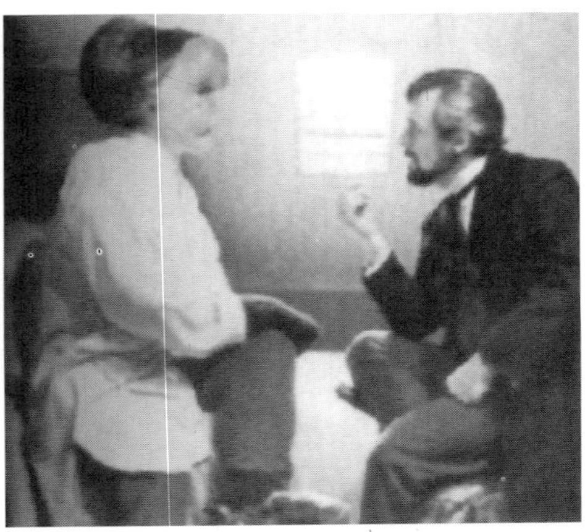

THE ELEPHANT MAN
Paramount, 1980
prod: Jonathan Sanger *dir:* David Lynch *scr:* Christopher DeVore, Eric Bergren, Lynch
w: John Hurt, Anthony Hopkins, Anne Bancroft, Freddie Jones.
r: 125 mins

ERASERHEAD
Libra, 1977
prod/dir/scr: David Lynch
w: John Nance.
r: 100 mins

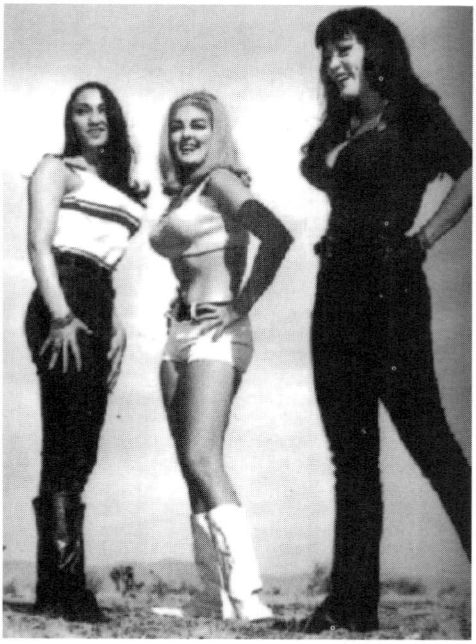

FASTER, PUSSYCAT, KILL! KILL!
(aka *Leather Girls* aka *Mankillers* aka *Pussycat*)
Russ Meyer Associates, 1965
prod: Russ and Eve Meyer *dir:* Russ Meyer *scr:* Jack Moran
w: Tura Satana, Haji, Lori Williams.
r: 84 mins

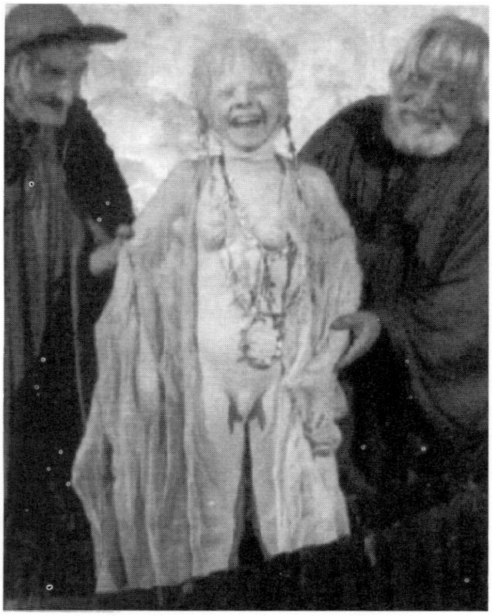

FELLINI-SATYRICON
United Artists, 1969
prod: Alberto Grimaldi *dir:* Federico Fellini *scr:* Fellini, B Zapponi, Brunello Rondi
w: Martin Potter, Capucine, Pasquale Baldassare, Hiram Keller.
r: 129 mins

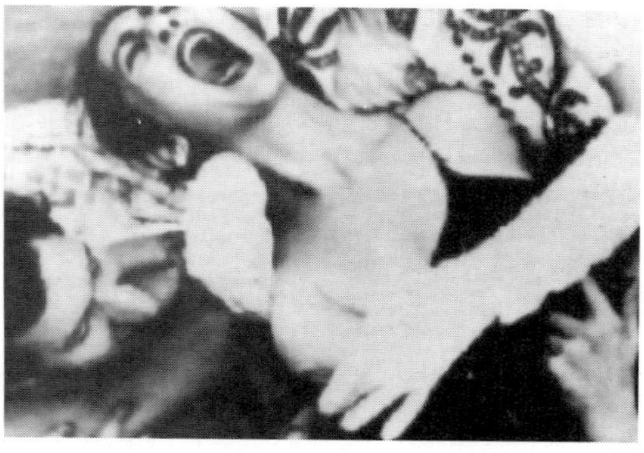

FLAMING CREATURES
USA, 1963
prod/dir/scr: Jack Smith
r: 43 mins

FREAKS
(aka *Forbidden Love* aka *Nature's Mistakes* aka *The Monster Show*)
MGM, 1932
prod/dir: Tod Browning *scr:* Willis Goldbeck, Leon Gordon, Edgar Allan Woolf, Al Boasberg
w: Harry and Daisy Earles, Olga Baclanova, Henry Victor, Johnny Eck, Violet and Daisy Hilton, Prince Randian, Angelo Rossitto.
r: 64 mins

HOUSE OF THE DAMNED
20th Century Fox, 1963
prod/dir: Maury Dexter *scr:* Harry Spalding
w: Merry Anders, Richard Crane, Richard Kiel.
r: 63 mins

IT'S A SMALL WORLD
Eagle Lion, 1950
prod: Peter Scully *dir:* William Castle *scr:* Otto Schreiber
w: Paul Dale, Will Geer.

MAD LOVE
MGM, 1935
prod: John W Considine Jnr *dir:* Karl Freund *scr:* PJ Wolfson, John L Balderston
w: Peter Lorre, Colin Clive, Frances Drake.
r: 70 mins

THE MAN WHO LAUGHS
Universal, 1927
prod: Carl Laemmle *dir:* Paul Leni *scr:* J Grubb Alexander
w: Conrad Veidt, Mary Philbin, Olga Baclanova.
r: 92 mins

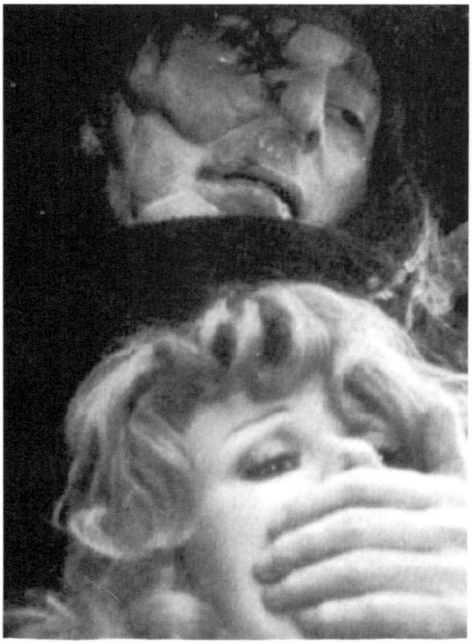

THE MUTATIONS
Columbia, 1973
prod: Robert Weinbach *dir:* Jack Cardiff *scr:* Garson Raye
w: Donald Pleasance, Tom Baker, Michael Dunn, Julie Ege.
r: 92 mins

MONDO CANE
(aka *A Dog's Life*)
Italy, 1964
prod/dir: Gualtiero Jacopetti
r: 105 mins

THE MYSTERY OF THE WAX MUSEUM
Warner Brothers, 1933
prod: Henry Blanke *dir:* Michael Curtiz *scr:* Don Mullany, Carl Erickson
w: Lionel Atwill, Fay Wray.
r: 77 mins

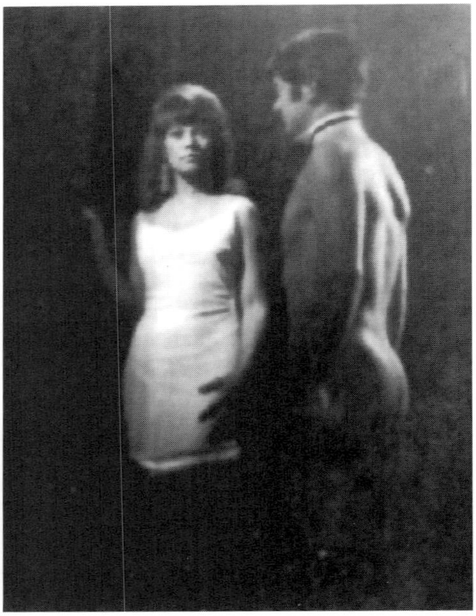

NECRONOMICON
(aka *Succubus*)
Trans-American, 1968
prod: Adrian Hoven *dir:* Jesse Franco *scr:* Pier A Caminneci
w: Janine Reynaud, Howard Vernon.
r: 91 mins

NIGHT TIDE
AIP, 1961
prod: Aram Kantarian *dir/scr:* Curtis Harrington
w: Dennis Hopper, Linda Lawson, Bruno Ve Sota, Luana Anders, Cameron Parsons.
r: 84 mins

NIGHTMARE ALLEY
20th Century Fox, 1947
prod: George Jessel *dir:* Edmund Goulding *scr:* Jules Furthman
w: Tyrone Power, Joan Blondell.
r: 111 mins

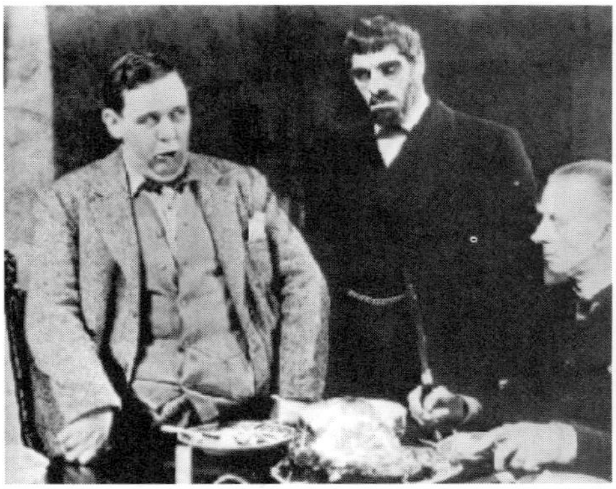

THE OLD DARK HOUSE
Universal, 1932
prod: Carl Laemmle Jnr *dir:* James Whale *scr:* Ben Levy
w: Boris Karloff, Charles Laughton, Ernest Thesiger, Gloria Stuart.
r: 75 mins

LOS OLVIDADOS
(aka *The Young And The Damned*)
Ultramar, 1950
prod: Oscar Dancigers *dir:* Luis Buñuel *scr:* Buñuel, Luis Alcoriza
w: Alfonso Mejía, Roberto Cobo, Miguel Inclán, Efrain Arauz.
r: 88 mins

PEEPING TOM
(aka *Face Of Fear*)
Anglo-Amalgamated/Astor, 1960
prod: Michael Powell, Albert Fennell *dir:* Michael Powell *scr:* Leo Marks
w: Karl Boehm, Anna Massey, Shirley Ann Field, Michael Powell.
r: 109 mins

THE PENALTY
Goldwyn, 1920
prod: Sam Goldwyn *dir:* Wallace Worsley *scr:* Charles Kenyon
w: Lon Chaney, Claire Adams.

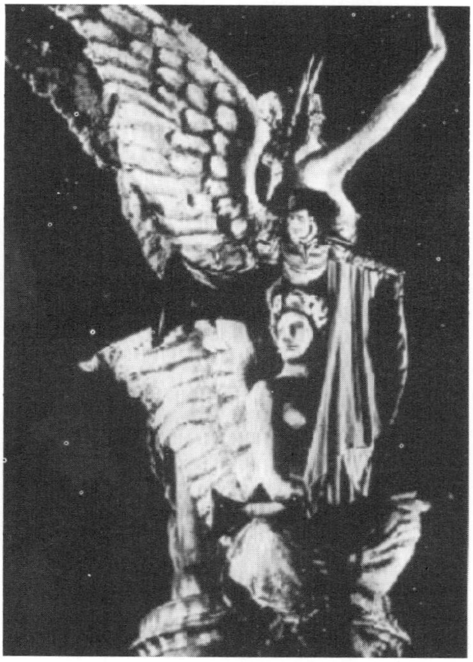

THE PHANTOM OF THE OPERA
Universal, 1925
prod: Carl Laemmle *dir:* Rupert Julien *scr:* Raymond Schrock, Elliot J Clawson
w: Lon Chaney, Mary Philbin, Norman Kerry.
r: 94 mins

PSYCHO
Paramount, 1960
prod/dir: Alfred Hitchcock *scr:* Joseph Stefano
w: Anthony Perkins, Janet Leigh, Vera Miles.
r: 109 mins

THE RAVEN
Universal, 1935
prod: David Diamond *dir:* Louis Friedlander *scr:* David Boehm, Jim Tully
w: Bela Lugosi, Boris Karloff.
r: 61 mins

SANTA SANGRE
Italy, 1989
prod: Claudio Argento *dir:* Alejandro Jodorowsky
scr: Alejandro Jodorowsky, Claudio Argento, Roberto Leoni
w: Axel Jodorowsky, Guy Stockwell, Thelma Tixou, Blanca Guera.

SHE FREAK
(aka *Alley Of Nightmares*)
Sonney-Friedman, 1966
prod/scr: David F Friedman *dir:* Byron Mabe
w: Claire Brennen, Lee Raymond.
r: 87 mins

SPIDER BABY
(aka *The Liver Eaters* aka *Cannibal Orgy*)
AGP, 1964
prod: Paul Monka, Gil Lasky *dir/scr:* Jack Hill
w: Lon Chaney Jnr, Carol Ohmart, Sid Haig.
r: 80 mins

TANIN NO KAO
(aka *The Face Of Another*)
Toho, 1967
prod/dir: Hiroshi Teshigahara *scr:* Kobo Abe
w: Tatsuya Nakadai, Mikijiro Hira.
r: 124 mins

TEXAS CHAINSAW MASSACRE
Bryanston, 1974
prod/dir: Tobe Hooper *scr:* Kim Henkel, Hooper.
w: Gunnar Hansen, Marilyn Burns, Jim Siedow.
r: 83 mins

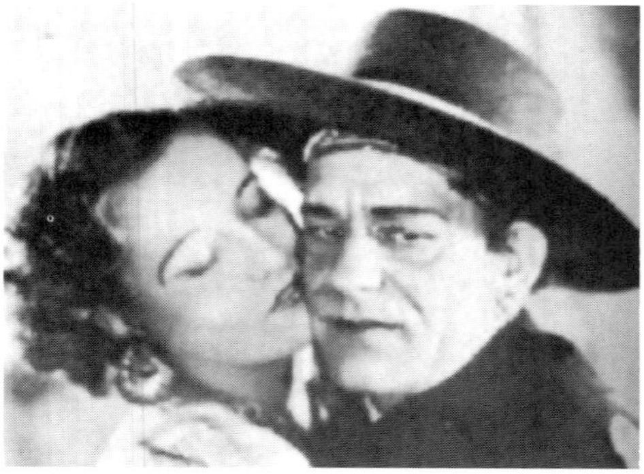

THE UNKNOWN
MGM, 1927
prod/dir: Tod Browning *scr:* Waldemar Young
w: Lon Chaney, Joan Crawford.

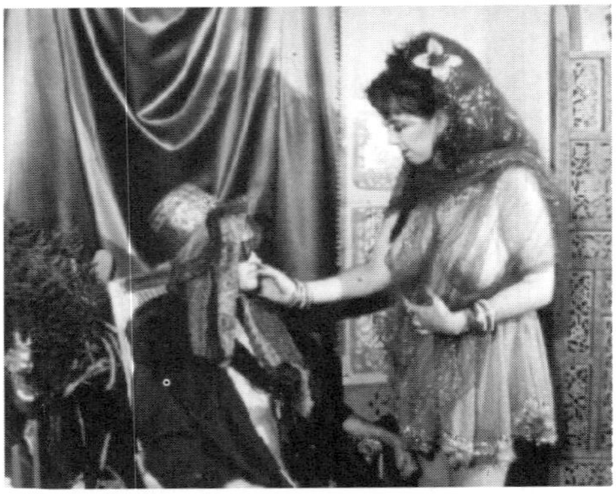

WAR IS MENSTRUAL ENVY
Penetration Films, 1990
prod/dir/scr: Nick Zedd
w: Kembra Pfahler, Annie Sprinkle, Nick Zedd.

WIZARD OF GORE
Mayflower, 1970
prod/dir: Herschell Gordon Lewis *scr:* Allen Kahn, Alison Downe
w: Ray Sagar, Sherry Carson.
r: 96 mins

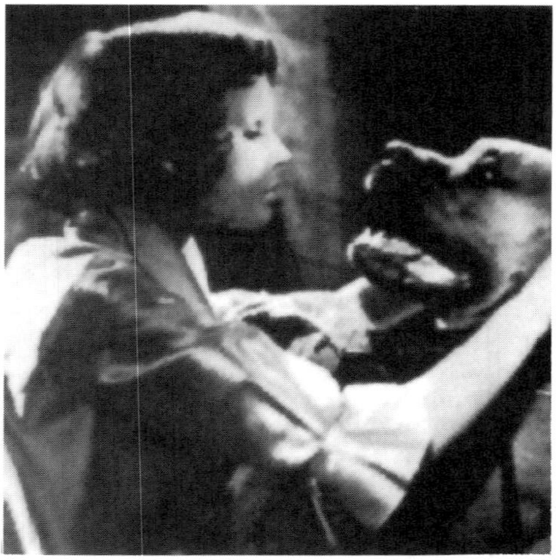

LES YEUX SANS VISAGE
(aka *Eyes Without A Face* aka *Horror Chamber Of Dr Faustus*)
Lopert, 1959
prod: Jules Borkon *dir:* Georges Franju *scr:* Franju, Jean Redon, Claude Sautet, Pierre Boileau, Thomas Narcejac
w: Edith Scob, Pierre Brasseur, Alida Valli.
r: 95 mins

INDEX OF FILMS

Page numbers in italics indicate an illustration

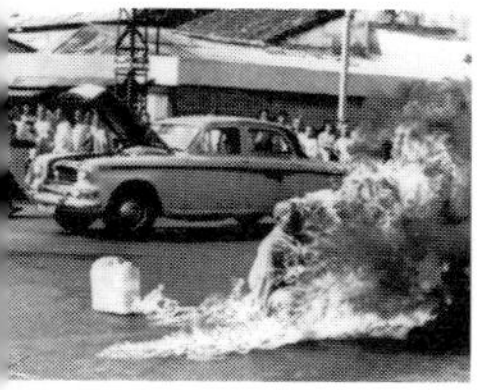

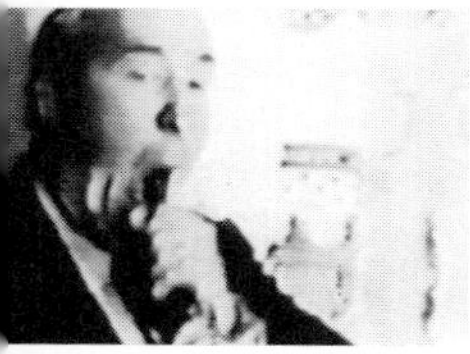

1 KILLING FOR CULTURE *Kerekes & Slater*

Killing For Culture is a definitive investigation into the urban myth of the "snuff movie". Includes: FEATURE FILM – from *Peeping Tom* to *Videodrome* and beyond; MONDO FILM – from *Mondo Cane* to present day 'shockumentaries'; DEATH FILM – from *Faces Of Death* to real deaths captured on film such as live-TV suicides, executions, and news footage

Illustrated by stunning photographs from cinema, documentary and real life, **Killing For Culture** is a necessary book which examines and questions the human obsession with images of violence, dismemberment and death, and the way our society is coping with an increased profusion of these disturbing yet compelling images from all quarters. Includes filmography and index.

"Well-researched and highly readable, Killing For Culture *is a must-have."*
– FILM THREAT

CINEMA/CULTURE Trade Paperback 1 871592 20 8 169 x 244mm 288 pages £14.95

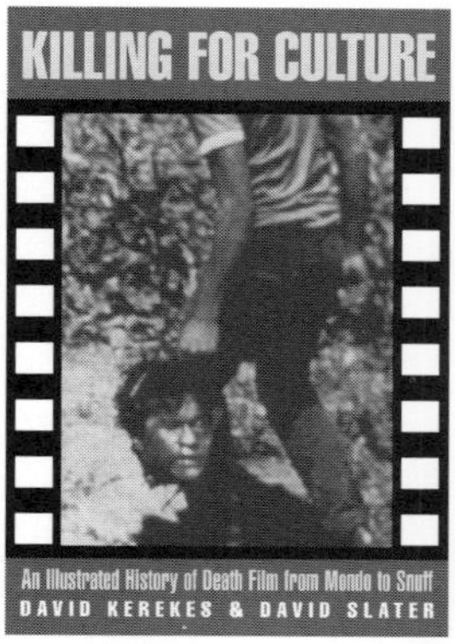

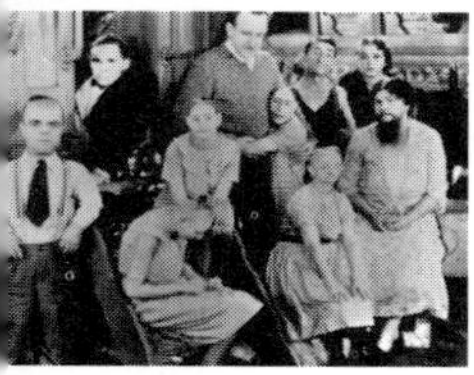

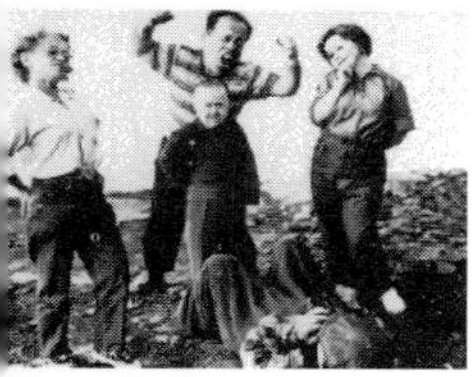

2 INSIDE TERADOME *Jack Hunter*

Freakshows – human anomalies presented for spectacle – have flourished throughout recorded history. The birth of the movies provided a further outlet for these displays, which in turn led to a peculiar strain of bizarre cinema: Freak Film. **Inside Teradome** is a comprehensive, fully illustrated guide to the roots and development of this fascinating, often disturbing cinematic genre.

Including: Teratology: freaks in myth and medicine; the history of freakshows, origins of cinema; influence of sideshows on cinema; use of human anomalies in cinema; freaks and geeks; bizarre cinema: mutilation and other fetishes; illustrated filmography; index; over 350 photographs. From the real-life grotesqueries of Tod Browning's *Freaks*, to the modern nightmare vision of *Santa Sangre*, **Inside Teradome** reveals a twisted thread of voyeuristic sickness running both through cinema and the society it mirrors.

CINEMA/CULTURE Trade Paperback 1 871592 41 0 169 x 244mm 256 pages £14.95

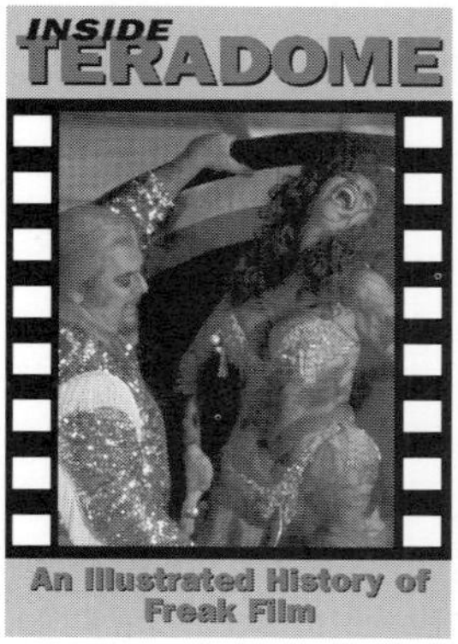

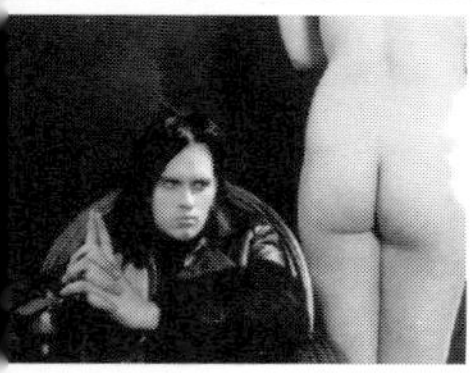

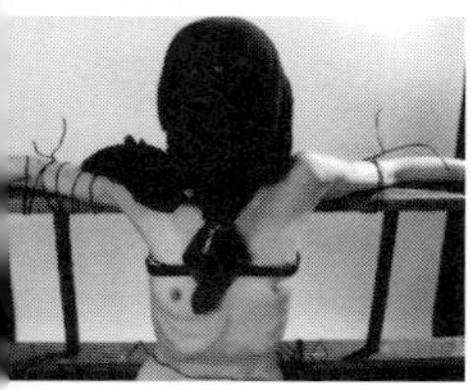

3 DEATHTRIPPING *Jack Sargeant*

Deathtripping is an illustrated history, account and critique of the "Cinema Of Transgression", providing a long-overdue and comprehensive documentation of this essential modern sub-cultural movement. Including: A brief history of underground/trash cinema: seminal influences including Andy Warhol, Jack Smith, George and Mike Kuchar, John Waters. Interviews with key film-makers, including Richard Kern, Nick Zedd, Cassandra Stark, Beth B, Tommy Turner; plus associates such as Joe Coleman, Lydia Lunch, Lung Leg and David Wojnarowicz. Notes and essays on transgressive cinema, philosophy of transgression; manifestos, screen-plays; film index and bibliography.

Heavily illustrated with rare and sometimes disturbing photographs, **Deathtripping** is a unique guide to a style of film-making whose impact and influence can no longer be ignored.

CINEMA/CULTURE Trade Paperback 1 871592 29 1 169 x 244mm 256 pages £11.95

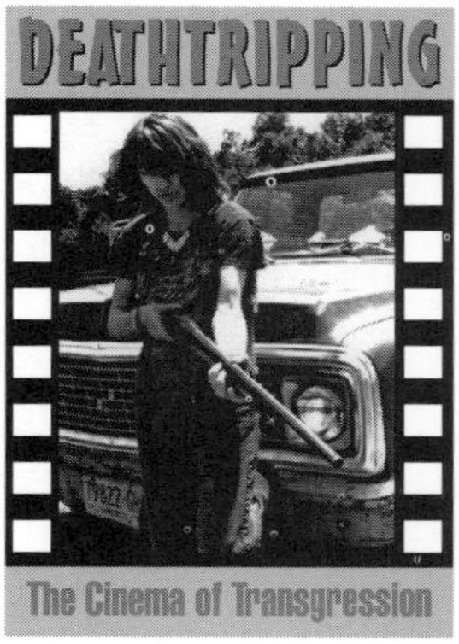

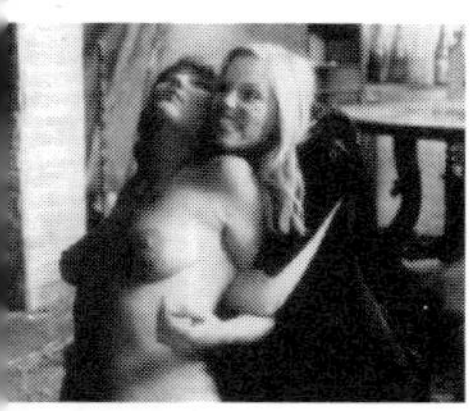

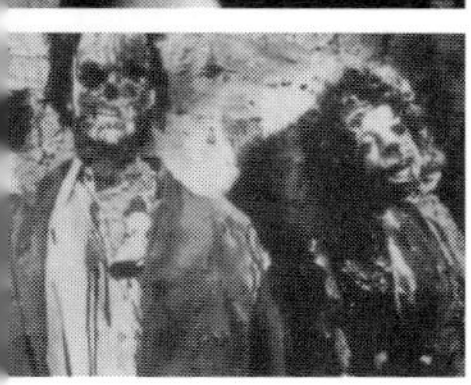

4 FRAGMENTS OF FEAR *Andy Boot*

Fragments Of Fear is an illustrated history of an often neglected film genre: the British Horror Movie. The book examines a wide range of British horror films, and the stories behind them, from the early melodramas of Tod Slaughter right through to Hammer and their rivals Tigon and Amicus, plus mavericks like Michael Reeves, sex/horror director Peter Walker and more recent talents such as Clive Barker, director of *Hellraiser*. Films discussed range in scope from the sadism of *Peeping Tom* to the mutant SF of *A Clockwork Orange* and the softcore porn/horror of Jose Larraz' *Vampyres*.

With plentiful illustrations, author Andy Boot unravels a tangled history and discovers many little-known gems amid the more familiar images of Hammer, including a wealth of exploitational cinema, to establish the British horror movie as a genre which can easily stand up to its more lauded American counterpart in the depth and diversity of its scope.

CINEMA Trade Paperback 1 871592 35 6 169 x 244mm 288 pages £12.95

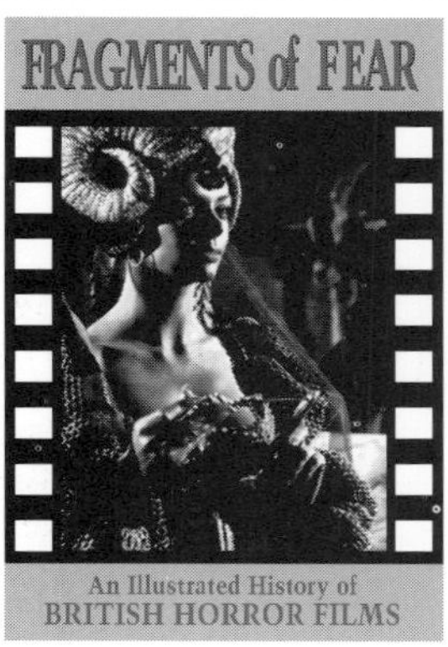

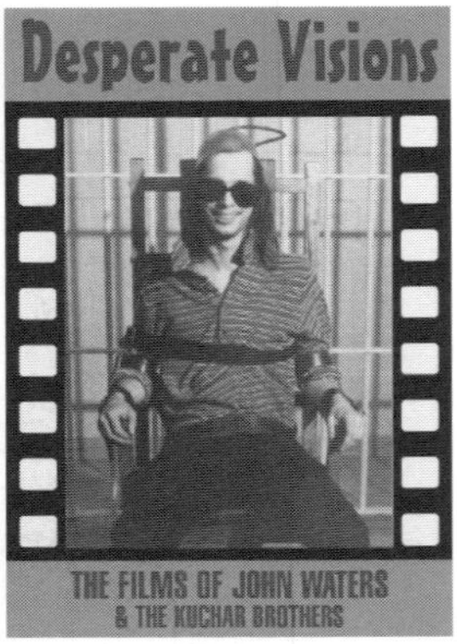

5 DESPERATE VISIONS *Jack Stevenson*

John Waters is the notorious director of *Pink Flamingos, Female Trouble, Desperate Living* and *Hairspray,* amongst other cult movie classics.

Desperate Visions features several in-depth interviews with Waters, as well as with members of his legendary entourage including Divine, Mary Vivian Pearce, Mink Stole and Miss Jean Hill. George & Mike Kuchar are the directors of such low-budget/underground classics as *Sins Of The Fleshapoids* and *Hold Me While I'm Naked.* Their visionary trash aesthetic was a great influence on the young John Waters.

Desperate Visions includes extensive interviews with the Kuchars, as well as a comprehensive assessment of their career and influence. Also included is a unique feature on actress Marion Eaton, star of the gothic porn epic *Thundercrack!.*

With many rare photographs, filmography and index, **Desperate Visions** is an essential introduction to the wild world of John Waters, and to the outrageous camp/underground film tradition which his movies exemplify.

CINEMA/CULTURE Trade Paperback 1 871592 34 8 169 x 244mm 256 pages £14.95

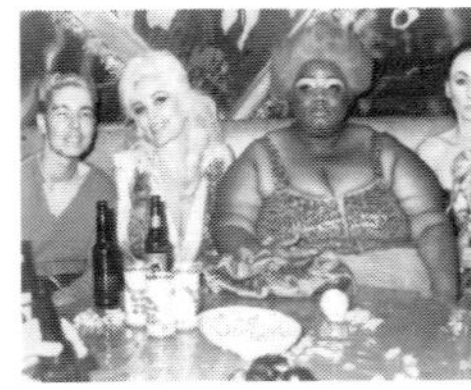

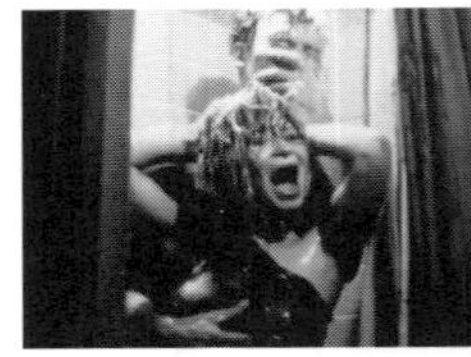

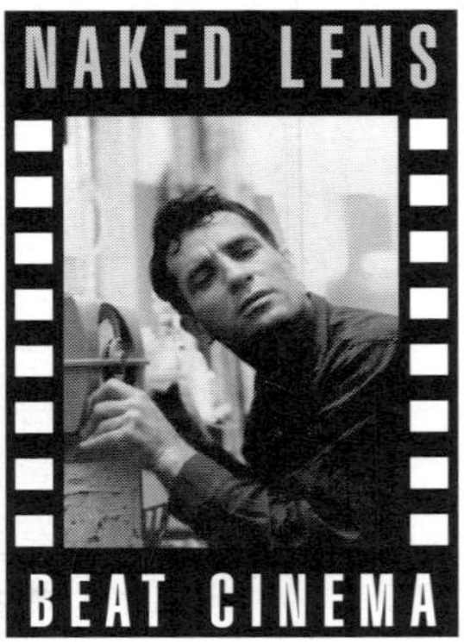

6 THE NAKED LENS *Jack Sargeant*

The Naked Lens is a vital collection of essays and interviews focusing on the most significant interfaces between the Beat writers, Beat culture and cinema; films by, featuring, or inspired by: WILLIAM S BURROUGHS • ALLEN GINSBERG • JACK KEROUAC • CHARLES BUKOWSKI • BRION GYSIN ANTHONY BALCH • RON RICE JOHN CASSAVETES • ANDY WARHOL • BOB DYLAN • KLAUS MAECK • GUS VAN SANT *& many others*

Including interviews with writers such as Allen Ginsberg, directors such as Robert Frank and actors such as Taylor Mead; plus detailed examination of key Beat texts and cult classics such as *Pull My Daisy, Chappaqua, Towers Open Fire* and *The Flower Thief*; verité and performance films such as *Shadows, Don't Look Back* and *Wholly Communion*; B-movies such as *The Subterraneans, Beat Generation* and Roger Corman's *Bucket Of Blood*; and Hollywood-style adaptations from *Heart Beat* and *Barfly* through to Cronenberg's *Naked Lunch.*

CINEMA/BEAT CULTURE Trade Paperback 1 871592 67 4 169 x 244mm 288 pages £12.95

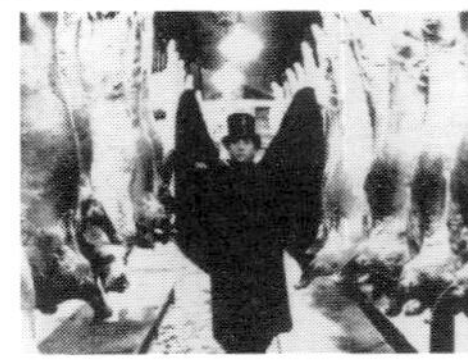

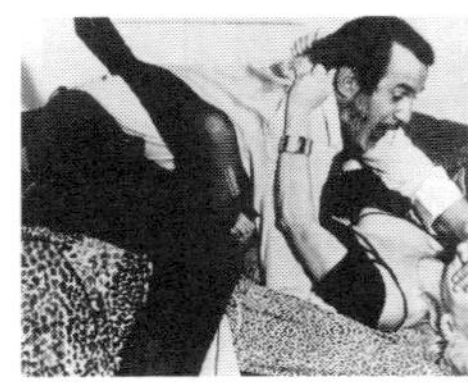

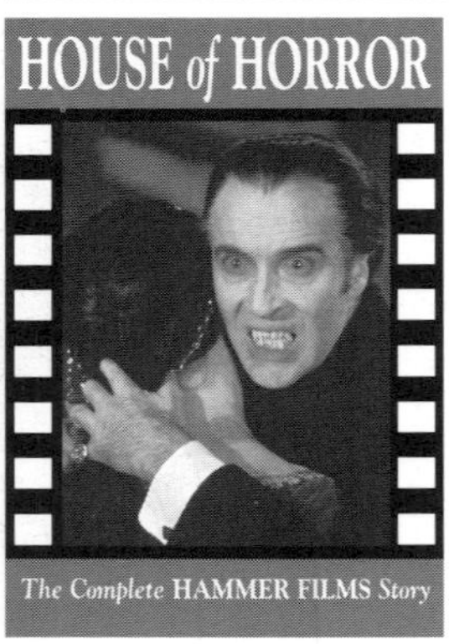

7 HOUSE OF HORROR *Jack Hunter*

HAMMER FILMS remains one of the most successful and legendary of all British film companies. Their name is synonymous with gothic horror throughout the world.

House Of Horror traces the complete history of Hammer, from its early origins through to its golden era of classic horror movies, and presents a comprehensive overview of Hammer's importance and influence in world cinema.

House Of Horror includes interviews with Hammer stars Christopher Lee and Peter Cushing, detailed analysis of all Hammer's horror and fantasy films and their key directors, and dozens of rare and exciting photographs and posters; plus a fully illustrated A–Z of key Hammer personnel from both sides of the camera, a directory of unfilmed projects, a complete filmography, and full film index. **Third, expanded edition**

CINEMA Trade Paperback 1 871592 19 4 169 x 244mm 224 pages £12.95

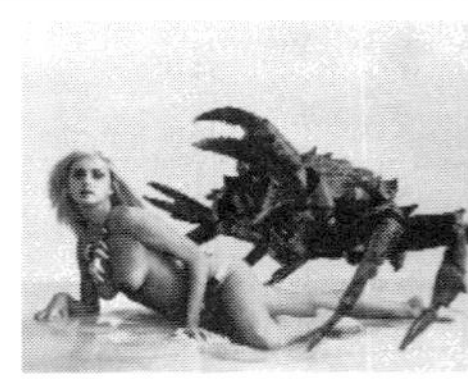

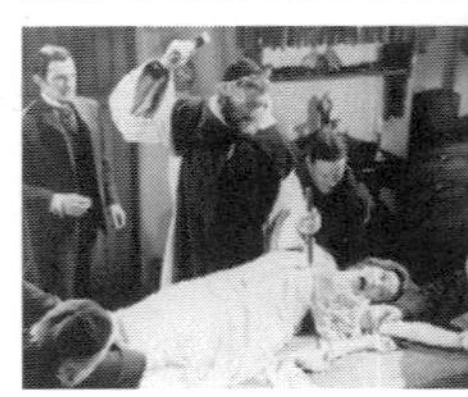

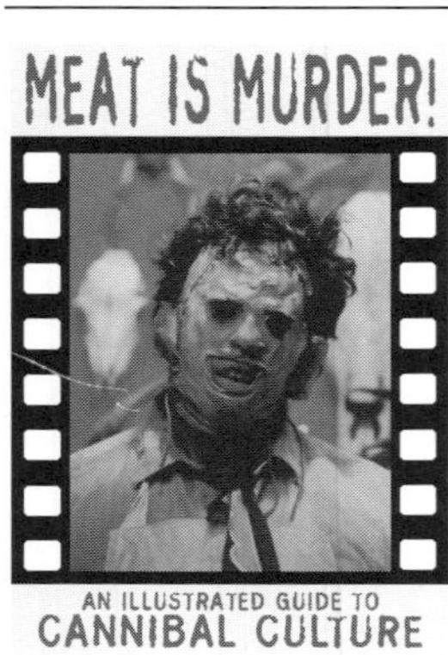

8 MEAT IS MURDER! *Mikita Brottman*

Violent death, murder, mutilation, eating and defaecation, ritualism, bodily extremes; cannibalism combines these crucial themes to represent one of the most symbolically charged narratives in the human psychic repertoire.

As a grotesque figure of power, threat, and atavistic appetites, the cannibal has played a formidable role in the tales told by members of all cultures – whether oral, written, or filmic – and embodies the ultimate extent of transgressive behaviour to which human beings can be driven.

Meat Is Murder! is a unique and explicit exploration of the stories that are told about cannibals, from classical myth to contemporary film and fiction, and features an in-depth illustrated critique of cannibalism as portrayed in the cinema, from mondo and exploitation films to horror movies and arthouse classics. It also details the atrocious crimes of real life cannibals of the modern age, such as Albert Fish, Ed Gein, Jeffrey Dahmer and Andrei Chikatilo.

CINEMA/CULTURE Trade Paperback 1 871592 90 9 169 x 244mm 208 pages £14.95

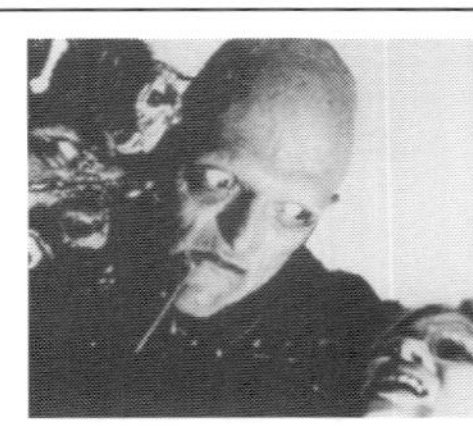

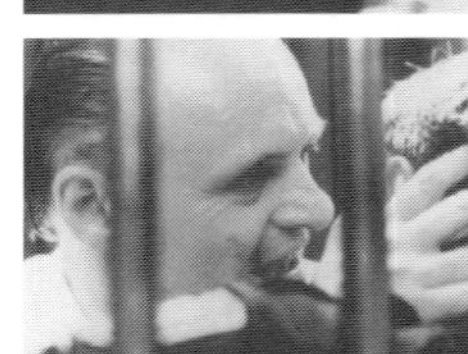